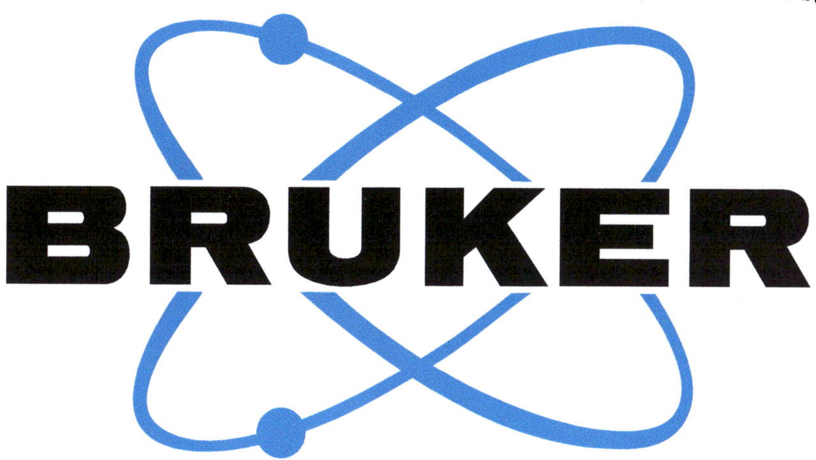

Exhibitors of IWMPI 2019

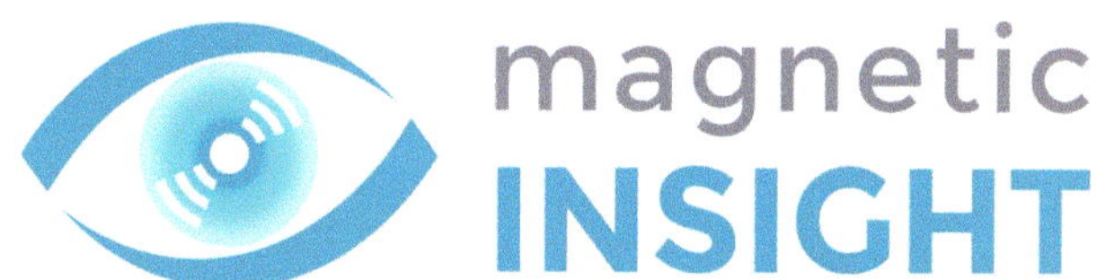

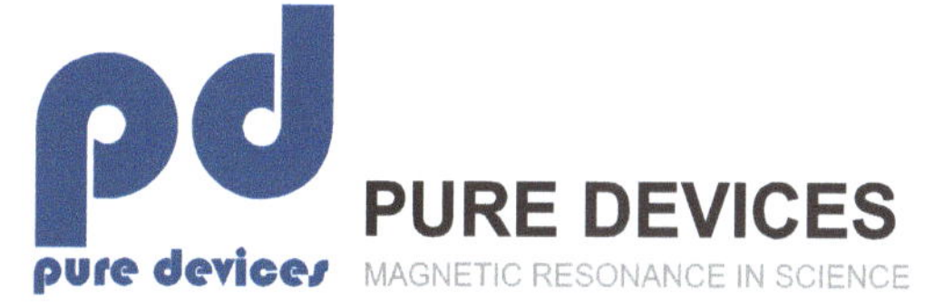

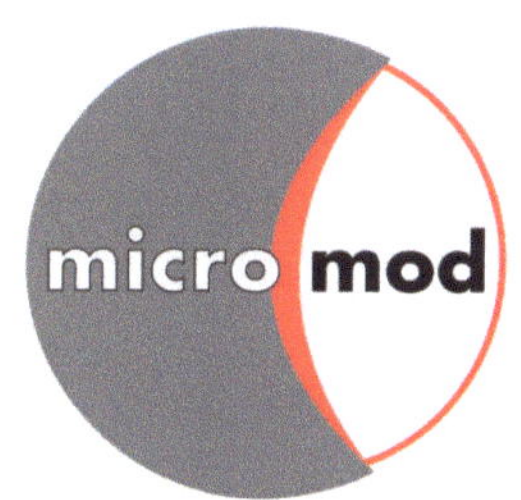

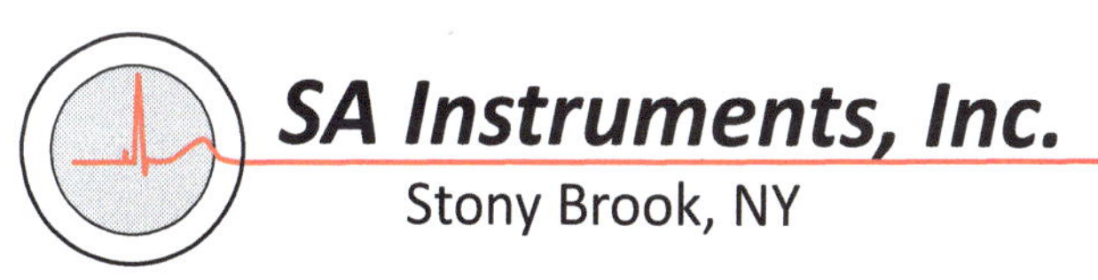

Endorsements of IWMPI 2019

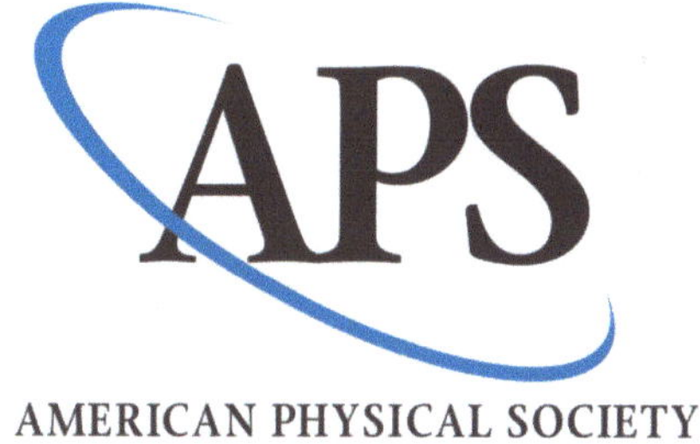

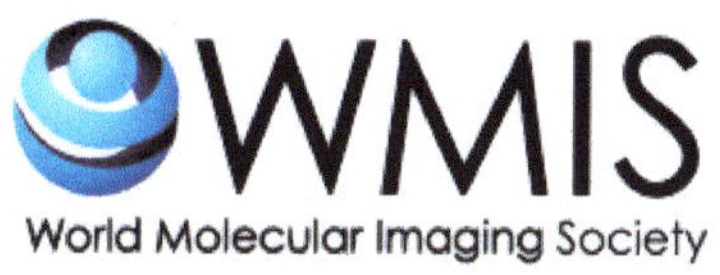

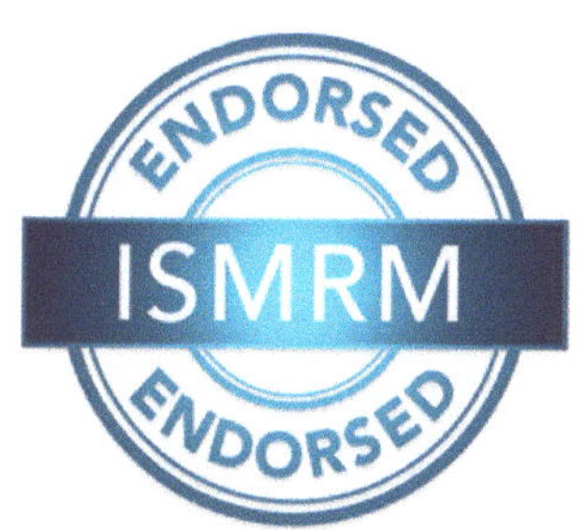

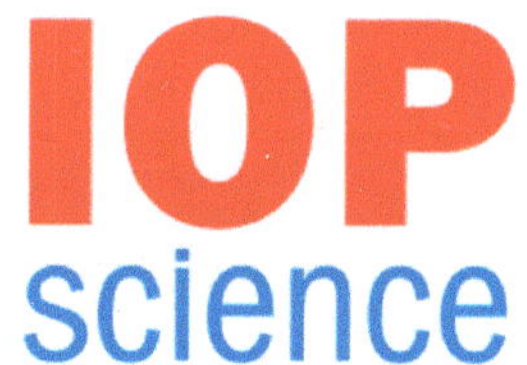

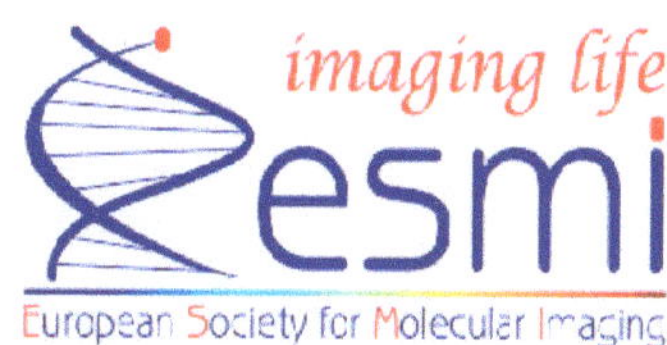

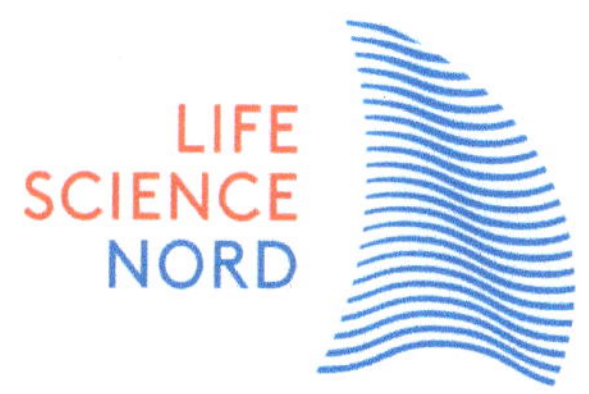

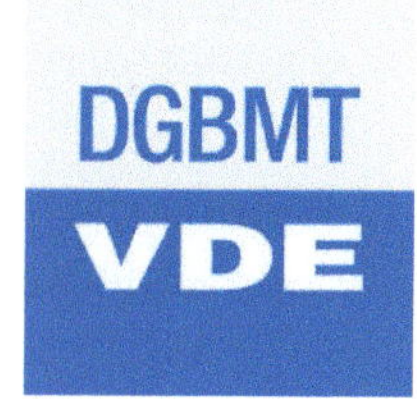

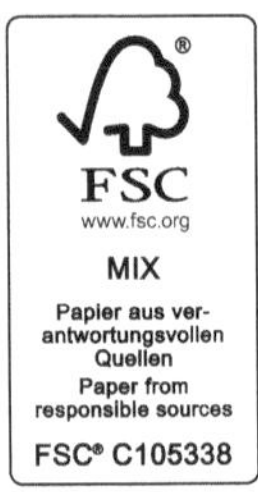

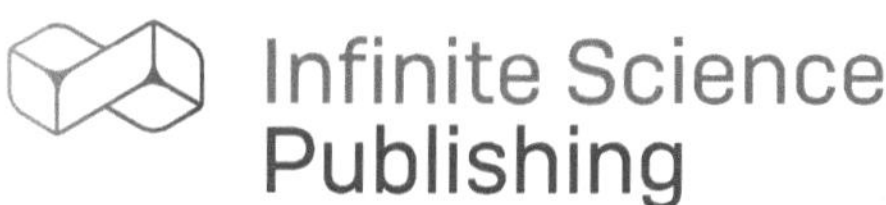

Infinite Science
Publishing

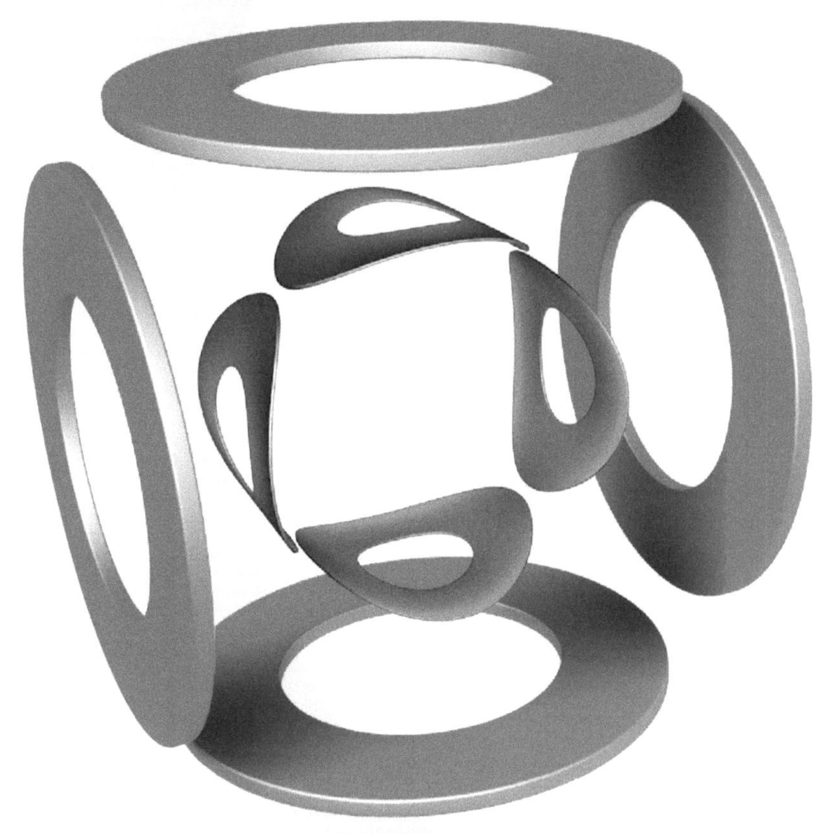

9th International Workshop on

Magnetic Particle Imaging
IWMPI 2019

March 17–19, 2019 | New York, USA

Book of Abstracts

Youssef Wadghiri, Alexey Tonyushkin, Lawrence Wald,
John Weaver, Tobias Knopp, and Thorsten M. Buzug (Eds.)

Welcome Message from the Conference Chair,

On behalf of the organizing committee for the International Workshop on Magnetic Particle Imaging (IWMPI), I am honored and delighted to welcome all of you to the 9th annual workshop hosted at the New York University (NYU) School of Medicine and NYU Langone Health (NYULH) in New York, NY USA.

The IWMPI (www.iwmpi.org) is the premier international platform for this new medical imaging modality and creates an opportunity to gather attendees to meet and exchange ideas in this emerging field. The 9th IWMPI workshop, Sunday, March 17 to Tuesday, March 19, 2019 will continue this tradition by attracting researchers, developers, manufacturers, users and suppliers of material with direct relevance and importance to this growing field.

By way of introduction, I am Youssef Zaim Wadghiri, member of the Faculty NYU School of Medicine (Department of Radiology) and Chair of the 9th IWMPI. I am supported by my three co-chairs Drs. Alexey Tonyushkin (University of Massachusetts, Boston, MA USA); Lawrence L. Wald (Harvard Medical School & Massachusetts General Hospital Charlestown, MA USA) and John B. Weaver (Geisel School of Medicine at Dartmouth, Hanover, NH USA). Our U.S.-based team is supported by Dr. Thorsten M. Buzug (University of Lübeck (Lübeck, Germany) as the Program Chair and Dr. Tobias Knopp (Technical University of Hamburg, Germany) as the Publication Chair of IWMPI.

As the hosting site of this exciting scientific forum, I cannot imagine a better symbolism than hosting this workshop in New York. While our great city is often referred as the "Big Apple", its other nickname, the "City of Lights", may be more appropriate in the current context, thanks to the past and present history of New York City.

It is worthwhile noting that the city of many lights was the battle ground of the biggest technology race between DC and AC that shaped the transmission and distribution power industry in the 19th century. Thomas Edison opened the first generating DC station in September 1882 on Pearl Street in lower Manhattan. Only a few miles away, all of the creative work of Nikola Tesla and his numerous contributions in wireless transmission took place in his laboratory located on East Houston. While the location of the 9th IWMPI workshop is within walking distance to more popular sites such as the Empire State building or the United Nations headquarters, it is also neighboring Bellevue Hospital, which is the oldest public hospital in the United States, founded on March 31, 1736.

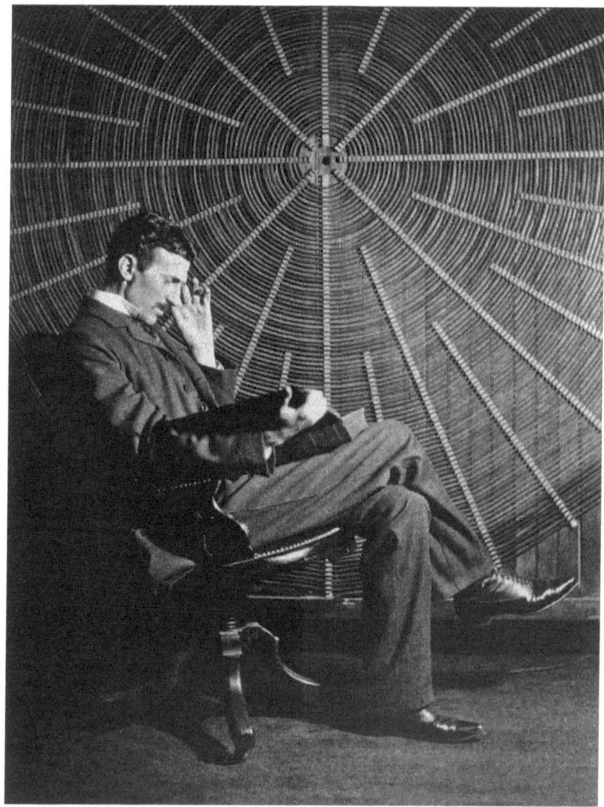

Portrait of Nikola Tesla in his laboratory at East Houston street in Manhattan few miles away from the New York University Medical campus where the 9th IWMPI is hosted.
From "Tesla's Important Advances," Electrical Review, 20 May 1896, 263.

For this year's IWMPI, we are excited to share with you that 106 abstracts that have been accepted from 14 countries, promising an interesting and dynamic conference. A comprehensive set of MPI topics will be presented at this conference including medical, pre-clinical, and non-medical applications. The areas of focus span the following topics: coil and field generator design, data acquisition and signal pre-processing, signal generation, amplification and filter design as well as magnetic field simulation and system modeling, magnetic particle spectroscopy (MPS), molecular imaging, nanoparticle development, particle physics and simulations, reconstruction methods, sequences, acquisition protocols and spatial coding, scanner geometries and system design. Both the quality and quantity of participants for the 9th year in a row is a true testament of the active and vibrant MPI research community.

I would like to thank Dr. Peter Caravan from the Athinoula A. Martinos Center for Biomedical Imaging, Department of Radiology, Massachusetts General Hospital (Charlestown, MA USA), for spontaneously accepting to give the Keynote lecture entitled "MPI: The Future of Biomedical Molecular Imaging?".

I would like to also acknowledge the help and support for our tutorial lectures by Jochen Franke, Product Manager for Magnetic Particle Imaging, System Engineering & Integration at Bruker BioSpin MRI (Ettlingen Germany); Klaas Bente at the German Federal Institute for Materials Research and Testing (BAM, Berlin, Germany); Steven Conolly, Professor of Bioengineering and EECS at UC Berkeley (Berkeley, CA USA); and Patrick Goodwill, Chief Technical Officer at Magnetic Insight (Alameda, CA USA).

Additionally, we would like to acknowledge the financial support of Bruker BioSpin GmbH at the partnership status as well as our other industrial participants including Magnetic Insight, Inc. (Alameda, CA USA); Pure Devices GmbH (Rimpar, Germany); MicroMod GmbH (Rostock, Germany); SA Instruments Inc. (Brookhaven, NY USA) for their financial contribution and participation as exhibitors at the IWMPI 2019.

I would like to express my gratitude to the leadership of the NYU Langone Health, NYU School of Medicine for facilitating the organization of this workshop and providing the needed resources to make this workshop a success. A big thank you goes to our local team Brianna Alvarez, Susana Esquenazi and Andrea Ohlsson from the Division of Advanced Research Technologies (DART) under the leadership of Assistant Dean Adriana Heguy, PhD, Senior Director Sheenah Mische, PhD and Director of Finance Tom Winner, MBA. My gratitude goes to my team at the Preclinical imaging laboratory, Orlando Aristizabal, Dina Ramadane, Zakia Ben You Gironda and Orin Mishkit who committed themselves to help on the ground and assist all of the attendees. And our organizing team cannot express enough thanks to Kanina Neideck of Infinite Science Conferencing, who's diligent and timely work in the background made the whole process seamless.

IWMPI is endorsed by the American Physical Society (APS), the International Society for Magnetic Resonance in Medicine (ISMRM), the World Molecular Imaging Society (WMIS), the European Society of Molecular Imaging (ESMI), and the German Life Science North Cluster and the German Society of Biomedical Engineering (DGBMT).

I look forward to welcoming you all to an exciting IWMPI 2019!

Youssef Zaim Wadghiri, PhD; IWMPI 2019 - Workshop Chair

Venue

New York University, NYU Langone Health
550 First Avenue
New York, NY 10016, USA

Date

March 17-19, 2019

Target Groups/Specialists Fields

Magnetic Particle Imaging (MPI) is a novel imaging modality that uses various static and oscillating magnetic fields to image the spatial distribution of superparamagnetic iron oxide nanoparticles (SPIOs) with high sensitivity, no tissue background, and no ionizing radiation. The method exploits the non-linear magnetization behavior of the SPIOs, and has shown great potential to surpass current in vivo imaging modalities in terms of sensitivity, safety, quantitation, and spatio-temporal resolution. MPI is well suited for clinical applications such as angiography, cancer imaging, and inflammation imaging; as well as research applications such as stem cell imaging and small animal imaging.

Workshop topics include (but are not limited to):

Application scenarios; Coil design; Data acquisition; Filter design; Imaging chain simulation; Magnetic field simulation; Magnetic particle spectroscopy; Nanoparticle development; Particle magnetization models; Reconstruction methods; Sequences and FFP trajectories; Spatial encoding; SAR and PNS simulations; Scanner topologies; Shielding and cooling; Signal amplification; Signal processing; Strong permanent magnets; System noise

Workshop Chair

Youssef Zaim Wadghiri   New York University, NYU Langone Health (USA)

Workshop Co-Chairs

Alexey Tonyushkin   University of Massachusetts, Boston (USA)
Lawrence L. Wald   Harvard Medical School, MGH, Boston (USA)
John Weaver   Dartmouth-Hitchcock Medical Center, Hanover (USA)

Workshop Program Chair

Thorsten M. Buzug   Universität zu Lübeck, Germany

Workshop Publication Chair

Tobias Knopp   Medical Center Hamburg-Eppendorf (UKE), Germany

Program Committee

Gerhard Adam	Medical Center Hamburg-Eppendorf (Germany)
Christoph Alexiou	University Medical Center Erlangen (Germany)
Meltem Asilturk	Akdeniz University, Antalya (Turkey)
Jörg Barkhausen	UKSH Lübeck (Germany)
Luis F. Barquin	University Cantabria, Santander (Spain)
Volker Behr	University of Würzburg (Germany)
Ayhan Bingolbali	Yildiz Technical University, Istanbul (Turkey)
Audrius Brazdeikis	University of Houston, (USA)
Jeff Bulte	John Hopkins University, Baltimore (USA)
Thorsten M. Buzug	University of Lübeck (Germany)
Steven M. Conolly	University of California, Berkeley (USA)
Nurcan Dogan	Gebze Institute of Technology, Kocaeli (Turkey)
Silvio Dutz	Technical University of Ilmenau (Germany)
Matthew Ferguson	LodeSpin Labs, Seattle (USA)
Dominique Finas	Magdeburg Clinic (Germany)
Patrick W. Goodwill	Magnetic Insight, Berkeley (USA)
Marc Griswold	Case Western Reserve University (USA)
Urs Häfeli	University of British Columbia, Vancouver (Canada)
Jens Haueisen	Technical University of Ilmenau (Germany)
Michael Heidenreich	Bruker Biospin (Germany)
Ulrich Heinen	Pforzheim University of Applied Sciences (Germany)
Hyobong Hong	Electronics and Telecommunications Research Institute (Korea)
Hui Hui	Chinese Academy of Sciences, Beijing (China)
Yasutoshi Ishihara	Meiji University, Tokyo (Japan)
Harald Ittrich	University Medical Center Hamburg-Eppendorf (Germany)
Peter Jakob	University of Würzburg (Germany)
Christer Johansson	RISE Research Institutes of Sweden (Sweden)
Fabian Kiesling	UKA Aachen (Germany)
Tobias Knopp	University Medical Center Hamburg-Eppendorf (Germany)
Tetsuo Kobayashi	Kyoto University (Japan)
Kannan Krishnan	University of Washington, Seattle (USA)
Wenzhong Liu	Huazhong University of Science and Technology (China)

Program Committee (cont'd)

Frank Ludwig	Technical University of Braunschweig (Germany)
Mauro Magnani	University of Urbino (Italy)
Michael Martens	Case Western Reserve University (USA)
M. del Puerto Morales	Instituto de Ciencia de Materiales de Madrid (Spain)
Kenya Murase	Osaka University (Japan)
Jan Niehaus	CAN Center für Applied Nanotechnology, Hamburg (Germany)
Stefan Odenbach	Technical University of Dresden (Germany)
Eva Olsson	Chalmers University of Technology, Gothenburg (Sweden)
Quentin Pankhurst	University College London (UK)
Ulrich Pison	Charité Universitätsmedizin Mitte, Berlin (Germany)
Anna Cristina Samia	Case Western Reserve University, Cleveland (USA)
Emine Ulku Saritas	Bilkent University, Bilkent/Ankara (Turkey)
Meinhard Schilling	Technical University of Braunschweig (Germany)
Jörg Schnorr	Charité Universitätsmedizin Mitte, Berlin (Germany)
Volkmar Schulz	RWTH Aachen (Germany)
Ludek Sefc	Charles University, Prague (Czech Republik)
Yasushi Takemura	Yokohama National University (Japan)
Saburo Tanaka	Toyohashi University of Technology, Aichi (Japan)
Michael Taupitz	Charité Universitätsmedizin, Berlin (Germany)
Bennie ten Haken	University of Twente, Enschede (Netherlands)
Tian Jie	Chinese Academy of Sciences, Beijing (China)
Alexey Tonyushkin	University of Massachusetts, Boston (USA)
Lutz Trahms	PTB Physikalisch-Technische Bundesanstalt, Berlin (Germany)
Youssef Z. Wadghiri	New York University (NYU) Langone Health (USA)
Lawrence L. Wald	Harvard Medical School Massachusetts General Hospital (USA)
John B. Weaver	Dartmouth-Hitchcock Medical Center, Lebanon (USA)
Oliver Weber	Philips Hamburg (Germany)
Antoine Weis	University of Fribourg (Switzerland)
Jürgen Weizenecker	University of Applied Sciences, Karlsruhe (Germany)
Frank Wiekhorst	PTB Physikalisch-Technische Bundesanstalt, Berlin (Germany)
Barbara Wollenberg	University Medical Center Lübeck (Germany)
Takashi Yoshida	Kyushu University, Fukuoka (Japan)

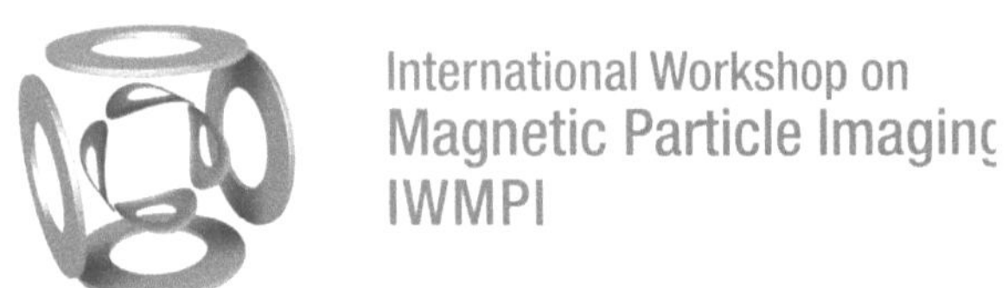

Technical Commitees

Organization

Infinite Science is in charge of marketing, registration and publication of IWMPI.

Infinite Science provides the platforms www.iwmpi.org

and the open access journal IJMPI www.ijmpi.org

Registration and Administration

Kanina Neideck

Managing Director

Infinite Science GmbH

MFC 1 - Technikzentrum Lübeck

Maria-Goeppert-Straße 1

D - 23562 Lübeck, Germany

Office: +49 451 5853 2900

Fax: +49 451 5853 2905

E-mail: neideck@infinite-science.de

E-mail: info@iwmpi.org

Local Chair

Youssef Zaim Wadghirir, PhD

Associate Professor of Radiology,

Director of Preclinical Imaging

NYU School of Medicine

New York University (NYU) Langone Health

660 First Ave 4th Floor Room 444

New York, NY 10016, USA

Office: (212) 263-3336

Fax: (212) 263-7541

E-mail Work: wadghiri@med.nyu.edu

Local Organization

Brianna Alvarez,

Susana Esquenazi,

Division for Advanced Research Technologies

NYU School of Medicine

Dina Ramadane,

Orin Mishkit,

Orlando Ariztizabal,

Zakia Gironda

Preclinical Imaging Laboratory

NYU School of Medicine

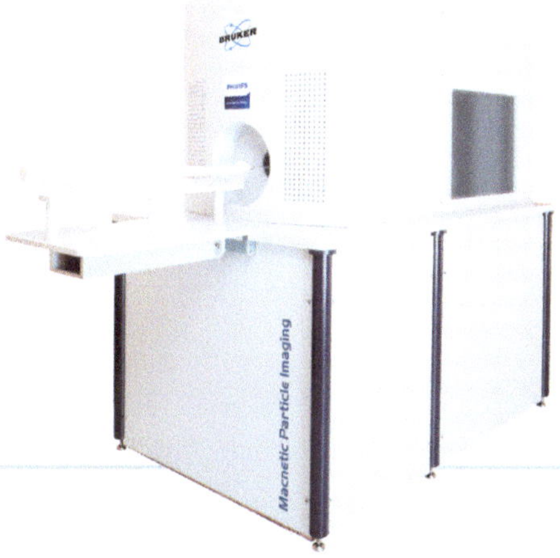

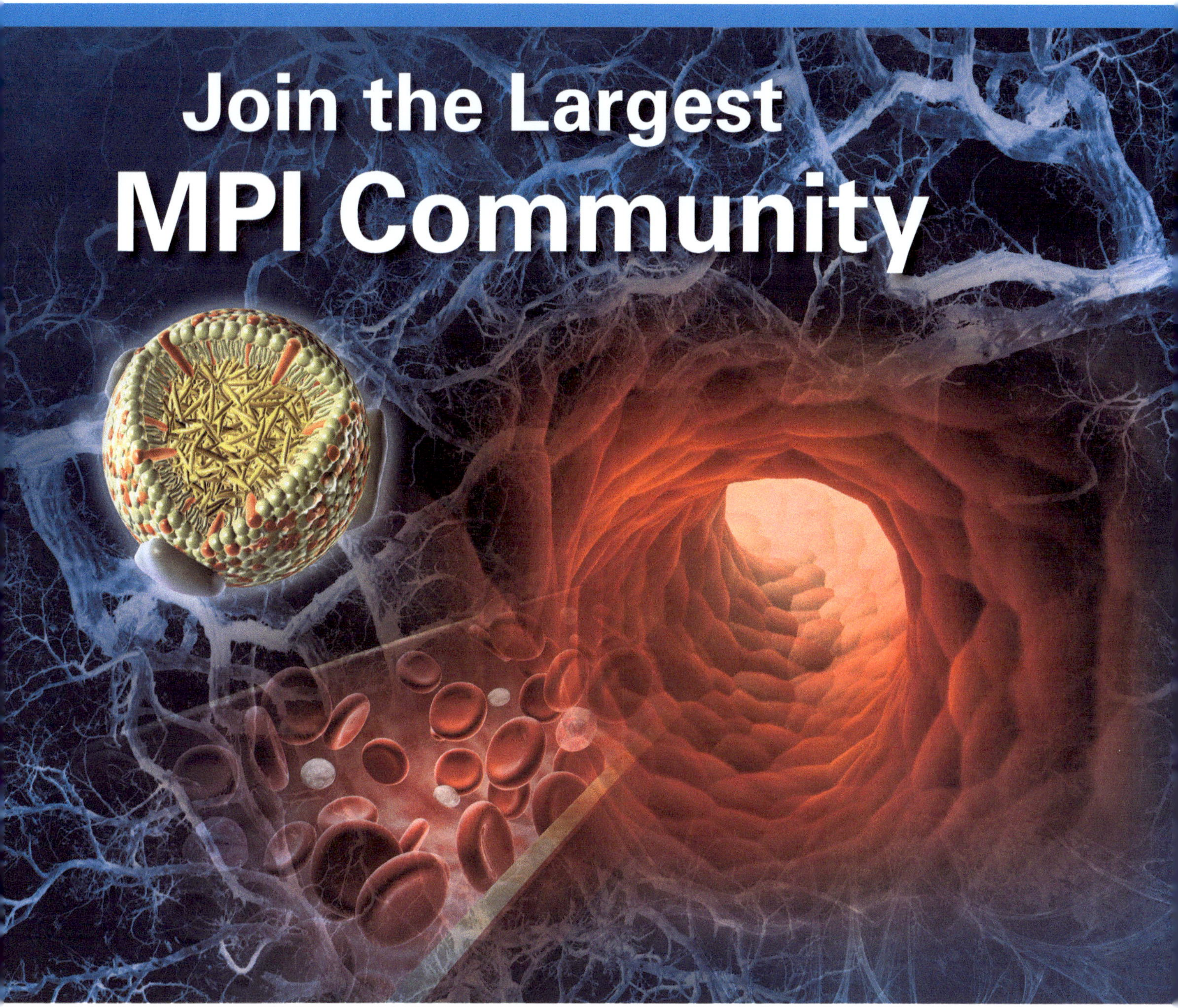

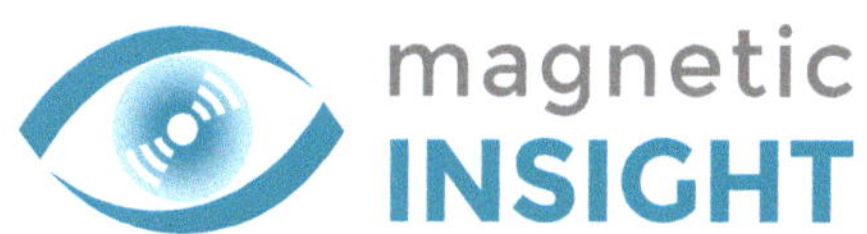

MAGNETIC PARTICLE IMAGING

MOMENTUM
MPI IMAGING SYSTEM

HYPER
LOCALIZED HYPERTHERMIA PLATFORM

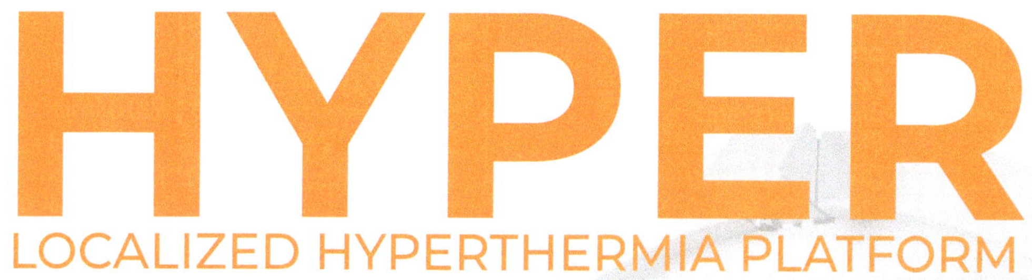

RELAX
PARTICLE RELAXOMETRY MODULE

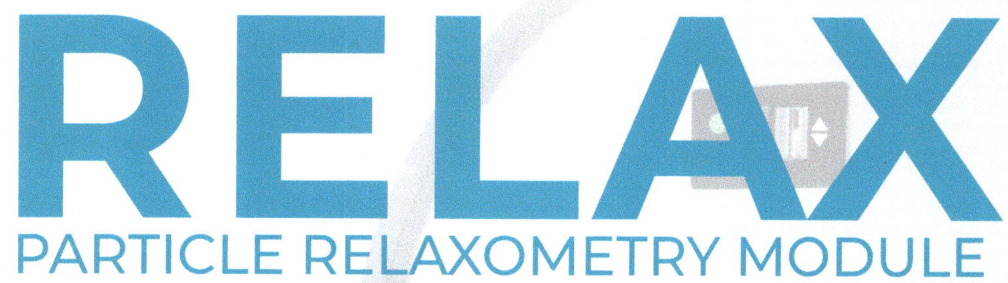

VIVOTRAX
SUPER-PARAMAGNETIC IRON OXIDE IMAGING TRACER

www.magneticinsight.com

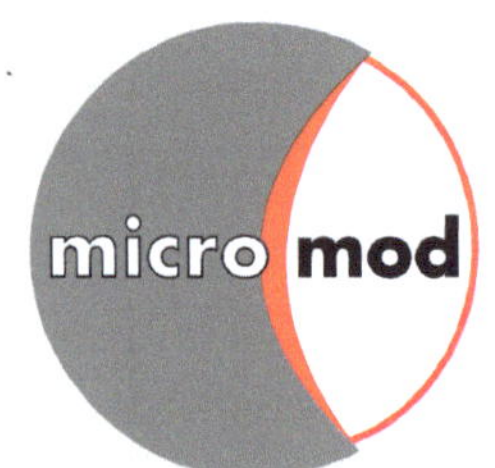

micromod Partikeltechnologie GmbH

More than **20 years** of experience in the production of chemically surface-functionalized and/or magnetizable micro- and nanoparticles

Our Magnetic Nanoparticle Classics

nanomag®-D

➡ **High-throughput nucleic acid separation**

➡ **Components in diagnostic kits and biosensors**

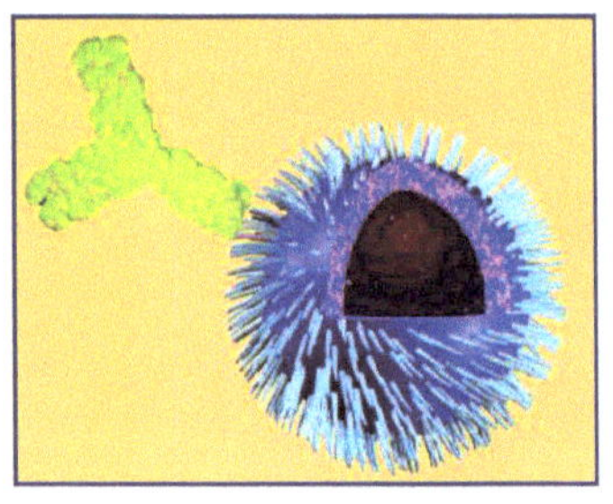

Viability assessment of Salmonella cells with nanomag®-D particles (E. Fernandez et al. Biosensors and Bioelectronics 2014, (52) 239-246.)

micromer®-M

➡ **High magnetomobility and selectivity for cell separation**

➡ **Components in biosensor and lab-on-chip applications**

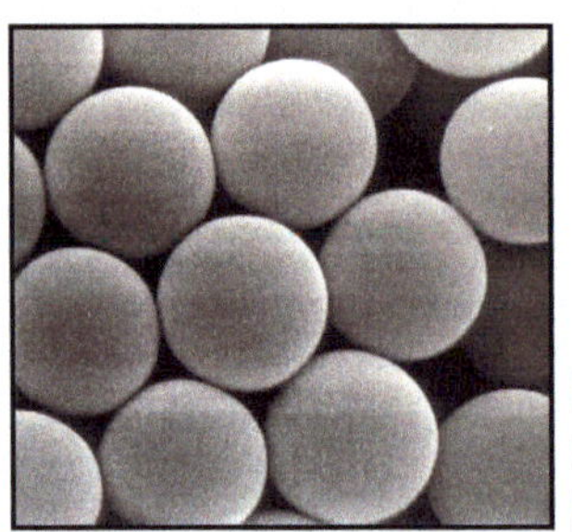

REM image of 3 μm micromer®-M particles

BNF particles

➡ **Tools for targeted MRI and hyperthermia applications**

➡ **Thermally blocked at room temperature**

➡ **Components in diagnostic kits and biosensors**

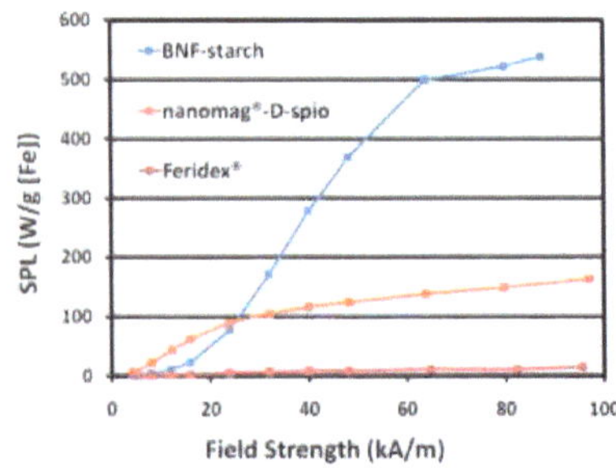

Comparison of heating rates of BNF particles, nanomag®-D-spio and Feridex® (D. Bordelon et al., *J. Appl. Phys.* 2011, 109 (12) 24904)

perimag®

➡ **Tracer for Magnetic Particle Imaging (MPI) and Magnetic resonance Imaging (MRI)**

➡ **Tools for hyperthermia applications**

➡ **Tracer for homing and tracking of stem cells in regenerative medicine**

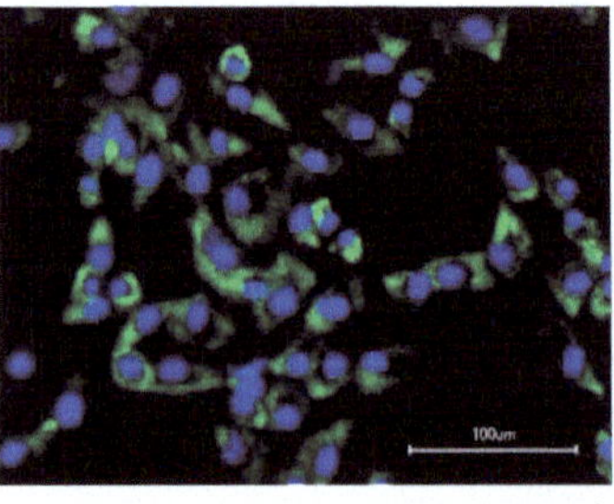

Labeling of hMSC with fluorescent perimag® (nucleus: blue; perimag® in cytoplasm: green) (T. Kilian et al. *Nanomedicine* 2016, 11 (15) 1957-1970)

micromod Partikeltechnologie GmbH

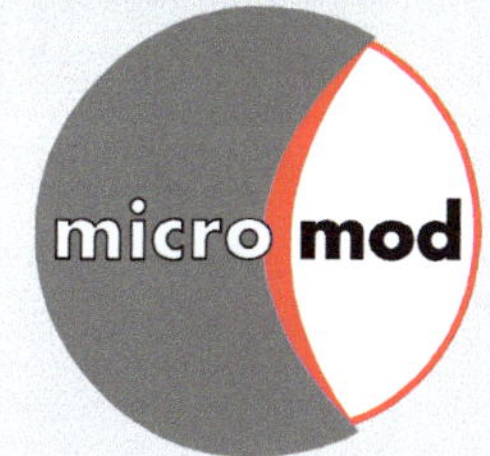

More than **20 years** of experience in the production of chemically surface-functionalized and/or magnetizable micro- and nanoparticles

A recent research highlight

synomag® - our new Nanoflower-shaped Magnetic Nanoparticles with Excellent Properties

➡ **as tracer for Magnetic Particle Imaging (MPI)**

➡ **as contrast agent for Magnetic Resonance Imaging (MRI)**

➡ **for hyperthermia applications**

➡ **as tool for biosensor and lab-on-chip applications**

Magnetic Particle Spectra:

Magnetic Particle Spectra (MPS) of 50 nm synomag®-D particles at 20 and 30 mT, amplitude of odd harmonics scaled to the amount of iron compared to Resovist®
(C. Grüttner *et al. Proceedings of IWMPI 2018*)

TEM images of synomag®-D:

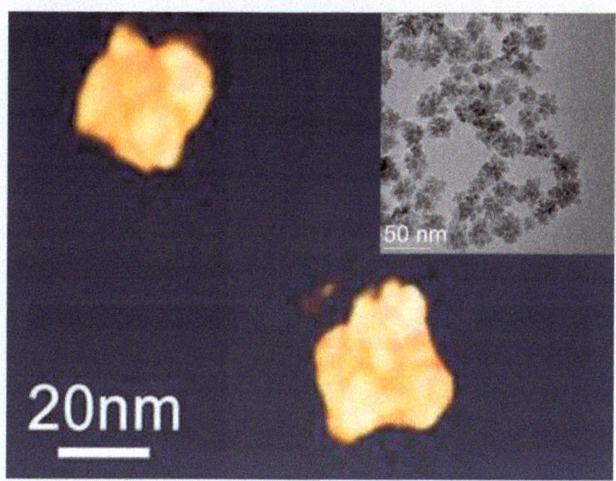

TEM tomography image of synomag®-D with a closer look at two particles viewed parallel to the electron beam direction
(L.J. Zeng, Chalmers University of Technology, Göteborg)

● **The amplitude A3 of the 3rd harmonic in the MPS spectrum of synomag®-D is more than twice as high as that of Resovist®.**

● **synomag®-D have a very high intrinsic loss power (ILP) of about 7 nHm2/kgFe**
(P. Bender et al., J. Phys. Chem. C, 2018, 122(5), 3068-3077).

Titles on Magnetic Particle Imaging
by Infinite Science Publishing

Herstellung und Charakterisierung superparamagnetischer Lacke
Inga Christine Kuschnerus
EUR 29,90

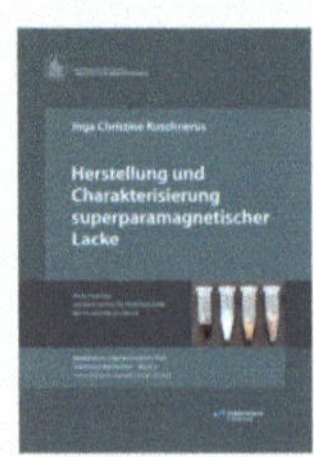

Optimierung der Permanentmagnetengeometrie zur Generierung eines Selektionsfeldes für Magnetic Particle Imaging
Matthias Weber
EUR 29,90

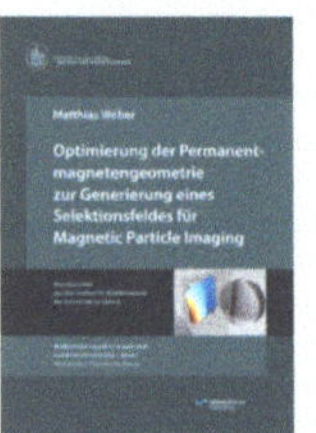

In-Silico Analysis of Superparamagnetic Nanoparticles
Henrik Rogge
EUR 59,90

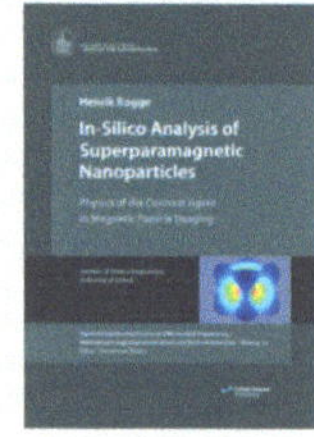

Compressed Sensing und Sparse Rekonstruktion bei Magnetic Particle Imaging
Anselm von Gladiß
EUR 49,90

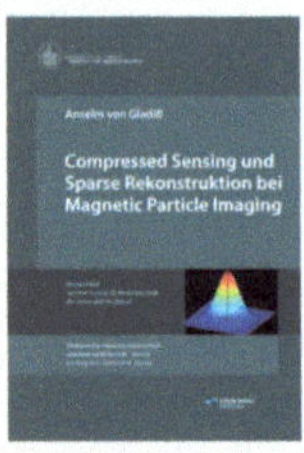

Beschleunigtes Magnetic Particle Imaging: Untersuchung des Einsatzes von Compressed Sensing für die Signalaufnahme
Nadine Traulsen
EUR 49,90

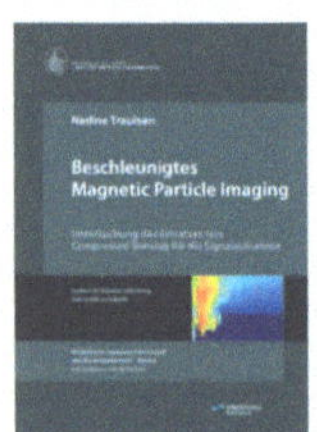

Implementation of a Magnetic Particle Imaging System for a Dynamic Field Free Line
Klaas Bente
EUR 39,90

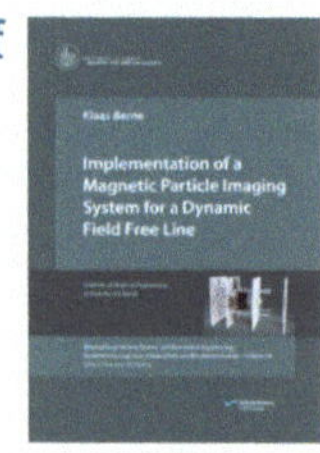

Power-Loss Optimized Field-Free Line Generation for Magnetic Particle Imaging
Matthias Weber
EUR 49,90

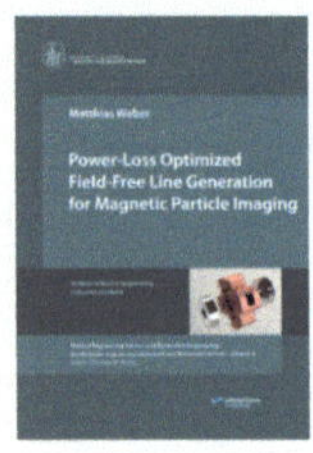

Elliptical Coils in Magnetic Particle Imaging
Christian Kaethner
EUR 49,90

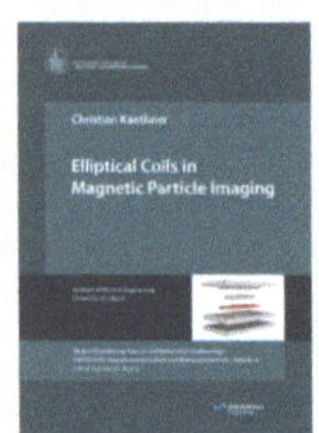

Automatische Bestimmung der Entfaltungsparameter bei der x-Space-Rekonstruktion für FFL-MPI
Steffen Bruns
EUR 19,90

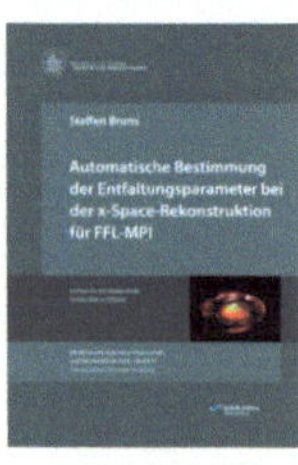

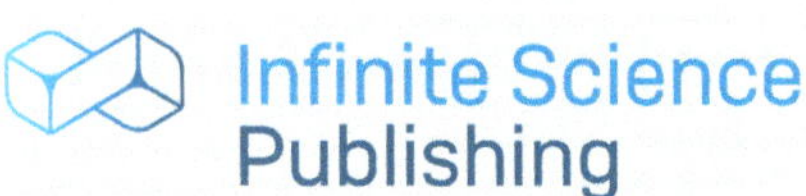
Infinite Science Publishing

https://books.infinite-science.de/mpi/

Infinite Science GmbH
MFC 1 | BioMedTec Wissenschaftscampus
Maria-Goeppert-Str. 1, 23562 Lübeck
book@infinite-science.de

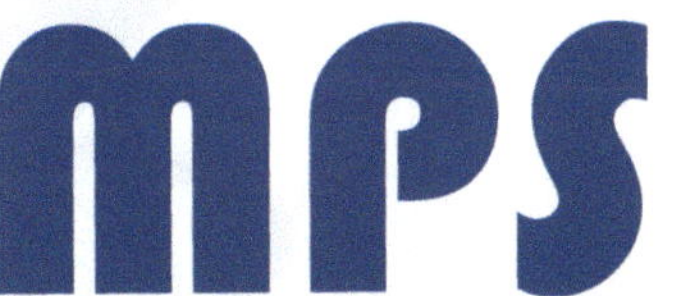

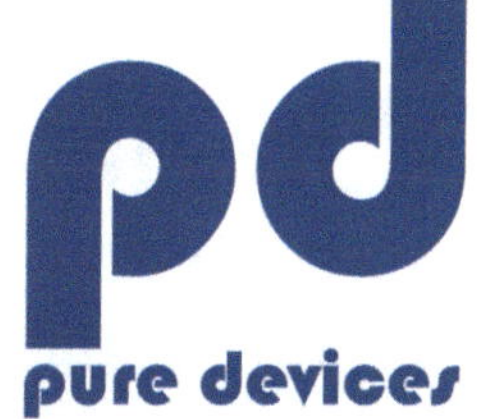

Magnetic Particle Spectrometer

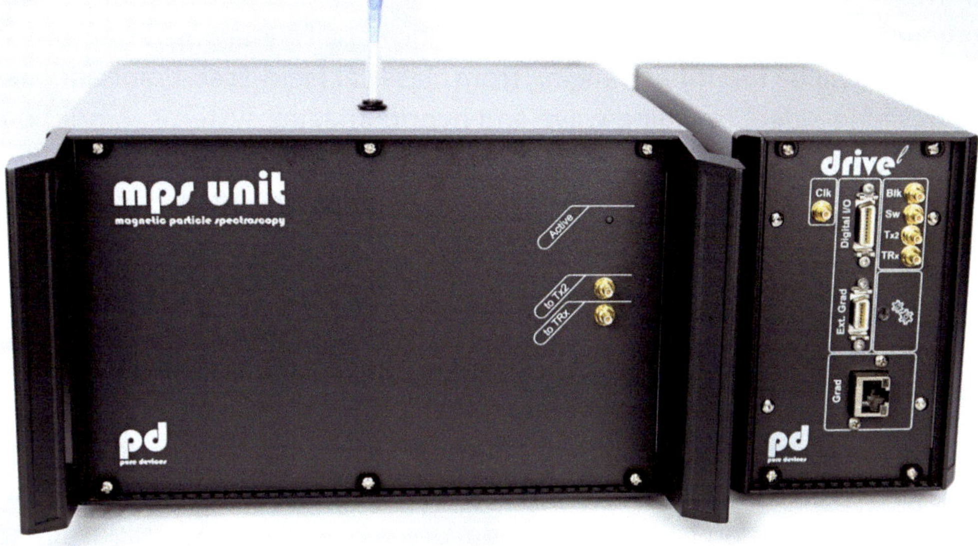

Characterization of

contrast agents
magnetic particles
MPI tracers
ferrofluides

Specifications

drive field: 0 - 30 mT
frequency: 20 kHz
bandwidth: 2.5 MHZ
test tubes: 6 mm

easy to set up

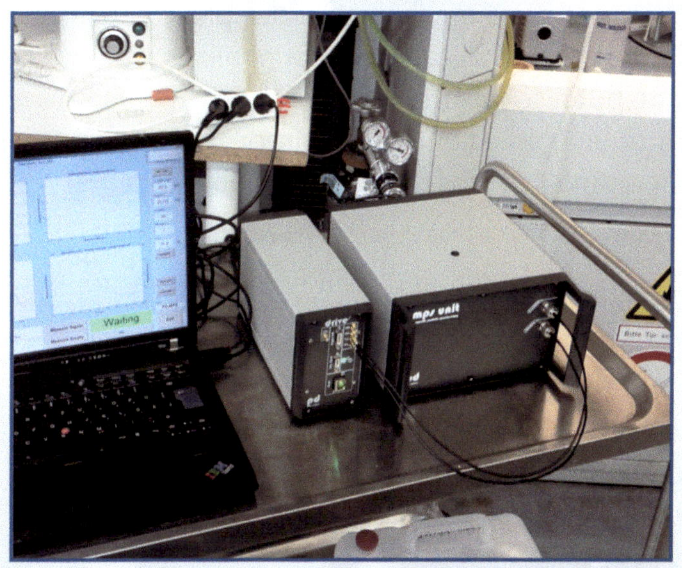

easy to operate

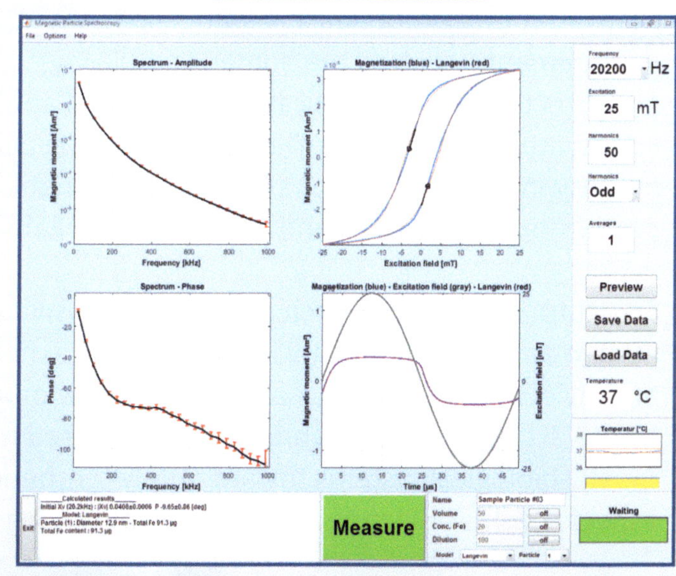

Pure Devices GmbH
Kettelerstr. 5-11
97222 Rimpar
GERMANY

www.pure-devices.com
info@pure-devices.com
Tel.: +49 (0) 9365 2069490
Fax: +49 (0) 9365 2069486

Tutorial

Lecture 1: Introduction into MPI Instrumentation and Image Reconstruction

Jochen Franke, Product Manager Magnetic Particle Imaging, System Engineering & Integration, Bruker BioSpin MRI, Germany

The scope of the first part of this tutorial is to present an overview of signal generation and spatial encoding schemes used nowadays in Magnetic Particle Imaging. State-of-the-art MPI scanner topologies will be identified ranging from classical Field-Free-Point and Field-Free-Line systems to single-sided, traveling-wave and hybrid imaging systems. A brief description of magnetic field components with their field requirements and their functionality will be highlighted. With the help of block diagrams, MPI system components of classical signal chains will be described and characterized.

The second part of this tutorial covers the basic introduction of state-of-the-art reconstruction techniques used in Magnetic Particle Imaging. At most, the differences and similarities between the frequency- and time-space reconstruction approach will be addressed. With this overview, advanced techniques such as enlarged field of view or multi-color reconstruction will be discussed. Model-based reconstruction approaches and the usage of complementary information from other modalities will lead to the outlook and discussion section.

For all topics addressed during this tutorial, scientific papers will be highlighted to provide in-depth training material.

Lecture 2: Introduction into Magnetomotion

Klaas Bente, German Federal Institute for Materials Research and Testing (BAM), Germany

Many motile microorganisms swim and navigate in chemically and mechanically complex environments, such as the human vascular system. These organisms can be functionalized and directly used for applications (biohybrid approach), but also inspire designs for fully synthetic microbots. The most promising designs of biohybrids and bioinspired microswimmers include one or several magnetic components, which lead to sustainable propulsion mechanisms and external controllability.

This tutorial addresses such magnetic microswimmers, which are often studied in view of certain applications, mostly in the biomedical field. First, propulsion systems at the microscale are reviewed and the magnetism of microswimmers is introduced. The presentation of state-of-the-art magnetic biohybrids and bioinspired microswimmers is structured gradually from mostly biological systems toward purely synthetic approaches. Finally, currently less explored aspects of this field ranging from in vivo imaging to swarm control are discussed.

Lecture 3: MPI Application Review in Diagnostics, Monitoring and Therapy

Steve Conolly, Professor of Bioengineering and Electrical Engineering and Computer Sciences, UC Berkeley, USA;
Patrick Goodwill, Chief Technical Officer, Magnetic Insight, USA

MPI research has expanded beyond hardware and groups are now working on applying MPI to solve problems in scientific research and medicine.

In the first half of this tutorial we discuss some of the latest animal research being tested on MPI systems around the world. These applications span immune and cell tracking, cancer imaging, brain perfusion imaging, gut bleed detection, and lung ventilation-perfusion imaging.

In the second half of this tutorial, we discuss combined MPI/RF hyperthermia. In traditional RF hyperthermia, the application of high frequency, high amplitude magnetic fields heats up nanoparticles in the sample. The heating can have myriad applications including heating tumors to therapeutic temperatures and releasing payloads of interest such as drugs. We discuss how combining RF hyperthermia with MPI gives new opportunities, including spatial control of the heating to millimeter-scales, and real-time monitoring of the therapeutic heat dose.

Contents

Poster Session 01

Session 03
Reconstruction, Theory, and Nanoparticle Physics II

Magnetic Insight – Lunch Session87

Session 04
Application I

Poster Session 02

Session 05
Application II

Session 06
Synthesis and Spectroscopy

Poster Session 03

Session 07
Application III

Bruker – Lunch Session 227

Session 08
Instrumentation II

Session 01: Instrumentation I

A Field-Free Line Magnetic Particle Imager for Functional Neuroimaging in Rodents

E. E. Mason[a,b*], **E. Mattingly**[b], **J. Franke**[d], **S. M. Bradley**[b], **C. Z. Cooley**[b,c], and **L. L. Wald**[b,c]

[a] Harvard-MIT Health Sciences & Technology, Cambridge, MA, USA
[b] MGH/HST A.A. Martinos Center for Biomedical Imaging, Dept. of Radiology, Massachusetts General Hospital, Boston, MA, USA
[c] Harvard Medical School, Boston, MA, USA
[d] Bruker BioSpin MRI GmbH, Ettlingen, Germany
[*] Corresponding author, email: ericamas@mit.edu

Abstract: MPI has been proposed as an alternative to fMRI for detecting cerebral blood volume (CBV) changes associated with brain activation. MPI directly detects injected superparamagnetic iron oxide nanoparticles (SPIOs) with high sensitivity and short scan times, making it a promising modality to fill this important research and clinical need. The functional MPI (fMPI) application requires a time-series of images with a temporal resolution of 5 s or less. This places specific demands that are mechanically difficult for conventional mechanically rotating field-free line (FFL) instruments, which do not allow continuous rotation. Here we present images from a rodent imager designed for continuous rotation time-series imaging.

I. Introduction

I.I. Background & Motivation

Magnetic Particle Imaging (MPI) has been investigated as a modality for functional neuroimaging, specifically for detecting hemodynamic modulations in response to functional brain activation [1, 2]. MPI directly detects superparamagnetic iron oxide (SPIO) nanoparticles [3], which do not cross the blood-brain barrier, and thus serve as a direct measure of brain blood volume. Cerebral blood volume (CBV) increases by 20% in activated regions of the brain, as is observed in fMRI studies that use SPIOs as an indirect reporter of blood volume [4]. MPI can detect the change in SPIO signal that directly reflects this change in CBV. Proof-of-concept experiments in our lab demonstrate single-sided detection of MPI signal changes corresponding to CBV changes in rodents during hyper/hypocapnia challenges [1]. However, this single-sided detector lacked spatial localization and is therefore impractical for activation studies. Expanding on this work, we present a full imaging system designed for functional CBV imaging in rodents. The system is a field-free line (FFL) MPI scanner with electrical and water slip-ring rotation to enable continuous time-series imaging. Here, we present our initial detection sensitivity results and first phantom images.

II. Material and Methods

II.I. System Details

Fig. 1A shows the overall system concept using 2" x 2" x 16" N48 NdFeB permanent magnets to produce the FFL along y', and diamond-shaped, water-cooled shift coils to sweep the FFL across the projection axis, x'. The solenoid drive and gradiometer receive hardware sit inside the copper tube bore. The FFL magnets and shift coils are rotated about the bore to acquire multiple projections.

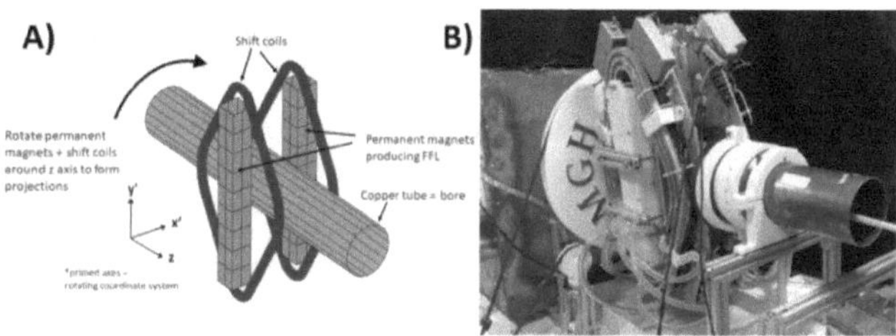

Figure 1: *A) Illustration of the small-bore imager design, showing the permanent magnets, electromagnet shift coils, copper tube bore, and coordinate system. **B)** Photo of the physical system.*

The drive and receive coils are similar to those used in the single-sided detector [1] but scaled to fit around a rodent head (5 cm-diameter clearance). The drive coil is a 12 cm long solenoid with two 41-turn layers, inner diameter 5.8 cm, and L=195 μH. It is wound with 16 AWG Litz Wire (New England Wire, Lisbon, NH) and produces 0.62 mT/A at the center of the imaging FOV (2 cm from end of coil). A 25 kHz drive signal is produced by an NI USB-6363 DAQ console (National Instruments, Austin, TX), amplified by an AE Techron 7224 power amplifier (Elkhart, IN), and filtered by a custom high-power low-pass filter. The drive coil and copper tube have a 2 cm spacing between them to reduce eddy currents in the tube below the level of the current density in the coil itself, and heating in the copper tube is less problematic than heating in the drive coil due to the reduced current density, better air cooling, significant copper mass, and conduction away from the source.

A gradiometer receive coil with 5 cm inner diameter is nested and epoxied inside the drive coil. Its two oppositely wound 20 AWG Litz wire coils (4 cm long, 66 turns each, 4 cm separation between them) provides first-order drive field cancellation. Unlike most MPI systems, only the $3f_0$ frequency is sampled. Receive circuit alterations to collect additional harmonics are underway. The receive chain includes a tuning/notch filter (73 dB attenuation between $3f_0$ and f_0), low-noise pre-amplifier (Stanford Research Systems SR560, Sunnyvale, CA) and high- and low-pass filtering with 40 kHz and 99.9 kHz cutoffs, respectively (SR650, Sunnyvale, CA), before console digitization (sampled with 500 kHz bandwidth).

The FFL is produced by two 2" x 2" x 16" NdFeB N48 magnets (each made of four 2" x 2" x 4" blocks), and has a gradient of approximately 3.5 T/m. The shift coils are 250-turn diamond-shaped coils wound with 14 AWG magnet wire. Each coil has DC resistance of 2.4 Ω and is water-cooled. The shift coils produce a 1.3 mT/A field across the region of interest. An image of the full system is shown in Fig. 1B.

III. Results

Fig. 2 shows sensitivity measurements taken with our FFL imager without image encoding. Samples of VivoTrax SPIOs (Magnetic Insight, Alameda, CA) of varying concentrations in 18 µL glass bulbs are inserted into the receive coil, 2 cm from its surface. The drive field is 18.4 mT at the sample location, produced with a 29.6 A, 25 kHz sinusoid. Each data point is acquired over 12 ms. The system detects 50 ng samples with SNR = 3.99.

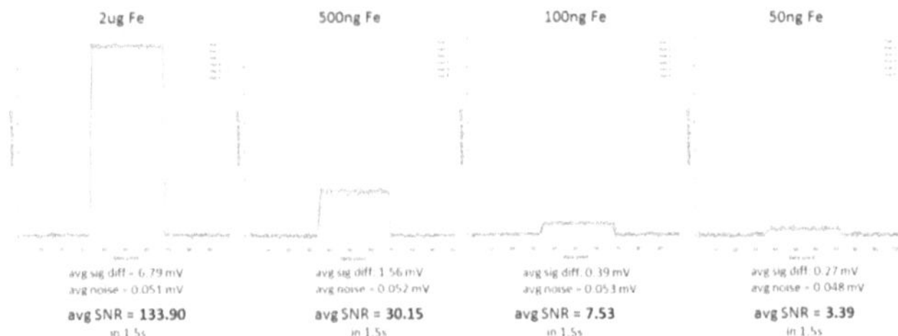

Figure 2: *Detection sensitivity data. No image encoding used. 18 uL bulb samples placed inside coil (center of one side of gradiometer). Drive field produced by 29.6 A (amplitude) 25 kHz current, producing 18.4 mT at sample location. Each data point is from a 12 ms burst pulse of drive, 1.5 s pause following. Preamp G=500. Linear drift removed in post-processing.*

Fig. 3C shows an image of two 18 µL bulbs (3 mm dia.) spaced by 1 cm and filled with 0.5 mg/ml Fe of VivoTrax SPIOs, 9 µg Fe per bulb. Each projection has 62 points, and 26 projections are used across 180°. The drive field is 12 mT at the sample location, produced with a 19 A sinusoid at 25 kHz. Each point in the projection is acquired with a 12 ms drive field pulse plus a 500 ms pause. A background signal measured at the start of the experiment is subtracted during projection acquisition. The image is reconstructed using an inverse radon transform, with no other post-processing. The FOV of the image is about 2 cm.

SNR is 92.7, and spatial resolution is 2-3 mm, calculated by minimizing the difference between the image and convolution of a Gaussian PSF with a 3 mm bulb.

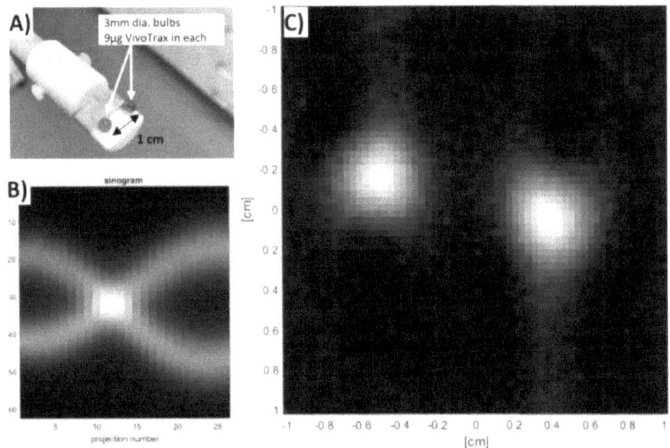

Figure 3: *A) Phantom is two 3mm diameter glass bulbs, each filled with 9 ug Fe VivoTrax SPIOs spaced 1 cm apart. B) Sinogram of projections. There are 62 points per projection, 26 projections covering 180°. Drive field is 12 mT, and each point in the projection comes from 12 ms drive pulse plus a 500 ms pause. Preamp G=100. The FFL gradient strength is approximately 3.5 T/m, and the shift coils cover a 2 cm FOV. C) Image of a two-bulb phantom. Image is reconstructed with an inverse radon transform. SNR = 92.7. Spatial resolution = 2-3 mm.*

IV. Discussion/Conclusion

We present detection sensitivity measurements and first images with our continuously rotating FFL MPI scanner. The system is currently capable of detecting 50 ng Fe. Two 3 mm dia. phantoms separated by 1 cm can be clearly distinguished and 9 µg Fe is seen with high SNR in the full image. Our next steps are to speed up the imaging time and fully utilize continuous rotation and produce time-series images, and finally to proceed to functional activation studies in rats.

ACKNOWLEDGEMENTS
Thank you to Suma Anand and Charlotte Sappo for their assistance with filter design, and to Simon Sigalovsky, Jason Jensen, Kieran Bradley, and Jack Hawk for their contributions to the mechanical components of the system.

AUTHOR'S STATEMENT
Funding for the work comes from NIBIB U01EB025121-02, NIMH R24106053, and NSF GRFP 1122374. Authors state no conflict of interest.

REFERENCES
[1] C. Z. Cooley, J. B. Mandeville, E. E. Mason, E. T. Mandeville, S. Anand, and L. L. Wald, "Rodent Cerebral Blood Volume (CBV) changes during hypercapnia observed using Magnetic Particle Imaging (MPI) detection," *Neuroimage.*

[2] E. E. Mason, C. Z. Cooley, S. F. Cauley, M. A. Griswold, S. M. Conolly, and L. L. Wald, "Design analysis of an MPI human functional brain scanner," *Int. J. Magn. Part. Imaging*, vol. 3, no. 1, 2017.

[3] B. Gleich and J. Weizenecker, "Tomographic imaging using the nonlinear response of magnetic particles," *Nature*, vol. 435, no. 7046, pp. 1214–7, Jun. 2005.

[4] J. B. Mandeville *et al.*, "Dynamic Functional Imaging of Relative Cerebral Blood Volume During Rat Forepaw Stimulation," *Magn. Reson. Med.*, vol. 39, no. 4, pp. 615–624, 1998.

Dynamic 2D Imaging with an MPI Scanner Featuring a Mechanically Rotated FFL

A. von Gladiss[a]*, J. Beuke[a], M. Weber[a,+], A. Malhotra[a], A. Behrends[a], A. Cordes[a], M. Stille[a], V. Behr[b], P. Vogel[b], K. Gräfe[a], Th. Friedrich[a], K. Lüdtke-Buzug[a], A. Neumann[a], M. Ahlborg[a] and T. M. Buzug[a]

[a] *Institute of Medical Engineering, University of Luebeck, Luebeck, Germany*
[b] *Department of Experimental Physics 5 (Biophysics), University of Wuerzburg, Wuerzburg, Germany*
[+] *now with: Magnetic Insight, Inc., Alameda CA, USA*
[*] *Corresponding author, email: {gladiss,buzug}@imt.uni-luebeck.de*

A Magnetic Particle Imaging scanner has been presented that features only one signal chain. A field free line is generated by permanent magnets and translated by an alternating homogeneous magnetic field in one direction. The gantry is rotated mechanically and thus, 1D projection images over 360° are acquired. 3D images have been acquired by rotating and translating a phantom stepwise. Here, 2D images of both static and moving phantoms are acquired by rotating the gantry continuously.

I. Introduction

Magnetic Particle Imaging (MPI) is a tracer-based medical imaging modality that has recently entered the preclinical evaluation phase [1]. It features high temporal resolution, superb sensitivity and has the potential of submillimeter spatial resolution. It is tailored for clinical application as neither ionizing radiation nor noxious tracer material are used. Current MPI scanners have a temporal resolution of down to few tens of ms for imaging a volume. 192 pg of iron could be detected using a Magnetic Particle Spectrometer. In an MPI scanner, 5 ng of iron could be imaged [2]. A spatial resolution in the submillimeter range has been claimed but could not be proven yet. A field free line (FFL) MPI scanner has been presented that focuses on sensitivity and spatial resolution [3]. Providing a magnetic gradient field of 5 T/m it may prove the claim for μm resolution in the field of MPI. Furthermore, it features an FFL that is supposed to increase the sensitivity of an MPI scanner [4]. A Halbach array geometry generates an FFL orthogonal to the bore direction of the MPI scanner (Fig. 1). The FFL is translated perpendicular to the bore direction using a homogeneous magnetic field, the drive field. The receive signal can be reconstructed into a 1D projection image. The gantry is rotated mechanically which rotates the FFL and the projection angle as well. A set of 1D projection images can be arranged as a sinogram and be reconstructed into a 2D image using filtered backprojection [5].

In [3], a 3D image has been acquired by simultaneously rotating and moving a vessel phantom in bore direction. Thus, the phantom has been sampled in a helical trajectory. In this work, a one dot phantom is imaged in 2D by rotating the gantry mechanically. Furthermore, dynamic 2D images of a moving two dot phantom are presented.

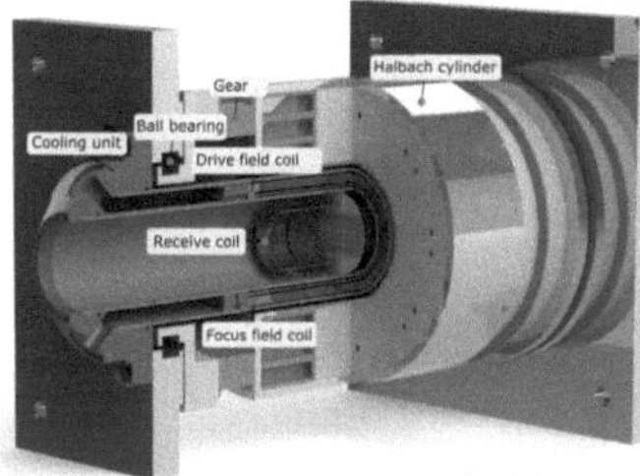

Figure 1: *Design of the FFL MPI scanner.*

II. Material and Methods

The FFL MPI scanner provides a field gradient of 5 T/m perpendicular to the FFL. A homogeneous drive field of 20 mT strength enables a 1D FOV of 8 mm length. By rotating the gantry mechanically using a motor, the angle of the 1D FOV is continuously varied. Photoelectric sensors keep track of the angular orientation of the gantry. The repetition time of the excitation field is 40 μs. The receive signals that are acquired at one angle are averaged and reconstructed into a 1D image. A regularization is used for reconstruction. The 1D images are arranged in a sinogram. The sinogram is reconstructed into a 2D image using filtered backprojection.

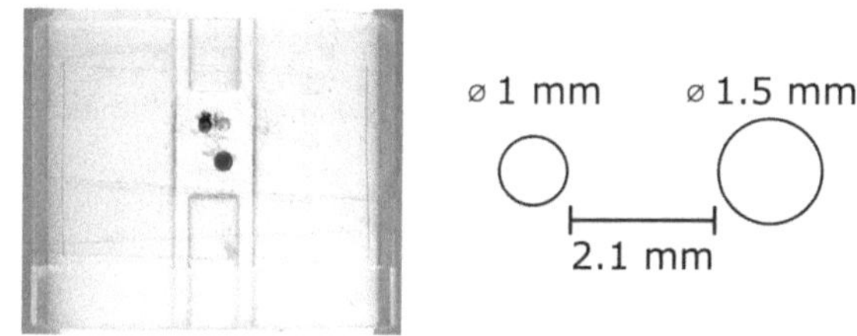

Figure 2: *Two dots of the phantom with a minimum distance of 2.1 mm and diameters of 1.5 mm and 1 mm have been filled.*

A one dot phantom (diameter of 3 mm) filled with 35 µl of undiluted Resovist (Bayer-Schering, Berlin, Germany) has been placed at two different fixed positions inside the scanner. During signal acquisition, the gantry has been rotated continuously over 360° with 10.8 rpm.

Another phantom consisting of two dots (diameters 1.5 mm and 1 mm) has been filled with 7 µl and π µl of undiluted Resovist (see Fig. 2). The rotation frequency of the gantry was 30 rpm. During the continuous signal acquisition, the phantom has been moved. An online reconstruction has been implemented to visualize the phantom position in real time.

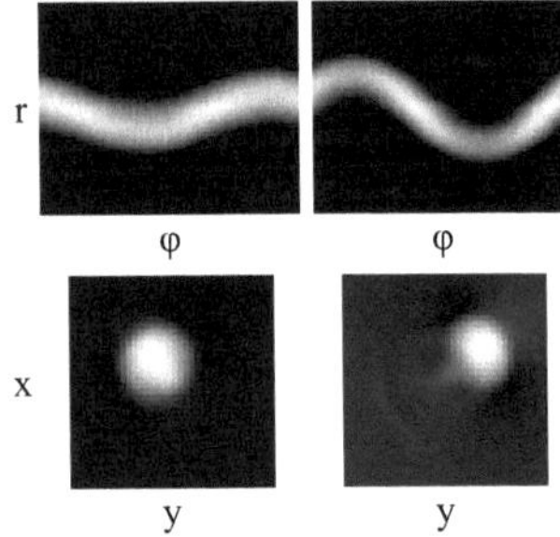

Figure 3: *Reconstruction results of a static phantom consisting of one dot with a diameter of 3 mm. The phantom has been placed at two different positions inside the FOV.*

III. Results

The reconstruction results of the one dot phantom are visualized in Fig. 3. The static phantom has been imaged at two different positions inside the FOV. Fig. 3 shows the sinograms that consist of reconstructed 1D projection images over 360 angular directions. The sinograms have been successfully reconstructed into 2D images.

Fig. 4 shows reconstructed images of the two dot phantom (see Fig. 2). The two dots can be identified in both the sinograms and images. During rotation #16, the phantom has been rotated quickly introducing motion artefacts. Streaking artefacts connecting the two dots can be seen.

IV. Discussion

The reconstructed images of the moving two dot phantom in Fig. 4 are noisier than the images of the static one dot phantom (see Fig. 3). As the rotation frequency of the gantry was about 3 times higher when imaging the two dot phantom, a smaller number of receive signal periods has been acquired for each angle decreasing the SNR. Furthermore, the two dot phantom features smaller diameters and volumes (factors 2 and 3 resp. 5 and 10) than the single dot phantom. Therefore, the dots contain smaller amounts of particles which results in a lower SNR. The detection slice thickness may be smaller than the length of the dots (4 mm). Then, the number of particles imaged is less than π µl indicating a high sensitivity of the scanner.

A minimum spatial distance of 2.1 mm can be clearly resolved. The reconstruction results indicate that a lower distance in µm range may be resolved as well.

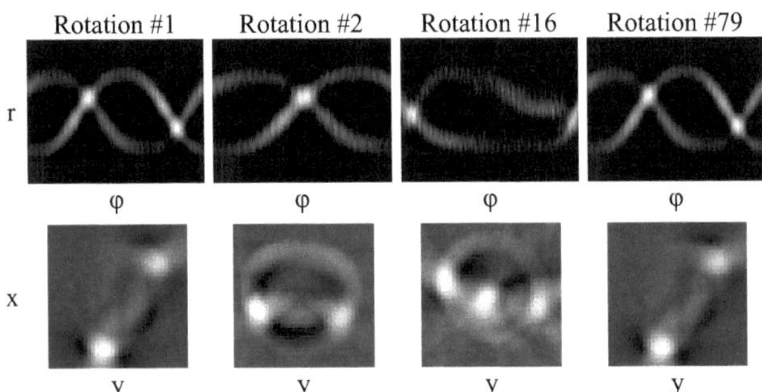

Figure 4: *Reconstruction results of a moving phantom consisting of two dots (diameters 1.5 mm and 1 mm).*

The temporal resolution of the images shown in Fig. 4 was about 0.5 Hz. The temporal resolution could be increased by increasing the rotation frequency of the gantry. Though, the SNR would drop as a fewer number of receive signal periods could be averaged for one angle. The sinogram may be updated with each new angle that has been acquired increasing the temporal resolution without decreasing the SNR. Furthermore, 2D images may be reconstructed using only half a rotation of the gantry increasing the temporal resolution by a factor of 2.

The streaking artefacts connecting the two dots may be caused by inconsistencies of the sinogram due to the regularization when reconstructing the 1D images. Data consistency parameters may be applied to reduce these artefacts. Furthermore, motion parameters may be estimated by applying data consistency parameters as well [6].

V. Conclusions

In [3], 3D images have been acquired by rotating and translating a phantom stepwise. The gantry did not move during the acquisition. Here, it has been shown that 2D images can successfully be acquired by rotating the gantry continuously. The movement of a phantom has been visualized. The reconstructed images indicate a high spatial resolution and sensitivity of the scanner. In the future, 3D images will be acquired by moving a 3D phantom through the FOV while the gantry is rotated continuously.

ACKNOWLEDGEMENTS

The authors thankfully acknowledge the financial support by the German Research Foundation (DFG, grant number BU 1436/9-1) and the Federal Ministry of Education and Research (BMBF, grant numbers 13GW0230B, 13GW0069A, 13GW0071D and 01DL17010A). The authors thank H. Schwegmann and D. Steinhagen for their technical support.

AUTHOR'S STATEMENT

The authors state no conflict of interest.

REFERENCES

[1] Gleich et al. *Nature*, 2005. doi: 10.1038/nature03808.
[2] Graeser et al. *Scientific Reports,* 2017. doi: 10.1038/s41598-017-06992-5.
[3] Weber et al. *IJMPI*, 2018. doi: 10.18416/IJMPI.2018.1811004.
[4] Weizenecker et al. *J. Phys. D*, 2008. doi: 10.1088/0022-3727/41/10/105009.
[5] Knopp et al. *Inverse Problems*, 2011. doi: 10.1088/0266-5611/27/9/095004.
[6] Yu et al., *IEEE Trans. Med. Imaging*, 2006. doi: 10.1109/TMI.2006.875424.

Design of a Preclinical Field Free Point/Field Free Line Hybrid MPI Scanner

A. R. Cagil[a,b*] and E. U. Saritas[a,b,c]

[a] *Department of Electrical and Electronics Engineering, Bilkent University, Ankara, Turkey*
[b] *National Magnetic Resonance Research Center, Ankara, Turkey*
[c] *Neuroscience Program, Sabuncu Brain Research Center, Bilkent University, Ankara, Turkey*
[*] *Corresponding author, email: cagil@ee.bilkent.edu.tr*

Abstract: − In this work, a preclinical field free line (FFL) magnetic particle imaging (MPI) scanner is proposed for imaging in projection format. The electromagnetical and mechanical simulations necessary for the design parameters of the scanner are conducted through finite element analysis in COMSOL. Furthermore, a novel "swap coil" configuration is proposed to allow electronical switching between FFL and field free point (FFP) modes, enabling to switch from projection format imaging to volumetric imaging.

I. Introduction

In magnetic particle imaging (MPI), field free line (FFL) scanner topologies achieve projection format imaging [1], similar to X-ray imaging. For this purpose, a gradient magnetic field is generated such that the field is near zero along a continuous line called a FFL [2-4]. This allows for the acquisition of the response from all SPIOs within the FFL at once, and provides significant improvements in terms of imaging speed, SNR, and detection sensitivity. However, projection images have the intrinsic disadvantage of lack of depth resolution. Previously, 3D projection reconstruction imaging was proposed via rotating the sample [3] or the FFL [5,6]. Here, we present an alternative approach with a preclinical hybrid 2D/3D MPI scanner that can swap between projection imaging via FFL mode and volumetric imaging via field free point (FFP) mode. This hybrid approach can enable rapid acquisition of a 2D projection image as a "localizer" to select a region of interest (ROI) for detailed 3D volumetric imaging.

II. Material and Methods

II.I. Permanent Magnet Choice and Placement

The dimensions, strength grade, and placement of magnets have a direct effect on the image quality and resolution in MPI. A sweep through dimensions of commercially available permanent magnets and placement options was performed. This search yielded an optimal design using $15\times10\times5$ cm^3 grade N42 magnets assembled into groups of 5 to form two larger $75\times10\times5$ cm^3 magnets. These two magnet structures are then placed 10 cm apart, North poles facing each other (see Fig. 1a). The resulting selection field gradient strengths in x- and z-directions are both 4.4 T/m at the center of the scanner, as shown in Fig. 2. The FFL lies along the y-direction, enabling projection format imaging onto the x-z plane. The deviations in gradient strengths are less than 10% within 5.3 cm and 4.2 cm diameters in x- and z-directions, respectively, suitable for preclinical imaging.

II.II. Supporting Frame Design

The geometric design of the scanner focused on the static stress and displacement simulations performed in Fusion 360. With our current choice of magnets, the supporting frame has to withstand forces of about 2500 N in the vertical direction and 1500 N in the horizontal direction, without any significant deformation or stretching. Here, a G10 composite was chosen as the supporting frame material, as it is a popular choice for enduring such large stresses with negligible deformation [7].

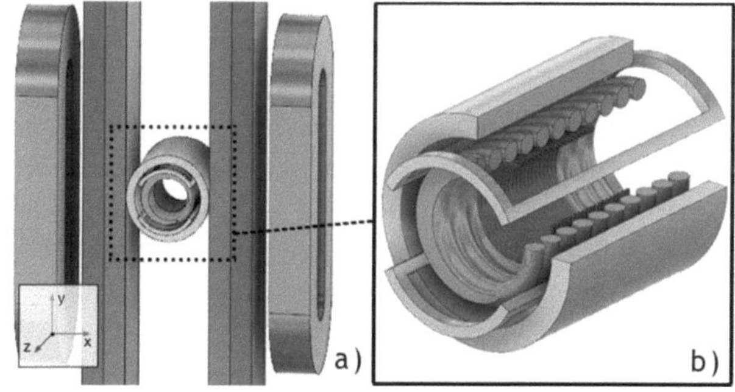

Figure 1: *Preclinical hybrid MPI scanner designed in this work. a) Overview of the scanner components. b) Close-up view of the bore. From periphery to center: Copper shield, FFL/FFP swap coil, transmit coil, and receive coil.*

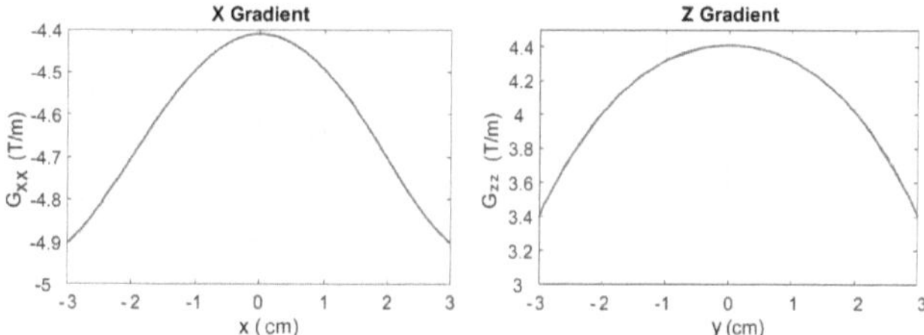

Figure 2: *Selection field gradients in x- and z-directions. The y-direction has zero gradient, as it corresponds to the FFL direction.*

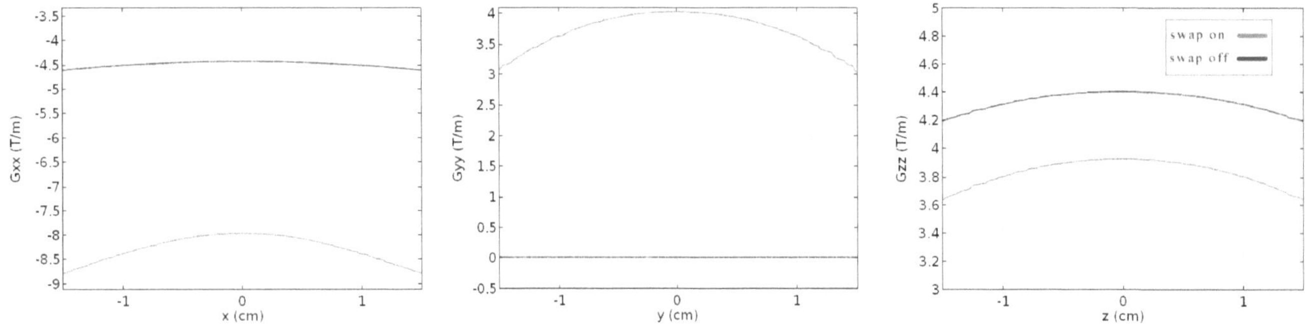

Figure 3: Selection field gradients within the bore with the FFL/FFP swap coil (i.e., the saddle coil) off or on.

II.III. Coils

The scanner is designed to achieve a drive field amplitude of 15 mT at 25 kHz along the z-direction, and a slow-shifting focus field of 115 mT along the x-direction. The coils aimed to minimize the power consumption. The movement of sample along the z-direction is designed to be achieved via a robotic arm. The copper shield was designed to balance between shield thickness and available bore radius. Finite element simulations were performed using COMSOL (COMSOL AB, Stockholm, Sweden). A novel electronic swapping between FFL and FFP modes can be realized through the use of a saddle coil (shown in Fig. 1b). Depending on the direction of the applied currents, this coil can either transform FFL into an FFP or flip the FFL such that it lies along the bore direction (when operating in non-gradient vs. gradient configurations, respectively).

III. Results

A finite elements analysis of the proposed coil arrangement was performed to demonstrate the FFL/FFP transition and to evaluate the suitability of the resulting fields for imaging. Figure 3 shows the selection field gradients near the center of the imaging bore when the swap coil is off and on. The increase in G_{xx} with the swap coil on is proportional to the swap coil current. This increased gradient strength will result in increased resolution along that direction during volumetric mode.

IV. Discussion

Simulation results show that the use of a saddle coil is a viable option for swapping between projection imaging and volumetric imaging. Note that the gradient strength of the volumetric mode can be varied using the saddle coil current only, and this can be used to zoom into a small ROI for targeted high-resolution imaging. The same feature may also prove useful for multi-resolution imaging [8]. A combined use case of first using the projection image as a "localizer" and then acquiring a higher resolution volumetric image from any selected region can help focus on a ROI to reduce the total scan time.

Reversing the current direction of the saddle coil results in the FFL flipping to lie along the bore direction (i.e., the z-direction). This mode enables projection imaging onto the x-y plane. This added feature can be utilized to design a scanner that can electronically switch projection planes to acquire rapid images in both x-z and x-y planes.

A drawback of the swap coil design is the high power of up to 20 kW (depending on the desired FFP resolution) needed to stay in the volumetric mode. As this power is dissipated within the bore, cooling becomes a necessity.

V. Conclusions

In this work, we have shown that a hybrid FFL/FFP scanner topology is feasible. This design can be utilized in achieving rapid projection imaging followed by 3D volumetric imaging using the same MPI scanner.

AUTHOR'S STATEMENT

Research funding: This work was supported by the Scientific and Technological Research Council of Turkey (TUBITAK 115E677). Conflict of interest: Authors state no conflict of interest.

REFERENCES

[1] B. Gleich and J. Weizenecker. Tomographic imaging using the nonlinear response of magnetic particles. *Nature*, 435(7046):1217-1217, 2005. doi: 10.1038/nature03808.

[2] J. Weizenecker, B. Gleich, and J. Borgert. Magnetic Particle Imaging using a Field Free Line. *J Phys D: Appl Phys*, 41(10):105009, 2008. doi: 10.1088/0022-3727/41/10/105009.

[3] P. W. Goodwill, J. J. Konkle, B. Zheng, E. U. Saritas and S. M. Conolly. Projection X-Space Magnetic Particle Imaging. *IEEE Trans Med Imaging*, 31(5):1076-1085, 2012. doi: 10.1109/TMI.2012.2185247.

[4] T. Knopp, M. Erbe, S. Biederer, T. F. Sattel, and T. M. Buzug. Efficient generation of a magnetic field-free line. *Med. Phys.* 37(7): 3538, 2010. doi: 10.1118/1.3447726.

[5] K. Bente, M. Weber, M. Graeser, T. F. Sattel, M. Erbe, T. M. Buzug. Electronic Field Free Line Rotation and Relaxation Deconvolution in Magnetic Particle Imaging. *IEEE Trans Med Imaging*, 34(2): 644-651, 2014. doi: 10.1109/TMI.2014.2364891.

[6] C. B. Top, S. İlbey, H. E. Güven. Electronically rotated and translated field□free line generation for open bore magnetic particle imaging. *Med. Phys.*, 44(12): 6225-6338, 2017. doi: 10.1002/mp.12604.

[7] P. W. Goodwill, K. Lu, B. Zheng and S. M. Conolly. An X-space Magnetic Particle Imaging Scanner. *Rev Sci Instrum*, 83(3):033708, 2012. doi: 10.1063/1.3694534.

[8] N. Gdaniec, P. Szwargulski and T. Knopp. Fast Multiresolution Data Acquisition For Magnetic Particle Imaging Using Adaptive Feature Detection. *Med. Phys.*, 44: 6456-6460. doi:10.1002/mp.12628

MPI meets CT: first hybrid MPI-CT scanner

Patrick Vogel [a,d], **Jonathan Markert** [a,c], **Martin A. Rückert** [a], **Stefan Herz** [d], **Benedikt Keßler** [c], **Kilian Dremel** [f], **Daniel Althoff** [f], **Matthias Weber** [e,+], **Thorsten M. Buzug** [e], **Thorsten A. Bley** [d], **Walter H. Kullmann** [c], **Randolf Hanke** [b,f], **Simon Zabler** [b,f], **Volker C. Behr** [a,*]

[a] Department of Experimental Physics 5 (Biophysics), University of Würzburg, 97074 Würzburg, Germany
[b] Department of Experimental Physics (X-Ray Microscopy), University of Würzburg, 97074 Würzburg, Germany
[c] Institute of Medical Engineering, University of Applied Sciences Schweinfurt, 97421 Schweinfurt, Germany
[d] Diagnostic and Interventional Radiology, University Hospital Würzburg, 97080 Würzburg, Germany
[e] Institute of Medical Engineering, University of Lübeck, 23562 Lübeck, Germany
[f] Fraunhofer Development Center X-ray Technology EZRT, 97074 Würzburg, Germany
[+] now with Magnetic Insight Inc., Alameda CA, USA
[*] Corresponding author, email: behr@physik.uni-wuerzburg.de

Abstract: Magnetic Particle Imaging (MPI) is a promising tomographic modality for fast as well as three-dimensional visualization of magnetic material. For anatomical or structural information an additional imaging modality such as computed tomography (CT) is required. In this contribution, the first hybrid MPI-CT scanner for multimodal imaging providing simultaneous data acquisition is presented.

I. Introduction

Magnetic Particle Imaging (MPI) can directly image the distribution of superparamagnetic iron-oxide nanoparticles (SPIONs) in three dimensions [1], but not from surrounding tissue. Thus, a combination with an additional tomographic modality allows for registering the particle signal and the anatomical information. Since MPI is based on the nonlinear response of SPIONs regarding time-varying magnetic fields, a combination with magnetic resonance imaging (MRI) is obvious [2, 3, 4]. Unfortunately, the incompatible hardware demands regarding field generation put both modalities at a disadvantage.

The combination of MPI with computed tomography (CT) implies certain challenges such as the usage of X-rays for imaging, which requires a 'free' view through the sample. Conventional MPI scanners are based on a closed-bore design providing an efficient generation of magnetic field gradients [5]. However, an MPI-CT hybrid system requires an open MPI concept, which could be provided by single-sided MPI approaches presented in the past, which demonstrate the general feasibility [6, 7] though the effort to realize such a single-sided MPI device is quite high.

In 2008 an MPI scanner concept was presented using a field free line (FFL) instead of a field free point (FFP) for encoding the volume of interest [8]. A common feature between CT and FFL-MPI is the acquisition scheme: Both technologies acquire projections. However, most FFL concepts are based on complex hardware designs for either electrical or mechanical rotation of the FFL or the sample and did not provide a direct view through the system [9, 10].

Recently, a concept for generating a static FFL utilizing Halbach rings [11, 12] was presented by Weber et al. [13]. Based on this concept, a novel FFL system is presented offering an open design to provide a 'window' for CT imaging.

II. Material and Methods

The hybrid MPI-CT scanner is based on the Micro-CT system "MetRIC", an inhouse scanner assembled on a sled-system providing a free adjustment of distances between X-ray source, sample holder, MPI-FFL-scanner and X-ray detector offering a flexible access to all parts (see Fig. 1 a).

The MPI-FFL scanner (Fig. 1 b) consists of two Halbach rings (k=1), both generating a magnetic field oriented in the plane of each ring. The rings are assembled along the z-axis facing each other with opposing magnetization directions, resulting in an FFL oriented in x-direction (see Fig. 1 c). The magnetic field gradient in z-direction is determined to 4.3 T/m. For projection imaging, an additional bisected solenoid generates a varying magnetic field (±100 mT) with an frequency of 10.25 kHz to deflect the FFL along the y-direction covering a cylindrical field-of-view (FOV) with a diameter of 39 mm. For a full 2D image the samples are assembled on a rotating holder offering a step-wise rotating around 360°. Both signals, MPI and CT, are acquired simultaneously within a 20 ms sequence.

III. Results

In Fig. 2 the results of a simultaneous MPI-CT measurement of a letter phantom are shown. The phantom is partially filled with mixtures of PeriMag and potassium iodide (KI) forming the letter "L" and PeriMag and H_2O completing the letter "E".

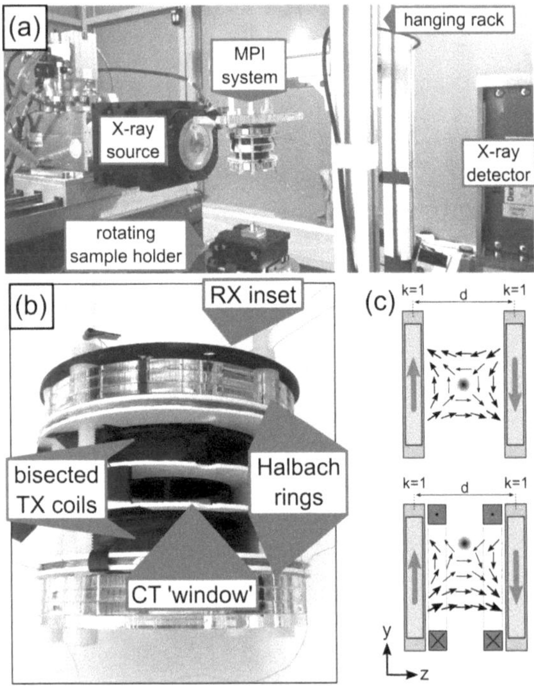

Figure 1: (a): *MPI-CT hybrid scanner: left the X-ray source, in the center the MPI scanner and on the bottom the rotating sample holder.* ***(b):*** *Fully assembled MPI-FFL scanner providing a CT "window".* ***(c)*** *FFL generation utilizing two Halbach rings and its movement for projection imaging.*

The MPI data is corrected and filtered using a custom reconstruction software [14] before generating a sinogram. Finally, both data sets, MPI and CT data, were reconstructed using a standard filtered backprojection algorithm.

IV. Discussion

There is no direct influence or interference between both modalities, MPI and CT, such as stray magnetic fields which could perturb the X-ray anode's focusing. This allows for truly simultaneous imaging, which is an enormous advantage compared to MPI-MRI hybrid scanners, that only allow sequential imaging due to incompatible magnetic field requirements.

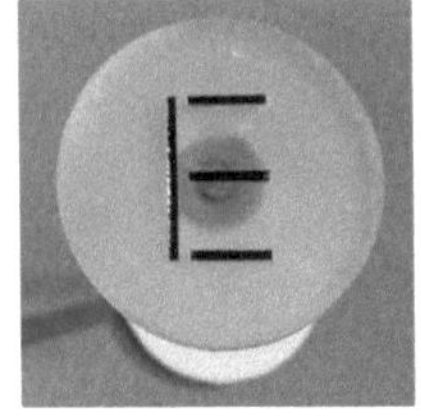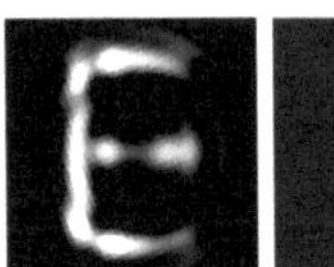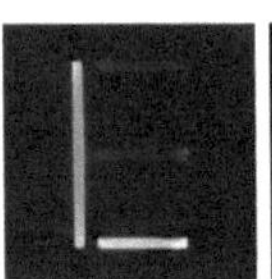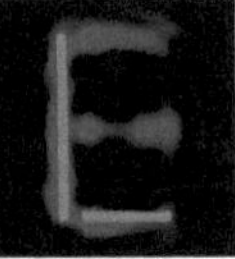

Figure 2: *Left: The phantom. Right: Results of simultaneous MPI- (left) and CT- (right) measurement as well as overlay of both.*

V. Conclusion

The first hybrid MPI-CT measurements are presented allowing simultaneous MPI and CT imaging of bimodal samples. A novel concept based on Halbach arrays is used for generating a static field free line featuring a strong magnetic field gradient. The newly developed MPI component offers an open design providing a CT 'window' for unobstructed transmission of X-rays and simultaneous imaging. Hence, the SPION distribution (MPI) as well as the anatomical information of the surrounding material (CT) can be visualized simultaneously and fast. Combination of the highly sensitive tracer-based imaging method of MPI with the exact visualization of anatomical structures of CT can be a basis for improving diagnostic accuracy in preclinical imaging.

ACKNOWLEDGEMENTS
We thank Dr. Henrik Teller and Dr. Cordula Grüttner (MicroMod) for providing PeriMag samples.

AUTHOR'S STATEMENT
Research funding: The author states no funding involved. Conflict of interest: Authors state no conflict of interest.

REFERENCES
[1] B. Gleich and J. Weizenecker. Tomographic imaging using the nonlinear response of magnetic particles. *Nature*, 435(7046):1217-1217, 2005. doi: 10.1038/nature03808.

[2] P.Vogel, et al., MRI Meets MPI: A Bimodal MPI-MRI Tomograph, *IEEE TMI*, Vol. 33: 1954-1959, 2014

[3] P. Vogel, et. al., Traveling Wave Magnetic Particle Imaging, *IEEE TMI*, vol. 33(2), pp. 400-7, 2014. doi: 10.1109/TMI.2013.2285472

[4] J. Franke, et al., System Characterization of a Highly Integrated Preclinical Hynrid MPI-MRI Scanner, *IEEE TMI*, vol. 35(9), pp. 1993-2004, 2016. doi: 10.1109/TMI.2016.2542041

[5] T. Knopp, et al., Magnetic Particle Imaging: From Proof of Principle to Preclinical Applications, *Physics in Medicine & Biology*, vol. 62(14):R124. 2017.

[6] K. Gräfe, et al., 2D Images Recorded with a Single-Sided Magnetic Particle Imaging Scanner, *IEEE TMI*, vol. 35(4), pp. 1056-1065, 2016, DOI: 10.1109/TMI.2015.2507187.

[7] A. Tonyushkin, Single-Sided Field-Free Line Generator Magnet for Multidimansional Magnetic Particle Imaging, *IEEE Trans. Magn.*, vol. 53(9):5300506, 2017. Doi: 10.1109/TMAG.2017.2718485

[8] J. Weizenecker, et al., Magnetic particle imaging using a field free line, *J. Phys. D: Appl Phys.*, 41 (105009) : 3pp, 2008. doi:10.1088/0022-3727/41/10/105009

[9] K. Bente, et al., Electronic field free line rotation and relaxation deconvolution in magnetic particle imaging, *IEEE TMI*, vol. 34(2), pp. 644-51, 2015. doi: 10.1109/TMI.2014.2364891

[10] P.W. Goodwill, et al., Projection X-space Magnetic Particle Imaging, *IEEE TMI*, vol. 31(5), pp. 1076-85, 2012. doi:10.1109/TMI.2012.2185247.

[11] K. Halbach, "Design of permanent multipole magnets with oriented rare earth cobalt material", *Nucl. Instr. Meth. Phys. Res*, 169: 1-10, 1980. doi:10.1016/0029-554X(80)90094-4

[12] H. Raich and P. Blümler, Design and construction of a dipolar Halbach array with a homogeneous field from identical bar magnets: *NMR Mandhalas. Concepts Magn. Reson. B Magn. Reson. Eng*, 23B(1): 16–25, 2004. doi: 10.1002/cmr.b.20018.

[13] Matthias Weber, et al., Novel Field Geometry featuring a Field Free Line for Magnetic Particle Imaging, *International Journal on Magnetic Particle Imaging*, vol 4(2):1811004, 2018. DOI:10.18416/IJMPI.2018.1811004

[14] P. Vogel, et al., Low latency Real-time Reconstruction for MPI Systems, *IJMPI*, vol. 3(2):1707002, 2017. Doi: 10.18416/ijmpi.2017.1707002

1D Multi-Frequency MPI by passive and active Drive Field Feed-Through Compensation

D. Pantke [a,*], N. Holle [a], A. Mogarkar [a], S. Reinartz [b], V. Schulz [a]

[a] *Department of Physics of Molecular Imaging, Institute for Experimental Molecular Imaging, RWTH Aachen University, Aachen, Germany*
[b] *Department of Diagnostic and Interventional Radiology, Uniklinik RWTH Aachen, Aachen, Germany*
* *Corresponding author, email: dennis.pantke@pmi.rwth-aachen.de*

Abstract: Besides imaging the distribution of superparamagnetic iron oxide nanoparticles, magnetic particle imaging (MPI) promises access to (local) functional parameters as temperature or viscosity. Using particle excitation at multiple frequencies is one promising approach to get access to functional information and carries further potential to increase spatial resolution and sensitivity. In this work, a novel one-dimensional multi-frequency MPI scanner is presented. It is enabled by a combined passive and active drive field feed-through compensation approach. The potential of spatial resolution enhancement has been demonstrated. The device shall be used to investigate the potential of measuring functional parameters in future studies.

I. Introduction

Conventional Magnetic Particle Imaging (MPI) devices quantitatively determine the spatial distribution of superparamagnetic iron oxide nanoparticles (SPIONs) *in-vivo* [1]. Although current scanners offer high temporal resolution, there is still potential to enhance spatial resolution and sensitivity. Besides imaging SPIONs another useful feature of MPI is measuring functional parameters as viscosity or temperature of particles' local environment. Continuous *in vivo* access to these parameters would be highly beneficial for a variety of medical applications as nanomedicine, cell tracking or magnetic hyperthermia. One promising approach to measure functional parameters is particle excitation at multiple frequencies or at other than sinusoidal waveforms [2-4]. Furthermore, it potentially increases spatial resolution due to a higher number of available harmonics. Current MPI systems use frequency-selective components in their signal chains as resonantly powered transmit coils or narrow band-stop filters to remove the drive field feed-through from the received signal. However, these approaches are incompatible with broadband excitation and application of different waveforms. Therefore, we propose using a combined passive and active drive field feed-through compensation approach and present a novel one-dimensional multi-frequency MPI (mf-MPI).

II. Materials and Methods

Passive compensation of the drive field feed-through was realized by inductive decoupling of separate transmit (TX) and receive (RX) solenoid coils made of Litz wire in a gradiometer coil design (Fig. 1 left). Compared to the coil design presented in [5], the RX coil L_R can be moved along the x-axis to allow fine tuning and the bore diameter is 33 mm. The TX coil was wound on top of the RX coil and is subdivided in three sections. The peripheral segments of the TX coil L_C are wound in two layers and the opposite direction to the central segment L_T. To calculate the winding pattern, a thin-wire approximation that computes the mutual inductance was used. Fine tuning was performed by connecting the coils to a network analyzer and adjusting the x-position of the RX coil until the power transfer between TX and RX was minimized. In contrast to [5], a reference measurement without L_C was subtracted from the measured power transfer.

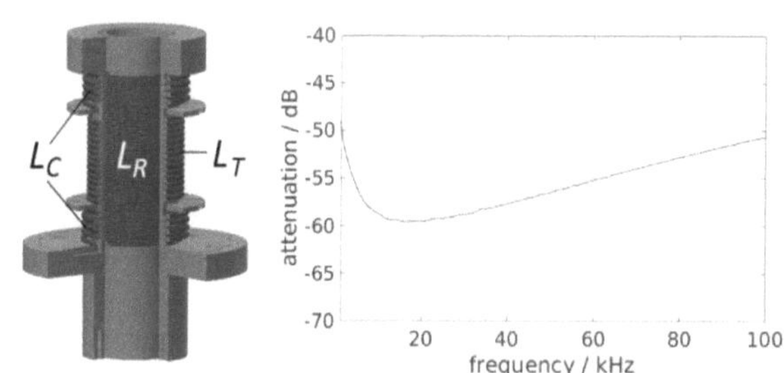

Figure 1: *Left: CAD sketch of gradiometer coil design for passive compensation. Right: Broadband feed-through attenuation by passive decoupling.*

A shielded low-loss transformer is used to actively apply a compensation signal to remove the drive field feed-through remaining from the passive compensation stage. The signal chain of the proposed 1D multi-frequency MPI can be seen in Fig. 2. Drive field and active compensation signals are generated by a remote controlled Keysight 33512B function generator. The drive field signal is amplified by a power amplifier AE Techron 7796. The residual feed-through is amplified by a Stanford research systems pre-amplifier model SR560 and then digitized by an Adlink PCIe-9852 analog-to-digital converter. An active compensation control was implemented that allows to minimize the peak of the feed-through in the frequency spectrum.

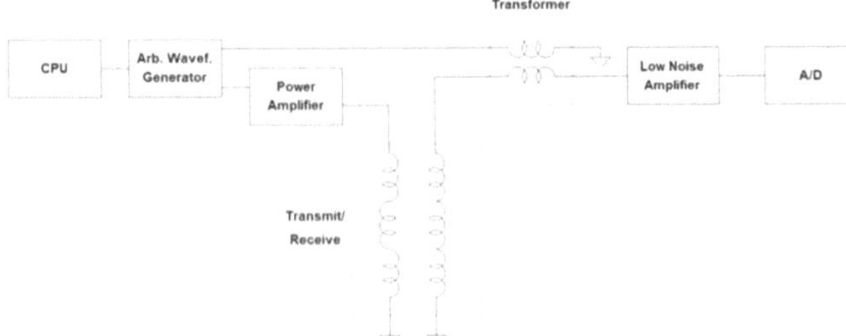

Figure 2: Signal chain of the proposed one-dimensional multi-frequency MPI.

To prove the concept and functionality of the proposed multi-frequency MPI and demonstrate the gain of spatial resolution, phantom images with excitation frequencies of 7, 10 and 13 kHz were acquired. They were compared to images, for which all three sets of data were used in a joint reconstruction (JR) method. The phantom consists of two samples longitudinally aligned along the x-axis of the bore. The dimensions of the samples are 1x1x2 mm (x,y,z) corresponding to 2 µl each. The distance between the sample centers is 2 mm. Perimag® with an iron concentration of 8 mg/ml was used. While the single-frequency images were averaged 6 times, the joint-reconstructed image was averaged only 2 times to ensure comparability. The scanners gradient field along the x-axis is 0.7 T/m and generated by permanent neodymium magnets. The applied sinusoidal drive field was 7 mT. For each frequency, system matrices with a grid of 0.5 mm and a drive field strength of 7 mT were acquired with a 4 µl Perimag® delta sample. For all image reconstructions the Kaczmarz method with 50 iterations was used and all frequency components besides the harmonics of the excitation signals were omitted. No regularization was used.

III. Results

The attenuation by inductive decoupling is depicted in Fig. 1, right. In the frequency range up to 100 kHz, the attenuation is between -50 and -59 dB. By active compensation, further reduction of the residual feed-through by -73 dB ± 10 dB in average for frequencies up to 20 kHz was measured. In total, attenuation values up to -132 dB were achieved. The line profile along the x-axis after reconstruction using only the single frequencies and all frequencies (left) and the respective grey value images (right) of the phantom are shown in Fig. 3.

IV. Discussion

The combined passive and active compensation approach attenuates the drive field feed-through by up to -132 dB and allows 1D-imaging applications with arbitrary frequencies up to 20 kHz. The magnetic field strength and applicable frequency range is currently limited by the performance of the power amplifier. Since no filter is used in the transmit chain, one must deal with harmonic power amplifier distortions, which are getting more prominent with increasing frequency and field strength. Currently, the

maximum drive field is approx. 10 mT at 10 kHz and 6 mT at 20 kHz. The active compensation approach can as well be used to suppress the mentioned amplifier distortions, as Zheng et al. have reported previously [6].

By using a joint reconstruction compared to using only single frequencies, the signal drop between the signal maxima of the samples is increased and the full width at half maximum (FWHM) of the signal maxima is decreased (Fig. 3). Thus, the spatial resolution was enhanced by using mf-MPI.

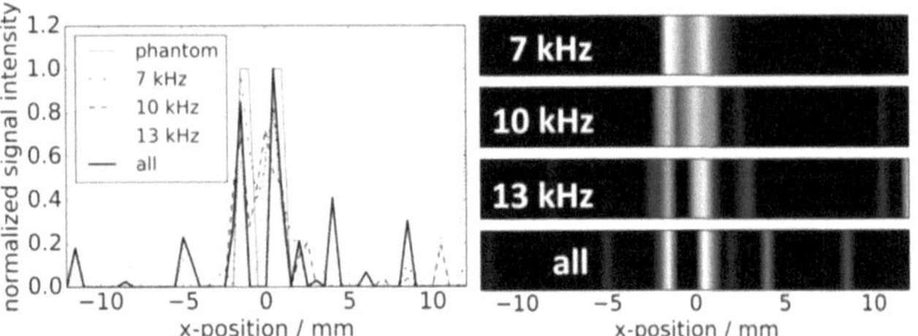

Figure 3: Line profile (left) and grey value images (right) of the phantom. The excitation frequencies were 7, 10, 13 kHz. The respective images were averaged 6 times. Additionally, a joint reconstructed image was generated, which was averaged only 2 times to ensure comparability. An enhanced spatial resolution can be observed in terms of increased signal drop between the signal maxima.

V. Conclusion

A novel one-dimensional multi-frequency MPI scanner enabled by using a combined passive and active compensation approach to attenuate the drive field feed-through was presented. In total, a combined passive and active compensation of up to -132 dB was achieved in a frequency range up to 20 kHz. First images were presented that demonstrate the potential of mf-MPI to increase spatial resolution. Furthermore, direct access to the first harmonic of the particle signal can be provided. In future projects [7], the presented mf-MPI scanner shall be used to investigate the potential of measuring functional parameters.

AUTHOR'S STATEMENT
The authors state no conflict of interest.

REFERENCES
[1] B. Gleich and J. Weizenecker. "Tomographic imaging using the nonlinear response of magnetic particles," *Nature*, 435(7046):1217-1217, 2005. doi: 10.1038/nature03808.
[2] C. Kuhlmann *et al.* "Drive-Field Frequency Dependent MPI Performance of Single-Core Magnetite Nanoparticle Tracers," *IEEE Transactions on Magnetics* 51, No. 2, 3-6, 2015.
[3] T. Viereck *et al.* "Dual-frequency magnetic particle imaging of the Brownian particle contribution," *Journal of Magnetism and Magnetic Materials* 427, 156-161, 2016.
[4] I.M. Perreard *et al.* "Temperature of the Magnetic Nanoparticle Microenvironment: Estimation from Relaxation Times" *Phys. Med. Biol.* 59, 1109-1119, 2014.
[5] D. Pantke *et al.* "Passive and Active Compensation of Drive Field Feed-Through for Multi-Frequency MPI", IWMPI 2018
[6] B. Zheng *et al.* "High-Power active Interference Suppression in Magnetic Particle Imaging", IWMPI 2013
[7] N. Holle *et al.* "Multi-parametric image reconstruction in Magnetic Particle Imaging", IWMPI 2019.

Magnet Assembly Design for a Human-Scale Functional Magnetic Particle Imager (fMPI)

E. E. Mason[a,b*], E. Mattingly[b], C. Z. Cooley[b,c], and L. L. Wald[b,c]

[a] *Harvard-MIT Health Sciences & Technology, Cambridge, MA, USA*
[b] *MGH/HST A.A. Martinos Center for Biomedical Imaging, Dept. of Radiology, Massachusetts General Hospital, Boston, MA, USA*
[c] *Harvard Medical School, Boston, MA, USA*
[*] *Corresponding author, email: ericamas@mit.edu*

Abstract: Magnetic Particle Imaging (MPI) is a quickly growing tracer-based imaging modality promising high sensitivity. Sensitive detection of hypercapnic manipulation of cerebral blood volume (CBV) was recently demonstrated, suggesting the potential of functional MPI (fMPI) for human neuroscience. Here, we detail the design of a field-free line (FFL) magnet capable of sweeping over a human head-sized volume. The magnet assembly consists of both permanent magnets and electromagnet coils and is designed to provide an FFL gradient of 1.22 T/m.

I. Introduction & Motivation

MPI is a high-sensitivity imaging modality with short scan times [1]–[3]. This, together with its ability to directly measure tracer Fe concentration and thus cerebral blood volume (CBV), makes it a promising technology for functional neuroimaging [4]. While fMRI can also image CBV modulation in response to neuronal activation, fMPI has the potential sensitivity advantages to enable study of more subtle activation and circuitry patterns and shift the focus of activation studies from group averages to the individual—a necessary step to clinical utility. The feasibility of detecting these CBV changes with MPI has been shown in rodents using a single-sided Magnetic Particle detector during hyper/hypocapnia-induced neural activation [6]. Here, we seek to scale up rodent-sized FFL devices for human use, and expand on our previous design analysis [4]. Our design uses NdFeB permanent magnets (PMs) to create the FFL, and hollow-conductor electromagnets (EMs) for shift fields to acquire the projections. The magnet assemblies must be rotated on a mechanical gantry to achieve projection imaging using power and water slip-ring technology to enable continuous time-series imaging as needed for functional studies.

II. Material and Methods

II.I. Basic System Concept

The overall concept of our fMPI system is shown in Fig. 1A. An FFL along y', produced by PMs, is swept by EMs across the projection axis, x'. A PM and EM together constitute a magnet assembly (MA). The MAs rotate about the patient to acquire projections.

II.II. Requirements for Human System

The design goal is the highest gradient strength producible with combinations of PMs, resistive EMs and iron, and shifting the FFL across a 20 cm FOV with less than 50 kW of heat dissipation. Resistive and eddy current heating is considered. The size constraints for the human system are detailed in Fig. 1B. Clearance of 42 cm allows for the human head and bore, and 18 cm from center of magnet to shoulder ensures the magnets will clear the shoulders.

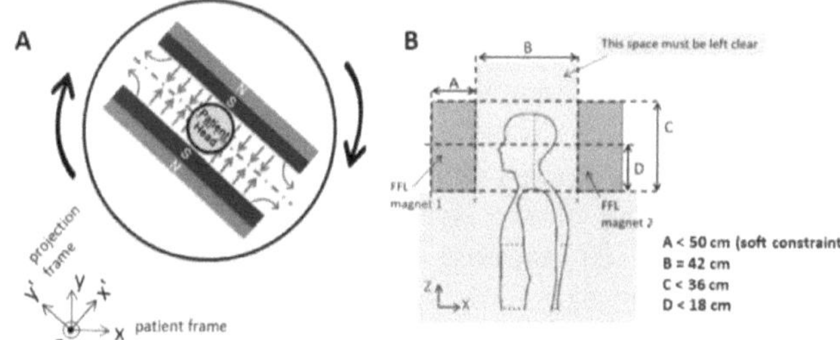

Figure 1: *A) Schematic of human system, indicating the static patient frame (xy) and the rotating gantry frame (x'y'), and the rotation of the FFL magnets about the bore. B) Size constraints for the magnet assemblies.*

II.III. Simulations & Analysis

Simulations of the PMs and EMs are done in COMSOL (COMSOL, Inc., Burlington, MA, USA) using a 3D Magnetic Fields physics. We compared using the windings solely to shift an FFL created by PMs (in which case only AC current is applied), or to produce the FFL as well as shift (requiring an AC and DC component to the EM current). We analyzed several windings, iron core shapes and sizes, as well as rare-earth block sizes, as illustrated in Fig. 2. We also analyzed the eddy current heating in the PM by the AC shift fields.

A highly parallelized water circuit cools the hollow-conductor EM. Computational Fluid Dynamics (CFD) analysis is done on the water manifold design using OpenFOAM's simpleFoam solver (OpenFOAM Foundation Ltd, London, UK) to confirm the even distribution of flow throughout the layers of wires.

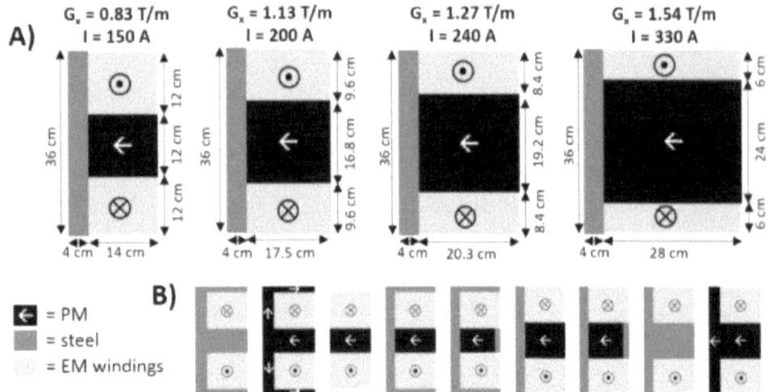

Figure 2: *Different geometries tested in COMSOL simulations (cross-section of single magnet assembly shown). A) Four variations of a given geometry with total number of turns and total height of 36 cm fixed, width variable. Current indicated is that needed to shift the FFL ±10 cm. B) A sampling of the tested geometries.*

III. Results: Current Design

III.I. Electromagnet (EM) & Water Manifold

AC current only will be applied to the EMs to simplify power requirements. The EM design uses 5 x 5 mm^2 square cross-section, insulated magnet wire with a 3 mm hollow channel for cooling water flow. Each EM will be wound in a racetrack shape, 16 turns and 26 layers. The coil will be broken into two sets of racetrack coils—a longer/outer racetrack (8 of the 16 turns) and an inner/shorter one (8 turns)—to create space for water manifolds and increase parallelization of the water cooling paths. The 26 layers of racetracks will be broken into 13 "pancakes." A pancake is a discrete assembly of two layers of windings (spiral in and spiral out), a water manifold block, and insulation between layers. The pancakes are stacked to form the racetrack assembly, and electrical current from one pancake to the next is passed through the water manifold. The pancakes will be clamped together mechanically. Each EM is estimated to have a resistance of 1.3 Ω, has inductance of ~400 mH, and will carry peak current of 250 A at 60 Hz. EM heating is estimated to be ~41 kW (RMS), so the number of parallel water cooling paths has been maximized. The manifold provides two parallel water circuits per pancake, with a total volumetric flow rate of 103 L/min, and a maximum pressure within the wires of 100 PSI, leading to an anticipated temperature increase of 11°C.

III.II. Permanent Magnet (PM) & Steel Backing

Each PM is a large block of rare earth NdFeB, with a total size of 16.8 x 18.1 x 96 cm^3, producing an FFL with (simulated) gradient strength of 1.22 T/m. However, for a solid PM of this size, eddy currents produced by the 150 mT, 60 Hz AC shift field are simulated to cause up to

59 kW of heating. To address this issue, the PM will be made up of smaller component NdFeB blocks, electrically insulated from one another. We aim to limit heating to 20°C over 1 hour to maintain the PM strength within 2% of its room-temperature value. We simulated eddy current heating for various component block sizes in a 150 mT, 60 Hz field, and determined that 2 x 2 x 6 cm^3 PM blocks will satisfy the constraint, with a 19.1°C temperature rise over 1 hour.

A 4 cm-thick back plate was chosen as the best yoke shape for enhancing the FFL gradient strength for this configuration. The plate will be broken up into strips or sheets to reduce eddy currents. A full magnet assembly is shown in Fig. 3.

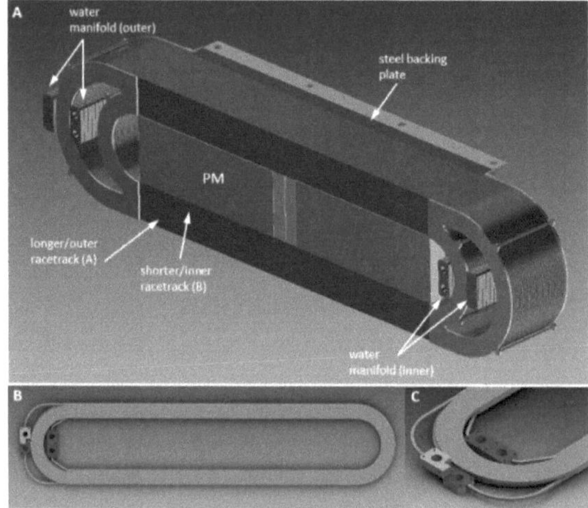

Figure 3: *CAD renderings of: A) one of the two magnet assemblies. The two racetrack coils (inner and outer), each made of 13 stacked "pancakes," comprise the EM; the PM fits inside the inner racetrack, B) a single pancake, consisting of two layers of 8 windings (spiral in and spiral out), a water manifold block, and insulation, and C) a close up of the water manifold block.*

IV. Discussion & Conclusion

We present the design of the magnet assemblies for producing and shifting a 1.22 T/m FFL sized for a human functional MPI system. The parallelization of the water cooling removes 41 kW of heat with an 11°C water temperature rise. The magnetic materials in the MAs are shielded from the 25 kHz excitation and higher harmonic pickup by a copper bore tube, which also serves to attenuate external interference. The next steps will be finalization of the designs, initiation of construction, and integration with the human-scaled rotating gantry.

AUTHOR'S STATEMENT
Funding for the work comes from NIBIB U01EB025121-02, NIMH R24106053, and NSF GRFP 1122374. Authors state no conflict of interest.

REFERENCES
[1] Gleich and Weizenecker, *Nature*, vol. 435, no. 7046, pp. 1214–7, 2005.
[2] M. Graeser *et al.*, *Sci. Rep.*, vol. 7, no. 1, pp. 1–13, 2017.
[3] Weizenecker *et al.*, *Phys. Med. Biol.*, vol. 54, no. 5, pp. L1–L10, 2009.
[4] Mason *et al.*, *Int. J. Magn. Part. Imaging*, vol. 3, no. 1, 2017.
[5] Mandeville *et al.*, *Magn. Reson. Med.*, vol. 39, no. 4, pp. 615–624, 1998.
[6] Cooley *et al.*, *Neuroimage*, vol. 178, 2017, pp. 713–720, 2018.

First human-sized Magnetic Particle Imaging Device for Cerebral Applications

M. Graeser[a,b], F. Thieben[a,b], P. Szwargulski[a,b], F. Werner[a,b], N. Gdaniec[a,b], M. Boberg[a,b], F. Griese, M. Möddel[a,b], P. Ludewig[c], D. van de Ven[d], O. M. Weber[e], O. Woywode[f], B. Gleich[g], T. Knopp[a,b]

a Section for Biomedical Imaging, University Medical Center Hamburg-Eppendorf, Hamburg, Germany
b Institute for Biomedical Imaging, Hamburg University of Technology, Hamburg, Germany
c Department of Neurology, University Medical Center Hamburg-Eppendorf, Hamburg, German
d Sensing and Inspection Technologies GmbH, Huerth, Germany
e Philips GmbH Market DACH, Hamburg, Germany
f Imaging Components, Philips Medical Systems DMC GmbH, Hamburg, Germany
g Research Laboratories, Philips GmbH Innovative Technologies, Hamburg, Germany
* Corresponding author, email: _ma.graeser@uke.de_

Abstract: In intensive care units, patients suffering from intracerebral hemorrhage or ischemic stroke cannot be monitored by imaging systems due to the demands of the scanning device like shielded rooms. In this work, we present the first MPI human head scanner, which can operate in unshielded environments. It is compact and flexible and can be integrated further to be a mobile, bedside device. The system demonstrates its capabilities in technical tests as well as on human sized phantoms.

I. Introduction

The determination of brain perfusion is an important task in diagnosis and treatment of intracerebral hemorrhage and ischemic stroke. After successful treatment, patients have a high risk of restenosis and rebleeding in the following days. The patient condition is currently controlled by motor tests, paralysis checks and ocular reaction. In addition, MRT or CT scans are performed if any sign of worsening is present. The transport to these imaging devices remains a risky and complex task, if patients are in narcosis or have to be

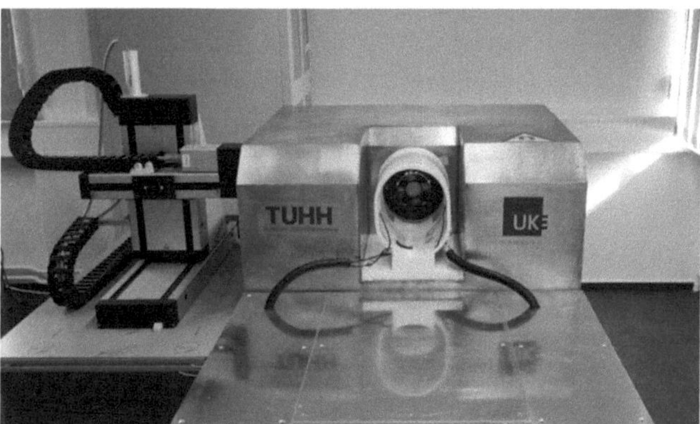

Figure 1: Picture of the developed brain imager. The system is self-shielded and can operate on without special requirements to the room infrastructure.

ventilated. An ideal solution would be to bring the imaging device into the ICU. However, the demands of MRT and CT for shielded rooms prevent that. Magnetic Particle Imaging (MPI) devices currently also operate within shielded rooms.

In contrast this is not due to protection of the environment from ionizing radiation or strong magnetic fields, but to protect the detector systems from disturbing signals. Upscaling of MPI systems to sizes fitting a human head is a complex task, but recent simulation results show the feasibility of human scale head scanners [1].

In this work we present the first MPI system tailored for brain applications, which is suitable for the work in unshielded environments and operates on a human scale. The system was designed to provide a gradient strength of 0.25 T/m and a drive field amplitude of 6 mT to reach a resolution below 1 cm. To determine perfusion parameter maps, it achieves a temporal resolution of 2 frames/second and provides a sensitivity of an iron mass of 2 µg or a concentration of 263 pmol/ml.

II. Material and Methods

Preclinical MPI scanners share a high gradient strength and high drive field amplitude to achieve a high resolution and a large field of view (FOV) [2]. However, brain perfusion defects caused by vessel occlusions normally exceed volumes of 50 ml [3]. Therefore, a resolution in the range of 1 cm is sufficient for detecting ischemic stroke and intracranial hemorrhage. In figure 2 the imaging concept of the system is shown. It is based on a selection field generator consisting of two coils mounted on a soft-iron yoke. The yoke amplifies the gradient and serves as structural support. It can be rotated by a servo motor and moved by a linear axis to position the FOV within the coil bore.

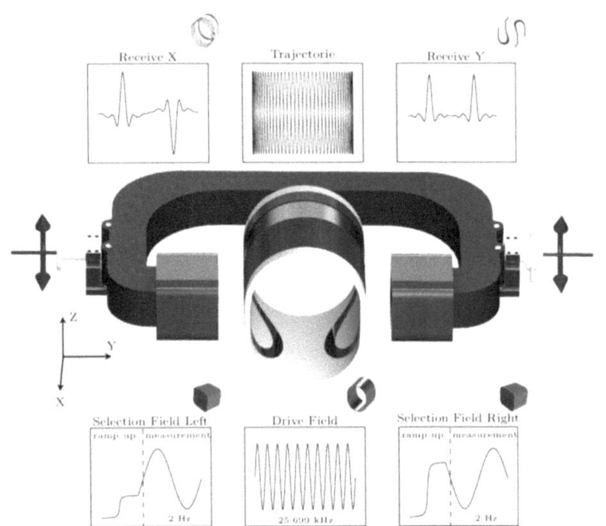

Figure 2: Imaging concept of the brain imager. The gradient field is generated by two coils, which share an iron yoke for field amplification and structural support. The yoke can be rotated and moved on a linear axis along the x-direction for slice selection. The drive field is generated by a ellipsoid like coil in x-direction. By varying the coil current on the selection field coils, an additional signal encoding in y-direction is achieved. The particle response is received by dedicated coils in x- and y- direction.

The coils are driven by dc currents producing a gradient of 0.25 T/m which is superimposed by sinusoidal currents of 2 Hz to shift the field free point along the y-axis. The soft-iron yoke is shielded from the drive field by a copper shield visible in figure 1 to prevent the generation of harmonics in the yoke. The drive field coil is generating a field of 6 mT/μ_0 to excite the particles. Together with the dynamic selection field, a Cartesian like trajectory is formed in the xy-plane. The particle response is recorded using dedicated receive coils in the x- and y-direction. Reconstruction is performed by frequency space reconstruction [4]. As tracer material perimag (micromod, Rostock, Germany) with an undiluted concentration of 8.5 mg/ml was used. The system performance was determined by sensitivity and resolution studies. The application scenario was tested using human-scale phantoms at clinical approved tracer concentrations.

III. Results

Using high concentration samples the system was able to achieve a resolution of 5 mm in x-direction, 6 mm in y-direction and 26 mm in z-direction. The sensitivity was measured to be 2 µg or 263 pmol/ml using perimag as tracer material. Figure 3 shows the reconstruction of a 3D phantom. As the dynamic part of the scanner images only the xy-plane the internal servo motor was used to move the field free point in z direction recording multiple slices for 3D imaging.

The human-scale phantom experiments proved that the system is able to image a perfusion deficit of a volume of typical ischemic strokes at clinical approved tracer concentrations.

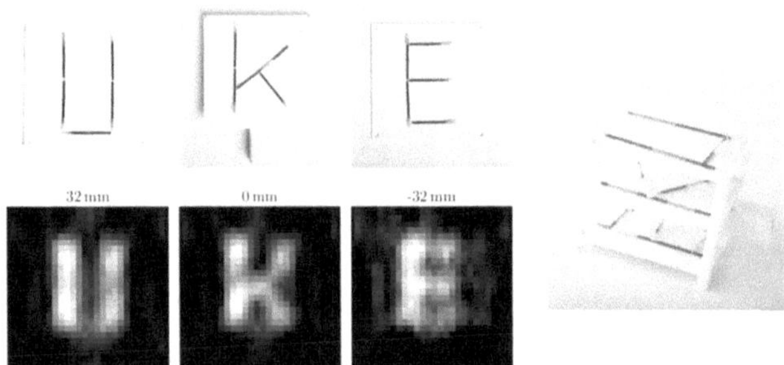

Figure 3:Reconstruction results of a 3D phantom using the internal servo for slice selection. The total measurement time was 6 s.

IV. Discussion

Within this work, we presented the first MPI imager on a human scale for brain applications. It showed high sensitivity, good spatial and temporal resolution while maintaining the possibility to operate within intensive care units. This enables to monitor stroke patients within the intensive care unit on a regular basis which was not possible till now. Assuming a maximal dose of 200 mg, which is within the range of approved iron oxide contrast agents, a surveillance time of 72 h can be achieved, while injecting a bolus every hour. In turn, the risk of patient transport and the workload of the medical staff can be reduced.

The next step is to show the capabilities of MPI in large animal studies. In advance, the field generator has to be modified to be in accordance to electrical safety for operating staff, which need to work next to the high voltage drive field coils. In addition, by improving the receiver circuits, it is expected to gain a factor of 10 in sensitivity based on scale rates derived in [5] and thus, reducing the dose necessary for imaging or improving the image quality while maintaining the surveillance time frame.

ACKNOWLEDGEMENTS
We thank MI Partners Eindhoven for technical assistance and the Insitute for Robotics and Cognitive Systems Lübeck for 3D printing the coil frame.

AUTHOR'S STATEMENT
Research funding: The project war funded by the German Research Fundation (KN 1108/2-1) and the German Federal Ministry of Education and Research (05M16GKA and 13XP5060B). Conflict of interest: Authors state no conflict of interest.

REFERENCES
[1] Mason, E. et al. Design analysis of an MPI human functional brain scanner. International Journal on Magnetic Particle Imaging 3, 2017. doi:10.18416/ijmpi.2017.1703008
[2] Panagiotopoulos N et al. Magnetic particle imaging: current developments and future directions, International Journal of Nanomedicine, 10(1), pp. 3097-3114, 2015. doi: 10.2147/IJN.S70488
[3] Sperber, C. and Karnath, H.-O. Topography of acute stroke in a sample of 439 right brain damaged patients. *NeuroImage: Clinical* 10, pp. 124 -128, 2016. doi: 10.1016/j.nicl.2015.11.012
[4] Knopp et al., Weighted iterative reconstruction for magnetic particle imaging, *Physics in medicine & biology* 55 (6), 1577 doi: 10.1088/0031-9155/55/6/003
[5] Graeser, M. et al. Towards picogram detection of superparamagnetic iron-oxide particles using a gradiometric receive coil. *Scientific Reports* 7, 6872, 2017. doi: 10.1038/s41598-017-06992-5

Keynote

MPI:
The Future of Biomedical Molecular Imaging?

Peter Caravan

Athinoula A. Martinos Center for Biomedical Imaging
Department of Radiology, Massachusetts General Hospital
149 Thirteenth St, Suite 2301
CHARLESTOWN, MA 02129 USA
Corresponding author, email: caravan@nmr.mgh.harvard.edu

Abstract

MPI shows great optimism for molecular imaging: potentially low cost device, shelf-stable molecular probes, no ionizing radiation, direct detection of the probe, and relatively high sensitivity for detection. Drawing upon other modalities, this lecture will describe the requirements for successful MPI applications. The ultimate utility of MPI is somewhat bounded by the need to utilize nanoparticle-based probes which are limited in their pharmacokinetic properties and biodistribution. Acknowledging and working within these constraints still leaves a broad field of impactful application. Here we will describe possible avenues for molecular probes that take advantage of this powerful emerging technology.

Curriculum Vitae

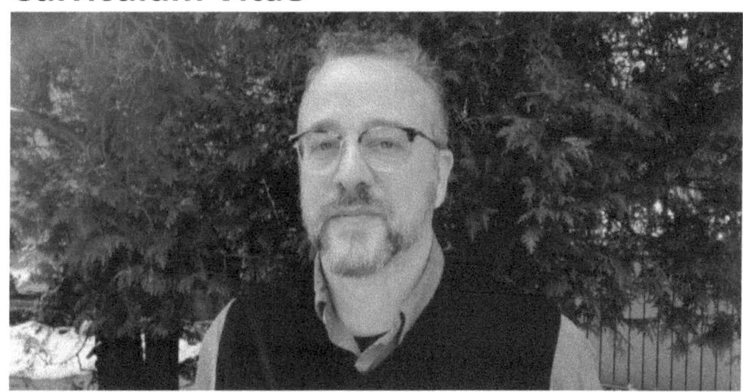

1997	PhD in Chemistry, University of British Columbia
1998	Post-doctoral fellow, Chemistry, Université de Lausanne
04/07-02/08	Instructor, Radiology, Harvard Medical School
02/08-09/13	Assistant Professor, Radiology, Harvard Medical School
10/13 -	Associate Professor, Professor, Radiology, Harvard Medical School
2014 -	Co-Director, Institute for Innovation in Imaging: Establish, direct, and manage translational imaging institute.

Fast temporal regularized reconstructions for magnetic particle imaging

C. Brandt[a]* and A. Hauptmann[b]

[a] *Department of Mathematics, Universität Hamburg, Hamburg, Germany*
[b] *Department of Computer Science, University College London, London, Great Britain*
* *Corresponding author, email:* *christina.brandt@uni-hamburg.de*

Abstract: Since the temporal resolution is high in MPI, there is only a slight change in the particle concentration from frame to frame. Therefore, it is reasonable to assume that the time derivative of the concentration obeys a certain regularity. We thus propose a regularization in space and time. We present a framework for real-time reconstruction in 4D MPI with a low-rank approximation of the system matrix and a truncated singular value decomposition in spatio-temporal domain. The presented method is able to achieve reconstruction times with 45 Hz that match the frame rate of MPI measurement systems.

I. Introduction

With potential frame rates of up to 45 Hz, MPI has the capability to visualize blood flow and enable instrument tracking in real-time. However, the reconstruction problem is ill-posed and there are no known analytic inversion formulas. Thus, to obtain an image one needs to solve a variational problem of the form

$$c^* = \underset{c}{\operatorname{argmin}} \|Sc - f\|_2^2 + \gamma \|c\|_2^2 , \tag{1}$$

where S denotes the measured system matrix, f is the Fourier transformed measured voltage and c denotes the corresponding vectorized particle concentration. The problem (1) is typically solved in an iterative way. Although recently, more adapted regularization methods based on a spatial correlation of the concentration have been proposed, there are no methods mentioned which uses the correlation of the frames in time. Instead, the minimization problem (1) is solved for each frame separately, i.e. for $f = f_k, k = 1, 2, ..., K$. An alternative to incorporate the correlation in time is to estimate the flow field directly [1] or the solve the joint image reconstruction and flow estimation problem jointly [2] leading the computationally expensive approaches. However, for monitoring purposes efficient methods are needed which allow real-time reconstruction.

In this paper we investigate a possibility to obtain spatio-temporal regularized reconstructions in real-time by first performing a matrix compression step on the system matrix and then computing a low-rank reconstruction with the well-established truncated singular value decomposition. We are able to obtain frame rates of up to 45 Hz in 4D, matching the speed of MPI measurement systems, with a sufficient image quality suitable for real-time tracking. We achieved this reconstruction rates with a system matrix $S \in \mathbb{R}^{M \times N}$ with $N = 25^3$ and $M = 13104$ and an implementation in MATLAB on a personal computer (Intel Core i5, 3.5GHz, 32 GB RAM).

I. Methods

II.I Spatio-temporal regularization

Since the temporal resolution is high in MPI, the particle concentration changes only slightly from frame to frame. Therefore, we can assume that the time derivative obeys a certain smoothness and we are searching for solutions which varying smoothly in time. Hence, we propose the following Tikhonov-type regularization method

$$c^* = \underset{c \geq 0}{\operatorname{argmin}} \int_0^T \|Sc - f\|_2^2 + \alpha \|\partial_t c\|_2^2 + \beta \|c\|_2^2 dt. \tag{2}$$

Here, ∂_t denotes the pixelwise time derivative which is evaluated pixelwise at each time point of $c_k = c(., t)$ by forward differences, i.e.

$$d_t c_k = \frac{c_{k+1} - c_k}{\Delta t} . \tag{3}$$

For simplicity, we set $\Delta t = 1$. In order to derive an efficient reconstruction scheme, we transform the problem into an equation with one quadratic penalty. Defining vectors $\bar{c} := (c_k, c_{k+1})^T$ and similarly for the data $\bar{f}$ and the system matrix $\bar{S}$, we choose a mapping

$$D_t \bar{c}_k = \begin{pmatrix} c_{k+1} - c_k \\ c_k \end{pmatrix} = v_k. \tag{4}$$

Instead of solving (2), we try to solve the minimization problem in v , i.e.

$$v_k^* = \underset{v}{\operatorname{argmin}} \|\bar{S} D_t^{-1} v - g\|_2^2 + \gamma \|v\|_2^2 . \tag{5}$$

Note that the two components of v_k are not coupled and that we obtain c_{k+1} by

$$c_{k+1} = v_{k,1} + v_{k,2} = c_k + d_t c_k. \tag{6}$$

II.II Low rank approximation

In order to obtain an online-reconstruction, we propose the following approach. First, we compress the system matrix in order to obtain a low-rank approximation A of the system matrix [3],[4]. For the combined matrix $C = \bar{A}D_t^{-1}$, we compute a truncated singular value decomposition (TSVD) of the largest s singular values to obtain a rank-s approximation of C. The resulting approximation of the pseudo inverse of C is used to solve the problem (5) such that we finally obtain the concentration via (6).

III. Results

We simulate a 2D setup with excitation frequencies 25kHz and 24 kHz in x and y direction with amplitude $18\text{mT}/\mu_0$ and gradient strength $2.75\text{T/m}/\mu_0$. The field of view (FOV) is of size 1.3 cm x 1.3 cm with pixel size of 0.32mm x 0.32 mm. We used the Langevin function for modeling the particle behavior and added additive Gaussian noise. The phantom consists of a ball (6 pixel diameter) moving from the left to the right hand side of the FOV with a velocity of 0.6 pixel per frame. The results are plotted in Figure 1. Because of the penalization of the time derivative, noise in the background of the reconstructed concentration is suppressed. Edges of the ball are preserved.

IV. Discussion

The presented approach based on a spatio-temporal regularization is able to improve the image reconstruction of objects in motion. It provides clear edges similar to total variation regularization and reduces the noise significantly. The approach can be used for 3D time-dependent measurements which will be discussed in the presentation. Here, the reconstruction is obtained by rates of 45 Hz in 4D MPI measurements. However, the reconstructed velocities still suffer from noise. A sparsity-promoting regularization such as the L_1-norm of the time derivative might further improve the reconstruction but comes with a higher computational cost and will be object of future research.

REFERENCES

[1] J. Franke, R. Lacroix, H. Lehr, M., Heidenreich, U., Heinen, and V. Schulz. MPI Flow Analysis Toolbox exploiting pulsed tracer information – an aneurysm phantom proof. *International Journal on Magnetic Particle Imaging, 3*(1) 2017.

[2] M. Burger, H. Dirks and C.Schönlieb. A Variational Model for Joint Motion Estimation and Image Reconstruction. SIAM Journal on Imaging Sciences, 11(1), 94-128 2018.

[3] J. Lampe, C. Bassov, J. Rahmer, J. Weizenecker, H. Voss, B. Gleich and J. Borgert. Fast reconstruction in magnetic particle imaging. *Physics in Medicine & Biology* 57(4):1113, 2012.

[4] T. Knopp and A. Weber. Local System Matrix Compression for Efficient Reconstruction in Magnetic Particle Imaging. Advances in Mathematical Physics, 2015, 2015.

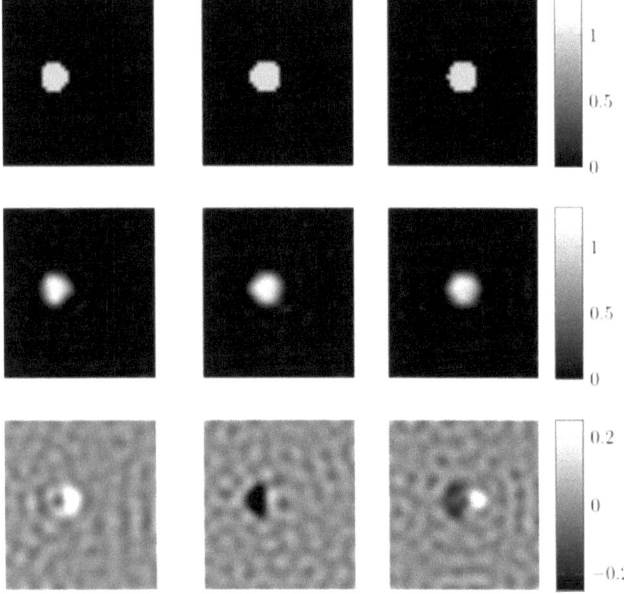

Figure 1: *Simulated phantom for frames k=8, 13 and 18 (first row) as well as reconstructions c_k (second row) and the corresponding time differences $v_{k,1}$.*

Spatio-temporal concentration reconstruction using motion priors in magnetic particle imaging

T. Kluth [a,*], **B. N. Hahn** [b], **C. Brandt** [c]

[a] Center for Industrial Mathematics, University of Bremen, Bibliothekstr. 5, 28359 Bremen
[b] Institute of Mathematics, University of Würzburg, Emil-Fischer-Str. 30, 97074, Würzburg
[c] Department of Mathematics, University of Hamburg, Bundesstr. 55, 20146 Hamburg
* Corresponding author, email: tkluth@math.uni-bremen.de

Abstract: In this presentation we address the dynamic concentration reconstruction problem in magnetic particle imaging. The tradeoff between the signal-to-noise ratio in the processed data used for the reconstruction and the concentration dynamics of the tracer requires sophisticated reconstruction techniques to avoid motion artifacts. We incorporate motion priors in the concentration reconstruction and as an extra we can obtain an estimate for a flow field.

I. Introduction

Magnetic particle imaging (MPI) allows for a rapid data acquisition with a high temporal resolution. For example, moving the FFP along a Lissajous trajectory allows short measurement times of approximately 21 ms for a small 3D volume. The signal-to-noise ratio (SNR) of the measurements can cause a loss in spatial resolution in the reconstruction. However, depending on the signal quality, the same time-periodic excitation (defining one *frame*) is repeated multiple times referred to as *multi-frame* scenario [6, 4]. To increase the SNR in the signal, the measurements are averaged over mutiple frames (*averaged multi-frame scenario*). In this setup the influence of the concentration dynamic is highly relevant and can cause motion artifacts in the concentration reconstruction degrading its spatial resolution as observed in [4]. For the special case of strictly periodic motion, several approaches are developed in [4] to collect data such that each state of the concentration can be reconstructed by averaging multiple motion corrected frames. In *in-vivo* experiments, it was further shown that even the necessary minimum number of frames requires the consideration of the temporal change of the concentration in the reconstruction due to the rapid heart beat of mice. This study reveals that concentration dynamics are an issue even though the data aquisition can be fast in MPI.

In this work we address the dynamic concentration reconstruction problem. An additional flow field is obtained by incorporating an optical flow constraint as a motion prior into the reconstruction process. We will discuss initial results and compare them to the existing standard approach.

II. Methods

Due to highly different time scales of the particles' mean magnetic moment $\bar{\mathbf{m}}$ and the concentration c, we are able to consider the following simplified setup for the dynamic concentration reconstruction problem (analogously formulated for multiple receive coils and including analog filters): Let $F_t : L^2(\Omega) \to \mathbb{R}$ with

$$F_t c = \int_\Omega -\mu_0 \mathbf{p}^R(x)^T \frac{\partial}{\partial t} \bar{\mathbf{m}}(x,t) c(x) dx$$

be the dynamic forward operator where $\mathbf{p}$ is the receive coil sensitivity. We then aim for solving

$$F_t c(t) = u(t), \quad t \in I = [0, T]$$

which is a highly underdetermined problem. Exploiting the temporal scale of the concentration motivates the assumption that c is piecewise constant with respect to $I_i := [t_i, t_{i+1}), 0 = t_1 < \ldots < t_i < \ldots < t_{N+1} = T$.

In this setup we can distinguish two existing approaches in MPI (frame length $T_{\text{FFP}} \leq T$). The (i) *single-frame* approach uses single frames for reconstruction which suffers from smaller SNR but motion artifacts may have a weaker influence ($I_1 = [0, T_{\text{FFP}}), \ldots$). The (ii) *block averaged multi-frame* approach which uses block averaged data $\bar{u}_i(t) = \frac{1}{M} \sum_{j=1}^{M} u(t + (j-1)T_{\text{FFP}} + (i-1)MT_{\text{FFP}})$ from M frames, which benefits from an enlarged SNR but suffers from motion artifacts ($I_1 = [0, MT_{\text{FFP}}), \ldots$). Here we consider a (iii) *multi-frame* approach which takes into account motion priors to obtain improved reconstructions on the temporal resolution of the single frame scenario. We introduce an optical flow constraint in the reconstruction process, i.e.,

$$\frac{\partial}{\partial t} c + \nabla c \cdot \mathbf{v} = 0$$

where $\mathbf{v} : \Omega \times I \to \mathbb{R}^3$ is a flow field which is simultaneously estimated. This approach is suitable for instrument tracking but it can also be used for flow estimation in reconstructed images in MPI [3].

A solution to the joint reconstruction problem is obtained by minimizing the following Tikhonov-type functional [1] for time-discrete concentration $\tilde{c} = (c_i)_{i=1}^{N}$ and flow field $\tilde{\mathbf{v}} = (\mathbf{v}_i)_{i=1}^{N}$ tuples with respect to $I_i \subset I$, $|I_i| = T_{\mathrm{FFP}}$, $i = 1, \ldots, N$, considering the discrete operators $A_i : L^2(\Omega) \to L^2(I_i)$, $c \mapsto (t \mapsto F_t c)$

$$
\begin{aligned}
J(\tilde{c}, \tilde{\mathbf{v}}) = \sum_{i=1}^{N} &\|A_i c_i - u_i\|_{L^2(I_i)}^2 + \alpha \|c_i\|_{L^2(\Omega)}^2 \\
&+ \beta(|v_{1,i}|_{BV(\Omega)} + |v_{2,i}|_{BV(\Omega)} + |v_{3,i}|_{BV(\Omega)}) \\
&+ \gamma \|c_{i+1} - c_i + \nabla c_{i+1} \mathbf{v}_i\|_{L^1(\Omega)};
\end{aligned}
$$

$BV(\Omega)$ is the space of functions of bounded variation. The minimization is done in an alternating iteration scheme yielding two convex sub-problems (solved with FlexBox [2]) for the fully discretized problem.

III. Results

We simulate a 2D setup with excitation frequencies 24.51 kHz and 26.04 kHz in x/y-direction with amplitude $12\mathrm{mT}/\mu_0$. Gradient strength is 2 T/m/μ_0 and the field of view with a size of 27 mm $\times$ 27 mm is discretized in pixels with size 1 mm $\times$ 1 mm. Measurements are simulated with pixel size 0.5 mm $\times$ 0.5 mm and additive Gaussian noise. Particle behavior is modeled by the equilibrium model (based on the Langevin function) which parameters can be found in [5, Table 1]. A counter-clockwise rotating phantom as used in the medium rotation per frame case in [4] is simulated. The averaged multi-frame reconstruction uses 30 subsequent frames. Single frame reconstructions are obtained via solely l^2-regularization (reg. ART with 10 iterations) and they are compared with optical flow constraint reconstruction in Figure 1. The multi-frame approach (iii) improves the reconstruction while the single frame approach (i) has background and motion artifacts.

IV. Discussion

The presented approach which incorporates motion priors is able to improve the reconstruction in the multi-frame scenario without the loss of temporal resolution. In contrast to the approach for periodic motion in [4] the presented approach does not require further measurements until each state of the concentration is measured several times for averaging. The approach can also be used for a 3D scenario which will be discussed in the presentation. Potential alternative motion models also suitable for flow estimation in MPI should take into account a mass conservation law which is beyond the present work and remains future research.

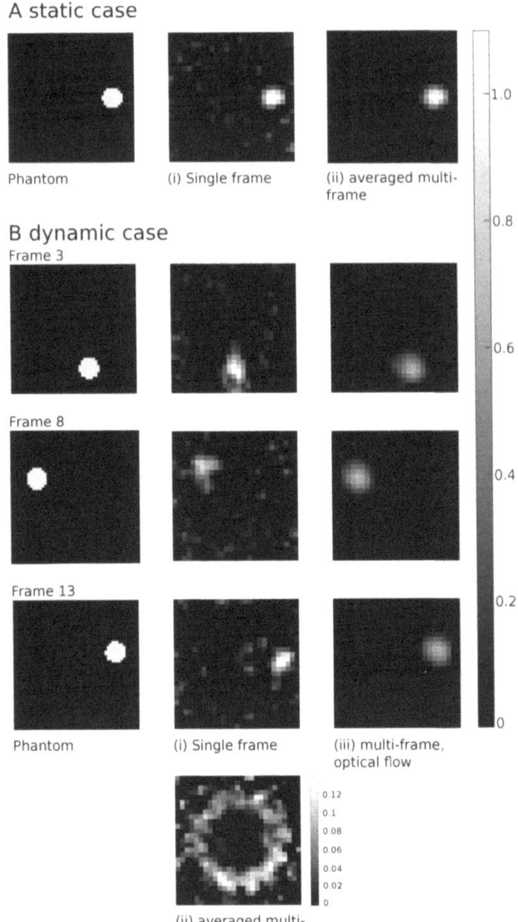

Figure 1: *Reconstructions are obtained for $\alpha = 1.14 \times 10^{-4}$ in cases (i) and (iii), $\alpha = 1.08 \times 10^{-5}$ in case (ii), and $\beta = 0.5$, $\gamma = 10$ in (iii). Regularization parameters stated for normalized operators.*

ACKNOWLEDGMENTS

T. Kluth is supported by the Deutsche Forschungsgemeinschaft (DFG) within the framework of GRK 2224/1. The authors thank M. Burger for guiding them to the FlexBox Toolbox.

REFERENCES

[1] M. Burger, H. Dirks, and C.-B. Schonlieb. A variational model for joint motion estimation and image reconstruction. *SIAM Journal on Imaging Sciences*, 11(1):94–128, 2018.

[2] H. Dirks. A flexible primal-dual toolbox. *arXiv preprint arXiv:1603.05835*, 2016.

[3] J. Franke, R. Lacroix, H. Lehr, M. Heidenreich, U. Heinen, and V. Schulz. MPI flow analysis toolbox exploiting pulsed tracer information â an aneurysm phantom proof. *International Journal on Magnetic Particle Imaging*, 3(1), 2017.

[4] N. Gdaniec, M. Schlüter, M. Möddel, M. G. Kaul, K. Krishnan, A. Schlaefer, and T. Knopp. Detection and compensation of periodic motion in magnetic particle imaging. *IEEE Transactions on Medical Imaging*, 36:1511–1521, 2017.

[5] T. Kluth and P. Maass. Model uncertainty in magnetic particle imaging: Nonlinear problem formulation and model-based sparse reconstruction. *International Journal on Magnetic Particle Imaging*, 3(2), 2017.

[6] T. Knopp and T. M. Buzug. *Magnetic Particle Imaging: An Introduction to Imaging Principles and Scanner Instrumentation.* Springer, Berlin/Heidelberg, 2012.

Experimental study on MPI motion artefacts

Markus Bujotzek[a], Heinrich Lehr[b], Timo Schwab[a], Dieter Gann[a], Jochen Franke[b] and Ulrich Heinen[a*]

[a] *Fakultät für Technik, Hochschule Pforzheim, Tiefenbronner Straße 65, 75175 Pforzheim, Germany*
[b] *Bruker BioSpin MRI GmbH, Rudolf-Plank-Str. 23, 76275 Ettlingen, Germany*
[*] *Corresponding author, email: ulrich.heinen@hs-pforzheim.de*

In this contribution, we explore the effective temporal resolution of time-resolved MPI on a preclinical MPI system and investigate the generation and nature of motion artefacts generated for fast-moving samples.

I. Introduction

Magnetic Particle Imaging (MPI) is a novel imaging technique that utilizes the magnetization signal of tracer materials containing superparamagnetic nanoparticles (MNPs) [1]. Various different setups of signal excitation and detection have been proposed and experimentally realized in a series of scanners [2]. In suitable setups, MPI is capable of delivering exceptionally high rates of 2D or even 3D image frames, providing an exciting opportunity to visualise fast dynamic processes in vivo such as a beating heart without the need for gating or triggering [3].

As in all time-resolved imaging modalities, object motion during data acquisition poses a risk of image artefacts. For MPI in particular, the images are computed from a continuous data stream, but are visualised as snapshots corresponding to individual points of time as defined by the scanner's repetition time. While in cinematographic movie capture a simple object blurring along the direction of motion occurs, a more complex type of motion artefacts must be expected for MPI depending on the interference between object movement and drive field trajectory. As MPI has been used for studying fast hemodynamics in previous studies [7], the reliability image sequences from fast moving contrast agents remains an issue of interest.

Recently, Gdaniec et al. introduced a methodology to fully recover unblurred high-resolution movies from samples exhibiting periodic motion at moderate speeds up to almost 7 Hz, and also successfully applied the technique to images of a beating mouse heart [4]. An alternative approach that does not rely on data periodicity was proposed in [5,6]. It is based on suppression of motion-induced spectral leakage. The applied filter was optimized to handle intensity modulations up to 33% percent of the frame rate, but no experimental verifications were provided in [5,6].

Here, we present a series of measurements on a point sample of Resovist moving at different speeds and along different paths. We study the correspondence between the true motion and its representation in the images reconstructed from unaveraged data and the onset of serious image artefacts

occurring for faster sample movement. Furthermore, we investigate whether the fidelity of the movie images can be improved by applying the spectral filters proposed in [6,7] to the raw data prior to image reconstruction.

II. Material and Methods

II.I. Movement of Point Sample

A sample tube filled with 8 µL of undiluted Resovist (Bayer Ch.-B. 810495) was mounted on a sample holder attached to a custom-made transmission gear that fits into the 120 mm free bore of a preclinical MPI scanner (Bruker BioSpin MRI GmbH, Ettlingen). The transmission gear (Fig. 1) can be configured either for a linearly oscillating movement along the scanner's Y axis or for a circular movement in the scanner's XY plane, where X corresponds to the bore axis and Z is aligned with the principal axis of the MPI selection field. By rotation of the transmission gear, additional movement modes such as linear motion along Z or rotation in the XZ plane or at intermediate angles are also available, although this option was not utilized in the present study. The sample holder can be clamped to the drive wheels at different radii of rotation to realize rotation diameters and/or translation distances between 1 and 20 mm. The transmission gear is driven via a rotating rod by an electric motor

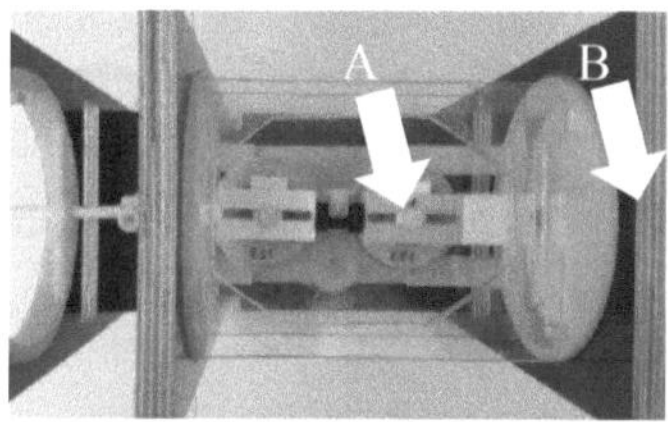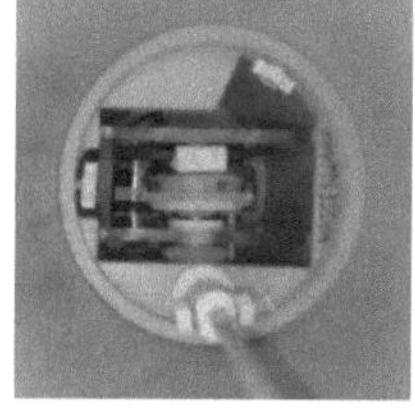

Figure 1: *Scanner insert for generating a well-defined sample movement. Left: Insert shown in a test mounting representing the scanner bore. The sample (arrow A) is placed in a holder unit which can either perform a rotary motion by clamping it to the rotating cogwheels visible underneath, or an oscillatory motion by allowing the wheel connectors to slide in the grooves. In the latter case lateral movement is prevented by an additional slider operating in the right groove of the mounting framework (arrow B) Right: Front view into MPI scanner with mounted motion insert.*

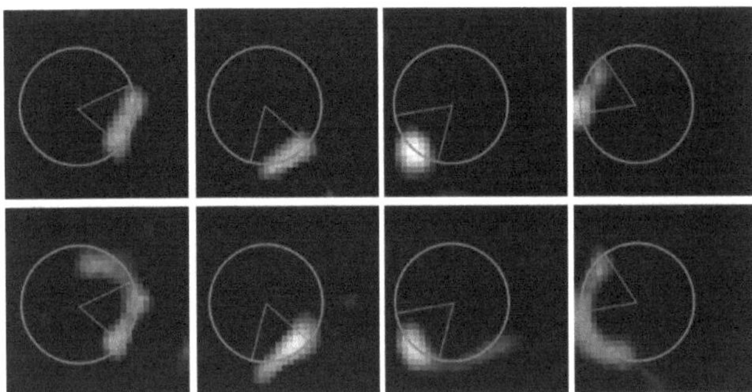

Figure 2: Four consecutive frames of an 8µl Resovist rotating at 8 rotations/second with a 10mm rotation radius. Top row: Reconstruction directly from raw data, Bottom row: Same frames reconstructed after applying a flat-top leakage-correction filter to the raw data. In each frame, the sample travels approximately 65°, This distance is indicated by two lines in each frame.

(Bühler 1.13.044.257) located outside the scanner bore, realizing oscillatory or rotatory motion at frequencies between 5 and 25 Hz. The speed of sample movement thus varies over two orders of magnitude between about 1.6 cm/s and 160 cm/s, covering most of the speed range for particles contained in physiological blood flows. The frequency of rotation is controlled by a pulse width modulation (PWM) controller (M171, Kemo Electronic). MPI signal perturbations caused by the PWM operated motor were suppressed by EMV shielding the entire drive unit using a grounded copper mesh. The exact sample position was monitored by an optical fork sensor and a cogwheel inside the drive unit synchronized to the sample movement. The monitoring signal was recorded together with the MPI signal for later verification.

II.II. MPI experiments

All MPI experiments were carried out using a 1.5 T/m selection field and drive field amplitudes of 12 mT in all three spatial directions. An offset between the center of sample rotation and the magnetic isocenter of approximately 10 mm was compensated by applying a 12 mT focus field in Z direction and a 2 mT focus field in Y direction, resulting in an effective 8 mm shift in Z direction and 2.7 mm in Y direction. For each combination of rotation frequency and diameter, 100 repetitions were captured, equivalent to a total scan time of 2.2 seconds. Background signals with an empty scanner bore were taken at regular intervals when the transmission gear was removed to establish a different mode or amplitude of movement.

II.II. Movie reconstruction

Prior to the experiments, an MPI system function with an isotropic resolution of 1 mm was acquired on a 32×32×16 grid using a 1 µl undiluted Resovist sample. To account for the spatial offset of the moving sample, an -8.7 mm focus field offset was applied in Y direction, and the coordinate grid was likewise shifted in the same direction. Movie reconstruction was performed by applying the regularized Kaczmarz algorithm to each acquired frame of the unfiltered

raw data using 30 iterations, a normalized regularization parameter λ=0.01 and 2427 frequency components from channels X and Y in the frequency range from 60-625 kHz above an SNR threshold of 15. An identical reconstruction was performed after application of a flat-top leakage correction filter covering 3 subsequent frames.

III. Results

As an example, Fig. 2 shows four consecutive frames of a point sample rotating at 8 Hz on a circle with 20 mm diameter ($v \approx 50 \; cm/s$), reconstructed both without and with data filtering. At this speed, first significant artefacts just start to arise. During each frame, the sample travels about 10 mm, or 65° as indicated in Fig. 2. While some frames show the point sample as a blurred arc, other frames almost exhibit a still image. At 25 Hz, the sample moves more than a semicircle during a single frame. All frames exhibit multiple intensity spots, some of which are no longer located on the actual trajectory, although the basic mode and speed of movement remains discernable in the most of the image sequence (data not shown here). As seen in Fig. 2, the image filtering proposed in [5,6] does not improve movie quality for fast movements but actually deteriorates the images. A positive effect at lower speeds is still being evaluated.

IV. Discussion

We conclude that MPI images of fast movement should be treated with caution, unless subframe averaging of periodic motion can be applied [4]. We attribute the failure of the leakage correction filter to the presence of modulation components outside the filter's suppression range.

V. Conclusions

We have experimentally established the creation and visual appearance of motion artefacts in time-resolved MPI for fast motions. Filtering based on non-periodic leakage-correction is insufficient for recovering unblurred images.

REFERENCES

[1] B. Gleich and J. Weizenecker. Tomographic imaging using the nonlinear response of magnetic particles. *Nature*, 435(7046):1217-1217, 2005. doi: 10.1038/nature03808.

[2] N. Panagiotopoulos et al., Magnetic Particle Imaging: current developments and future directions. *International Journal of Nanomedicine*, 10, 3097-3114, 2015, doi: 10.2147/IJN.S70488

[3] J. Weizenecker, B. Gleich, J. Rahmer, H. Dahnke, J. Borgert. Three-dimensional real-time in vivo magnetic particle imaging. *Physics in medicine and biology*, 54(5), L1-L10, 2009, doi: 10.1088/0031-9155/54/5/L01

[4] N. Gdaniec, M. Schlüter, M. Hofmann, K. Krishnan, A. Schläfer, T. Knopp. Detection and Compensation of Periodic Motion in Magnetic Particle Imaging, IEEE Transactions on Medical Imaging, 36(7), 1511-1521, 2017

[5] A. Weber, J. Franke, et. al. Artefact suppression in Time-Resolved Magnetic Particle Imaging, IWMPI 2016, Lübeck 2016

[6] A. Weber. Imperfektionen bei Magnetic Particle Imaging, Dissertation, Lübeck 2017, *Infinite Science Publishing*, 2017

[6] J. Sedlacik, A. Frölich et. al. Magnetic Particle Imaging for High Temporal Resolution Assessment of Aneurysm Hemodynamics, *PloS One*, 11(8), e0160097, 2016.

Multi-Patch Magnetic Particle Imaging of a Phantom with Periodic Motion

N. Gdaniec [a,b,*], P. Szwargulski [a,b], M. Möddel [a,b], M. Boberg [a,b], T. Knopp [a,b]

[a] *Section for Biomedical Imaging, University Medical Center Hamburg-Eppendorf, Hamburg, Germany*
[b] *Institute for Biomedical Imaging, Hamburg University of Technology, Hamburg, Germany*
* *Corresponding author, email: n.gdaniec@uke.de*

Abstract: Magnetic Particle Imaging of large objects is typically performed with the help of focus fields or by object movement. Because the different positions are acquired sequentially, the spatial resolution worsens with the number of acquired positions. We propose an imaging sequence and data processing steps to reconstruct an image from an object experiencing periodic motion with reduced motion artifacts. Feasibility is shown for phantom data.

I. Introduction

Magnetic Particle Imaging (MPI) is an imaging modality to determine the spatial distribution of superparamagnetic iron oxides with the help of static and dynamic magnetic fields [2]. MPI claims to be a fast imaging technique with a repetition time in the millisecond range for 3D volumes. Due to peripheral nerve stimulation and tissue heating, the extend of the field of view (FoV) is limited. Further techniques were presented to increase the imaging volume. This is commonly performed by spatially shifting the fields [4], or by shifting the objects [3]. These techniques have in common that they acquire different regions of the object in a temporal sequence, which reduces the temporal resolution. While this is not of importance for static objects (during the completion of one cycle), it becomes important for moving objects. For the special case of temporally repeating particle distributions a data sorting technique was proposed previously [1] for single patch sequences. We generalized the technique for multi-patch sequences and incorporated a flexible spectral leakage correction to account for different velocities of the object. We performed phantom measurements to show feasibility of the proposed method.

II. Material and Methods

II.I. Theory

The signal equation for a static object is given by

$$u_s(t) = -\mu_0 \int_\Omega p(r) \cdot \frac{\partial m}{\partial t}(r,t) c_s(r) d^3 r \qquad (1)$$

with the static concentration $c_s : \mathbb{R}^3 \to \mathbb{R}_+$, the coil sensitivity $p : \mathbb{R}^3 \to \mathbb{R}$, and magnetization $m : \mathbb{R}^3 \times \mathbb{R} \to \mathbb{R}$. For the special case of an object with periodic motion, the signal from later times equal the signal from the static object

$$u(t+nT) = u_s(t + (nT \mod T^R)), \qquad (2)$$

with the DF period T^R and the motion period T. With that we can define time intervals representing the same motion state by

$$\bigcup_{n=0}^{k} [t_s + nT, t_s + nT + \Delta t], \qquad (3)$$

with the time interval Δt for which the quasi-static approximation is fulfilled and the maximum number of repetitions k. The length of the time interval Δt depends on the motion profile and gives the maximum amount of data that can be used for reconstruction at each repetition. This width can be adapted in the reconstruction by choosing the window width for spectral leakage correction. The spectral leakage correction is a multiplication of the raw data signal from three subsequent DF cycles in time domain with a window function (e.g. Hann window) enforcing periodicity of the signal. The original window width $3T^R$ can be reduced to $\alpha 3T^R$ with $\alpha \in [0,1]$ to increase consistency of the data. For each point in time the patch position is determined by the imaging sequence such that the signal can be assigned accordingly and a joint reconstruction can be performed. The time intervals in Eq. 3 were calculated with the knowledge of the rotational frequency. The frequency is calculated individually from the raw data [1] of the subsequent DF cycles acquired at each patch position. The number of subsequent DF cycles at one patch position gives the minimum frequency that can be determined by a fourier analysis.

II.II. Experiments

Experiments were performed with the preclinical MPI scanner (Bruker). We used a 3D printed phantom holder with a diameter of 7 cm shown in Fig. 1 second column, first row and placed samples consisting of 10 µL perimag with a concentration of 50 mmol$_{Fe}$ L^{-1} in the holes. The phantom was rotated with a screw driver in the horizontal plane inside the scanner bore with two rotational frequencies.

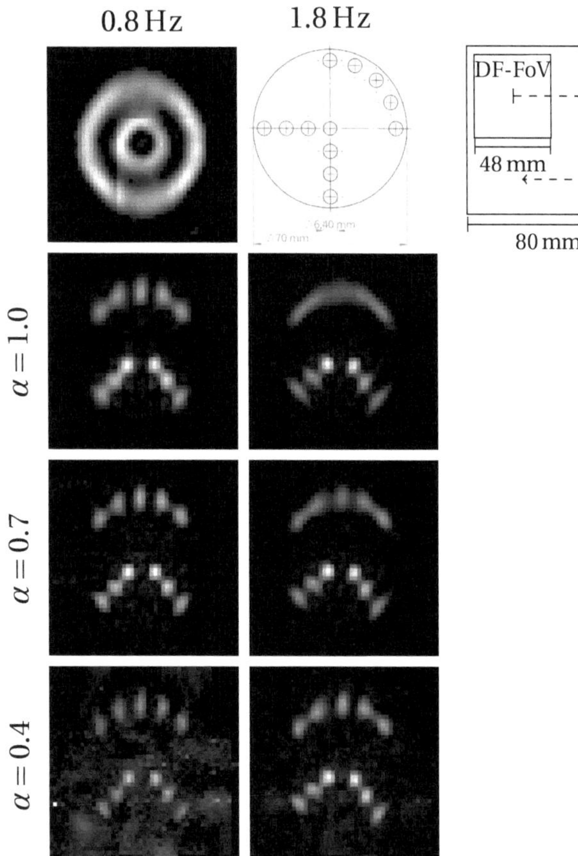

Figure 1: *Experimental results. A schematic image of the phantom is shown in the second column of the first row. A reconstructed image from a regular joint multi-patch reconstruction [4] is shown in the first column and a schematic overview of the scan sequence in the third column. The remaining rows show reconstructed images for frequencies of 0.8 Hz (first column) and 1.8 Hz (second column) for the indicated amount of data from a DF cycle.*

We used a focus field imaging sequence with a gradient strength of $0.5\,\mathrm{T\,m^{-1}}$ in the x- and y-direction and a DF amplitude of 12 mT. The four patches were shifted ±16 mm in x- and y-direction resulting in a FOV of ≈ 8 cm × 8 cm × 2.4 cm. At each patch position 200 subsequent DF cycles were acquired, followed by 7 DF cycles for the movement of the DF region to the next patch position, as schematically shown in the third column of Fig. 1. For the joint reconstruction, four system functions were acquired with the imaging parameters from the phantom experiment on a grid of size 33 × 33 × 27 covering a volume of 6.6 cm × 6.6 cm × 2.7 cm.

III. Results

The reconstructed images are shown in Fig.1. In the first row, a standard static multi-patch reconstruction of the four patches is shown with an averaging performed over all DF periods acquired for each patch. The rotating phantom results in circles in the final reconstructed image because the

temporal resolution is lost. The reconstruction incorporating a periodic motion of the object results in images shown in the second to fourth row of Fig.1. On the left for a frequency of 0.8 Hz and on the right for 1.8 Hz. The amount of a DF-cycle used for each repetition is given on the left for each row. For the lower frequency the quasi-static assumption is better preserved for one DF cycle, resulting in good image quality for $\alpha = 1.0$. For the higher frequency, the approximation is not fulfilled and motion artifacts appear. These can be reduced by lowering the amount of data used for reconstruction at each repetition. This reduces motion artifacts, but incorporates noise in the final image, limiting the minimum value of the window width α for a fixed total scan duration.

IV. Discussion

This work proposes a multi-patch imaging sequence and a data sorting algorithm for reconstruction of an object experiencing periodic motion. Regular multi-patch reconstruction techniques result in images with motion artifacts. With our approach, we were able to reproduce the shape of the phantom for different motion frequencies, while no prior knowledge about the frequency is necessary as far as enough subsequent data are available. The data sorting algorithm helps in reducing motion artifacts from periodic motion. The distortions in the final image at the patch boundaries are caused by field imperfections because we shifted the patches as far as possible to the boundaries resulting in a large FoV.

V. Conclusions

We were able to reconstruct images from an object experiencing periodic motion with a multi-patch imaging sequence with reduced motion artifacts.

AUTHOR'S STATEMENT
Research funding: The authors thankfully acknowledge the financial support by the German Research Foundation (DFG, grant number KN 1108/2-1) and the Federal Ministry of Education and Research (BMBF, grant number 05M16GKA). Conflict of interest: Authors state no conflict of interest. Informed consent: Informed consent has been obtained from all individuals included in this study.

REFERENCES
[1] N. Gdaniec, M. Schlueter, M. Hofmann, M. Kaul, K. Krishnan, A. Schlafer, and T. Knopp. Detection and compensation of periodic motion in magnetic particle imaging. *IEEE Transactions on Medical Imaging*, PP(99):1–1, 2017. ISSN 0278-0062. doi: 10.1109/TMI.2017.2666740.

[2] B. Gleich and J. Weizenecker. Tomographic imaging using the nonlinear response of magnetic particles. *Nature*, 435(7046):1214–1217, June 2005.

[3] P. W. Goodwill and S. M. Conolly. Multidimensional x-space magnetic particle imaging. *IEEE Transactions on Medical Imaging*, 30(9):1581–1590, Sept 2011. ISSN 0278-0062. doi: 10.1109/TMI.2011.2125982.

[4] T. Knopp, K. Them, M. Kaul, and N. Gdaniec. Joint reconstruction of non-overlapping magnetic particle imaging focus-field data. *Physics in medicine and biology*, 60(8):L15, 2015. doi: 10.1088/0031-9155/60/8/L15.

Pulsed MPI for Improved Resolution and Contrast

D. Hensley[*,a], Z. W. Tay[a], B. Zheng[a], J. Ma[a], N. Oude Booijink[a], P. Chandrasekharan[a], P. Goodwill[b], and S. Conolly[a,c]

[a] *Department of Bioengineering, University of California, Berkeley, United States*
[b] *Magnetic Insight, Inc., Alameda, United States*
[c] *Department of Electrical Engineering and Computer Sciences, University of California, Berkeley, United States*
[*] *Corresponding author, email: dwhensley@berkeley.edu*

Abstract: Magnetic Particle Imaging (MPI) is a promising new tracer-based imaging modality. Engineering efforts continue to probe current methods and new implementations. Here we describe the use of pulsed excitation waveforms, in contrast to continuous sinusoidal methods that currently predominate. We show how pulsed excitation can both overcome resolution limitations with current techniques due to magnetic relaxation and simultaneously provide high quality measures of relaxation information to potentially improve MPI molecular imaging contrast. We believe pulsed excitation techniques could initiate new and broad pulsed sequence development in MPI.

I. Introduction

The theory of superparamagnetic tracers predicts that MPI resolution and signal should improve as we increase the magnetic core size of our tracers. As depicted in (1), we have observed this only up to a point [1]. After about 25 nm, resolution and sensitivity typically degrade. This behavior is due to the long magnetic response times of larger tracers which acts like a low pass filter, degrading both resolution and signal-to-noise ratio. While magnetic relaxation can degrade performance relative to the steady-state ideal, it can also be a source of physiologic contrast leveraged in applications such as color MPI [2,3]. Better understanding magnetic relaxation in MPI is an active area of research.

Here we propose pulsed excitation waveforms that allow us to both mitigate the deleterious effects of relaxation on imaging resolution and quantify the relaxation processes in detail.

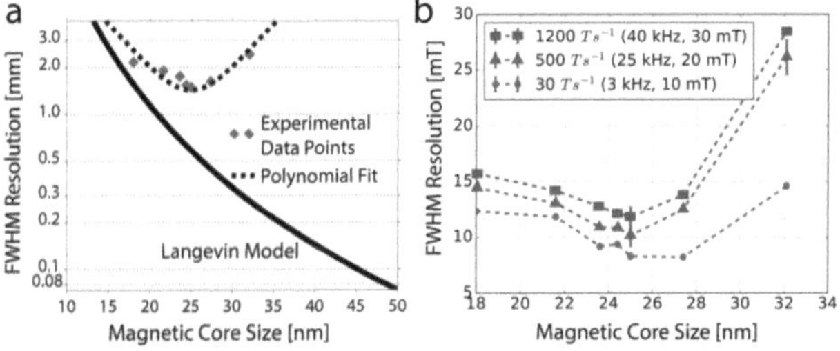

Figure 1: *Magnetic relaxation limits resolution with larger tracers in standard MPI. (a) Experimental data showing resolution (7 T/m gradient strength) as a function of tracer core size. Langevin theory predicts improved resolution with size indefinitely. In practice, relaxation-induced blurring leads to an optimum around 25 nm when using excitation frequencies in the range of 20-50 kHz. (b) Slowing down MPI sinusoidal excitation can partially mitigate this effect.*

II. Material and Methods

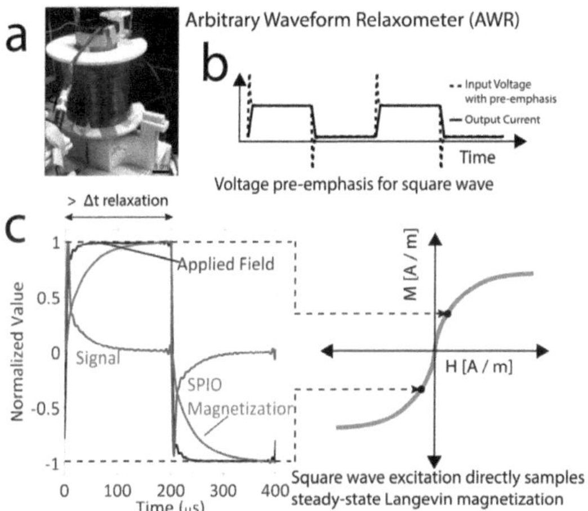

Figure 2: *Implementing pulsed excitation. (a) Arbitrary waveform relaxometer described in our previous work. (b) Exemplar pulsed waveform (square wave). (c) Experimental data with a single square wave period of excitation and depiction of how this relates to sampling the steady-state magnetization curve.*

Canonically, sinusoidal excitation waveforms (e.g., ~25 kHz and 20 mT) have been used in MPI [4], [5]. When the magnetic response time of a tracer is on the order of the period (e.g., ~40 microseconds), lossy relaxation blurring can noticeably degrade imaging resolution and signal. It is possible to slow the excitation sinusoid, as depicted in Fig. 1(b); however, this may not accommodate the particle's behavior without unacceptable losses to SNR. Furthermore, the frequency of resonant systems is not easily changed.

We propose using pulsed excitation waveforms such as the square wave of Fig. 2(b). Fig. 2(c) shows experimental MPI data taken with our arbitrary waveform relaxometer (AWR) [6] using square wave excitation. The tracer signal for each half-period is impulse response-like, per the tracer's magnetic relaxation properties. As in canonical MPI, we can grid these data to form images. A key constraint is that the quiescent hold time (half-period for a square wave) is long enough to ensure steady-state magnetization is reached.

II.I. Hardware

We used our previously described AWR [6] in this work. We typically use the AWR without a gradient field, which collapses the sample to a virtual point. Using a ramping bias field in addition to pulsed excitation, we can sample pulsed MPI point-spread functions (PSFs) in the magnetic field domain, which is equivalent to a 1D spatial PSF [6].

II.II. Software and Reconstruction

We used our standard x-space MPI pulse sequence and reconstruction software, modified to accommodate pulsed MPI excitation waveforms. We can grid both tracer mass PSFs and quantification of relaxation impulse responses (relaxation maps). For the former, we integrate the raw received signal associated with each half-period of pulsed excitation and grid this value to the known location (in physical or magnetic field space) of the FFR during that half-period. For relaxation maps, we grid a measured/fit value (*e.g.*, exponential time constant fit to the raw signal decay).

II.III. Experiments

For most experiments, we used a set of monodisperse tracers purchased from Imagion Biosystems with core sizes: 18.5, 21.6, 24.4, and 32.1 nm. Small samples (40 μL) were tested with both our canonical sinusoidal excitation (25 kHz, 20 mT) and square wave excitation scans (5 kHz, 1 mT). All scans were acquired in 0.5-0.7 seconds (with up to 25 averages) for the full -40 to +40 mT magnetic field of view. For viscometry experiments, a 33 nm tracer from LodeSpin Labs was used, and data was obtained using a steady-state recovery pulse sequence we developed.

III. Results

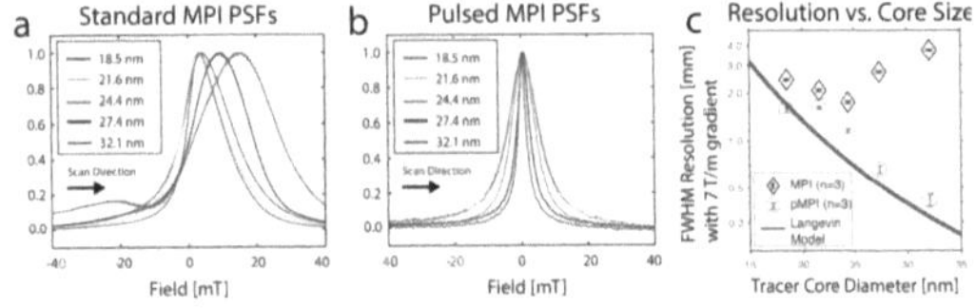

Figure 3: *Experimental comparison of 1D PSFs. (a) With standard sinusoidal excitation (25 kHz, 20 mT), tracers over ~25 nm perform poorly. (b) With square wave pulsed excitation (5 kHz, 1 mT), we see continuously improved resolution. (c) Pulsed MPI allows us to obtain high resolution with large tracers as the steady-state theory predicts (n indicates number of replicates).*

Fig. 3 shows results comparing square wave pulsed MPI with canonical sinusoidal MPI for tracers in the range of 18 – 32 nm. In the sinusoidal data, resolution and PSF shape degrade sharply after approximately 25 nm. In the pulsed MPI data, however, resolution continues to improve and

PSF shape is maintained with increasing size, realizing the promise of the steady state theory (Fig. 3(c)).

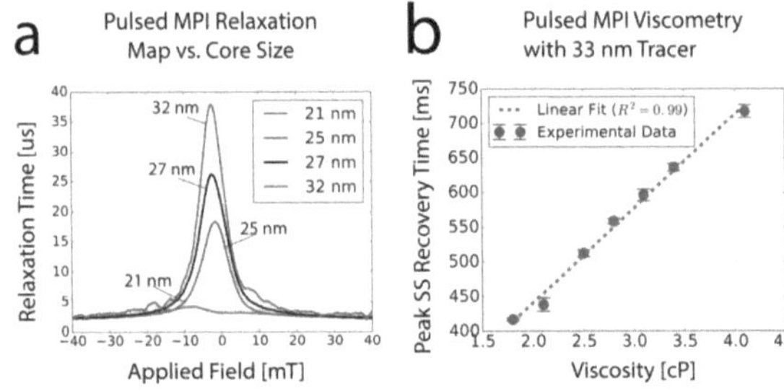

Figure 4: *Experimental pulsed MPI relaxation. (a) Relaxation maps: relaxation impulse response as a function of the total applied field. Larger tracers have more pronounced relaxation. (b) Viscometry using a steady-state recovery pulse sequence. We see a linear increase in relaxation time with increasing viscosity.*

Fig. 4 shows pulsed MPI used to experimentally quantify relaxation. In Fig. 4(a), we show 1D relaxation maps for tracers with different core sizes. In Fig. 4(b), we use a steady-state recovery pulse sequence to detect viscosity over a physiologically relevant range.

IV. Discussion

Pulsed excitation allows us to control how we encode relaxation phenomena in the MPI signal. We can use this to improve resolution, develop new types of images (relaxation maps), and detect physiologic variables such as viscosity. Pulsed MPI could lead to sophisticated pulse sequencing better able to exploit MPI physics for imaging purposes.

V. Conclusions

We have demonstrated new pulsed excitation methods in MPI. Pulsed MPI can unlock much higher resolution using large-core tracers and robustly measure tracer relaxation.

ACKNOWLEDGEMENTS

We thank Erika Vreeland and Matt Ferguson for help with custom tracers.

AUTHOR'S STATEMENT

Conflict of interest: D. Hensley and P. Goodwill are employed at Magnetic Insight, Inc., and D. Hensley, P. Goodwill, and S. Conolly hold stock.

REFERENCES

[1] Z. W. Tay, et al. The relaxation wall: experimental limits to improving MPI spatial resolution by increasing nanoparticle core size. *Biomedical physics & engineering express*, 3(3), p.035003. 2017.

[2] Rahmer, J., et al. (2015). First experimental evidence of the feasibility of multi-color magnetic particle imaging. *Physics in Medicine & Biology*, 60(5), 1775.

[3] D. Hensley, P. Goodwill, L. Croft, and S. M. Conolly, S. Preliminary experimental X-space color MPI. In *Magnetic particle imaging (IWMPI), 2015 5th international workshop on* (pp. 1-1). IEEE. 2015.

[4] B. Gleich and J. Weizenecker. Tomographic imaging using the nonlinear response of magnetic particles. *Nature*, 435(7046):1217-1217, 2005. doi: 10.1038/nature03808.

[5] P. Goodwill and S. M. Conolly. The X-space formulation of the magnetic particle imaging process: 1-D signal, resolution, bandwidth, SNR, SAR, and magnetostimulation. *IEEE transactions on medical imaging*, 29(11), pp.1851-1859. 2010.

[6] Z. W. Tay, et al. A high-throughput, arbitrary-waveform, mpi spectrometer and relaxometer for comprehensive magnetic particle optimization and characterization. *Scientific reports*, 6, p.34180. 2016.

Low Rank Approach to Sparse System Matrix Recovery for MPI

M. Grosser[a,b*] and T. Knopp[a,b]

[a] *Section for Biomedical Imaging, University Medical Center Hamburg-Eppendorf, Hamburg, Germany*
[b] *Institute for Biomedical Imaging, Technical University Hamburg, Hamburg, Germany*
[*] *Corresponding author, email: mi.grosser@uke.de*

Abstract: In Magnetic Particle Imaging, the time consuming measurement of a system function is required before image reconstruction. Reduction of measurement time has been achieved with the help of compressed sensing, which is based on the sparsity of the system function in some transform domain. In this work we demonstrate that the rows of a system function can be approximated by low-rank tensors. We develop a recovery method exploiting both the low rank of system function rows and the sparsity of their DCT coefficients. Experiments show that the proposed method yields system functions with increased accuracy and reduced noise.

I. Introduction

Magnetic particle imaging (MPI) is a very promising method, which allows imaging of the distribution of magnetic nanoparticles at both high spatial and high temporal resolution [1]. Prior to the actual imaging experiment, the system response needs to a measured in a time consuming calibration scan if multi-dimensional excitation patterns are used. The responses for all the imaging voxels are collected in the system matrix, which describes the mapping between particle concentration and the measured signal.

The scan time for this calibration can be reduced significantly by using compressed sensing techniques (CS) [2,3]. Such techniques exploit the fact that the rows of the system matrix become sparse after applying transformations such as a fast Fourier transform or a discrete cosine transform (DCT). In combination with an incoherent sampling pattern, CS allows to recover a complete system matrix from a highly undersampled measurement.

In this work we demonstrate that the rows of the system matrix can be approximated as low rank tensors. As an application of this knowledge, we develop a CS based system matrix recovery method, which exploits both sparsity in the DCT domain and aforementioned low rankedness (CSLR). Our tests show that the proposed method yields system matrices with reduced normalized root mean squared error (NRMSE) and reduced noise when compared to a standard CS reconstruction.

II. Material and Methods

II.I. Low Rank Expansion of the System Matrix

In Ref. [4], it has been shown that for ideal particles and an ideal MPI scanner, the patterns of the system matrix can be approximated by tensor products of Chebyshev polynomials. This suggests that patterns of a real scanner can be accurately

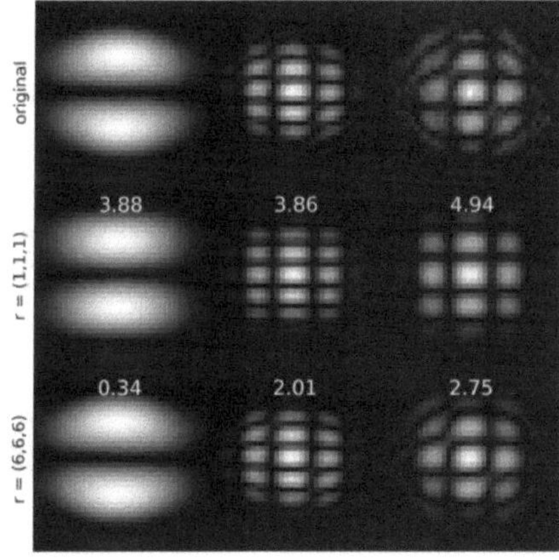

Figure 1: *Patterns of a 3d system matrix (top row) and their expansion with a generalized rank of (1,1,1) (middle row) and (6,6,6) (bottom row). Numbers in the patterns give the NRMSE in % with respect to the original pattern.*

approximated using a low-rank expansion. Such an expansion can be obtained by truncating the higher-order singular value decompositions (HOSVD) of the real- and imaginary part of the system matrix at a given (generalized) rank r [5]. This is shown in Fig 1., for selected patterns of a measured 3d system matrix.

II.II. Low Rank System Matrix Retrieval

For an efficient system matrix retrieval, we propose to augment the existing DCT-based CS problem with an additional low-rank constraint. Thus, for each matrix row s_k, we formulate the following optimization problem:

$$argmin_{s_k} \frac{1}{2}\|y_k - Ps_k\|_2^2 + \lambda\|\Phi s_k\|_1 + R_r(s_k). \quad (1)$$

Here y_k contains the measured points of the kth row of the system matrix and P denotes the corresponding sampling pattern. Φ is the 3d-DCT-II matrix. Finally, R_r denotes the characteristic function of the set of all tensors with a (generalized) rank not greater than r. The proximal map of R_r is approximated by thresholding the HOSVDs of the real- and imaginary part of the corresponding variable. For solving problem (1) we use the Split Bregman method [6].

II.III. Application to a 3d System Matrix
We tested our method on a 3d system matrix from the OpenMPIData repository (calibration measurement 6) [7]. Data and acquisition parameters can be found in Ref. [8]. All system matrix patterns with an SNR > 3 were chosen and subsampled with a Poisson disk pattern with a subsampling factor of 20. For comparison, system matrices were reconstructed with full rank and $r = (6,6,6)$, respectively.

III. Results
Reconstruction results of some representative system matrix rows are shown in Fig. 2. For the pattern on the left, the NRMSE is slightly increased in comparison to the CS reconstruction. However, there is no visual difference in image quality. For the other patterns, CSLR results in patterns with both reduced NRMSE and higher visual quality. For the CS reconstruction, 1584 out of 3175 were reconstructed with an NRMSE smaller than 5%. For CSLR the corresponding number is 1871. Finally, the average NRMSE over all matrix rows is 5.39 % for the CS reconstruction and 4.86% for the CSLR reconstruction

IV. Discussion
Our results show, that the low generalized rank of system matrix patterns is a strong prior for CS based system matrix recovery. Compared to a CS reconstruction, CSLR yields 287 (18.1 %) more patterns with a NRMSE smaller than 5%. This is beneficial because a larger number of system matrix rows can be used for image reconstruction.

As can be seen on the right sides of Figs. 1 and 2, constraining the rank of system matrix rows leads to a very efficient denoising. This is desirable with regard to image reconstruction, as it reduces the amount of noise.

It should be noted that the NRMSE values in this work are given with respect to a noisy measurement. Thus, they should be interpreted carefully. Notably, the reconstruction quality of some patterns obtained with CSLR, is likely to be higher than suggested by the NRMSE values provided.

In terms of numerical effort, the provided method is only slightly slower than a conventional CS reconstruction. This is caused by the fact that a HOSVD needs to be performed in each iteration of the solver. Note however, that for larger

system matrices, the contribution of the HOSVD to the reconstruction time becomes larger.

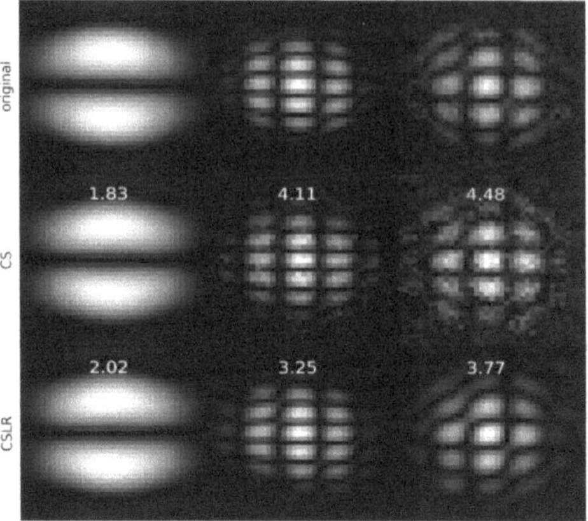

Figure 2: *Patterns of a 3d system matrix. The different rows show the original pattern (top row), reconstruction without low rank constraint (middle row) and reconstruction with a generalized rank of (6,6,6) (bottom row), respectively. Numbers in the patterns give the NRMSE in % with respect to the original pattern.*

V. Conclusions
In analogy, to the system matrix of an ideal scanner, real-life system matrices can be approximated accurately with a low-rank expansion. This knowledge was used to develop an efficient algorithm for sparse system matrix recovery. Tests on a 20-fold undersampled 3d system matrix show that the proposed method yields system matrices with a reduced NRMSE and increased SNR compared to a standard CS method. Note that a further reduction in measurement time could be achieved, by exploiting the symmetries of the system function, as was done in Ref. [3].

AUTHOR'S STATEMENT
Research funding: The author state no funding involved. Conflict of interest: Authors state no conflict of interest.

REFERENCES
[1] B. Gleich and J. Weizenecker. Tomographic imaging using the nonlinear response of magnetic particles. *Nature*, 435(7046):1217-1217, 2005. doi: 10.1038/nature03808.
[2] T. Knopp and A. Weber. Sparse reconstruction of the magnetic particle imaging system matrix. *IEEE transactions on medical imaging*, 32(8):1473-1480, 2013. doi: 10.1109/TMI.2013.2258029
[3] A. Weber and T. Knopp. Reconstruction of the magnetic particle imaging system matrix using symmetries and compressed sensing. *Advances in Mathematical Physics*, 2015, 2015. doi:10.1155/2015/460496
[4] J. Rahmer, et. al. Signal encoding in magnetic particle imaging:properties of the system function. *BMC medical imaging*, 9(1), 2009. doi: 10.1186/1471-2342-9-4
[5] G. Berqvist and E. G. Larsson. The higher-order singular value decomposition: Theory and an application [. *IEEE Signal Processing Magazine*, 27(3):151-154, 2010. doi: 10.1109/MSP.2010.936030
[6] T. Goldstein and S. Osher. The split Bregman method for L1-regularized problems. *SIAM journal on imaging sciences*, 2(2):323-343, 2009. doi:11.1137/080725891
[7] T. Knopp et al. Magnetic particle imaging data format. *arXiv preprint arXiv*, 1602.06072, 2016
[8] https://github.com/MagneticParticleImaging/OpenMPIData.jl

Background Removal by Mixing Factor based Filtering of the System Matrix

F. Lieb[a]* and H.-G. Stark[a]

[a] *Department of Engineering & Technomathematics, University of Applied Sciences, Aschaffenburg, Germany*
** Corresponding author, email: florian.lieb@h-ab.de*

Abstract: Removing the background of measured system matrices is currently done by subtracting empty scanner measurements taken during system matrix acquisition. In this work a filtering method based on mixing factors is proposed, which separates particle signal and background more efficiently without referring to background measurements anymore. Moreover, the proposed filter method leads to a novel SNR measure, which is unbiased by the background, entailing significantly less noisy and more detailed reconstruction results.

I. Introduction

In magnetic particle imaging the spatial concentration of magnetic nanoparticles is visualized by exploiting a priori knowledge of the relation between induced voltage and particle distribution. The spatial encoding is based on a field-free point shifted along a Lissajous trajectory. By placing delta samples at various discrete positions of the field-of-view, the relation between these spatial positions and the corresponding induced particle signal is determined. This collection is known as the measured system matrix (SM).

To be more precise, after applying a Fourier transform in the time domain, this collection leads to a matrix $S \in \mathbb{C}^{k \times l}$, with l corresponding to the spatial positions of the delta sample and k corresponding to the frequency index of the induced voltage. The desired particle concentration $c \in \mathbb{R}^l$ can then be obtained by solving the linear equation system

$$Sc = u, \qquad (1)$$

where $u \in \mathbb{C}^k$ is the Fourier transform of the measured particle signal. The system matrix can be background corrected by subtracting empty scanner measurements after system matrix acquisition [1]. For this purpose, the delta sample is frequently removed from the scanner and background measurements are taken. After acquisition, the background is linearly interpolated (BG_S) and subsequently subtracted from the system matrix, i.e., $S_{BGC} = S - BG_S$. Similarly, the measurement vector u is background corrected by subtracting empty scanner measurements (BG_u) taken before or after the recording of u, thus leading to $u_{BGC} = u - BG_u$.

In addition, for solving (1) only certain frequency components, i.e., a proper subset of the rows k of the system matrix, is considered [2]. This frequency selection is based on a signal-to-noise ratio (SNR), which supposedly filters out frequency components lacking particle information [1]. Non-static background components are removed by fixing a cutoff frequency, usually within the range of 80 kHz, removing all frequencies below this threshold [1].

This procedure has some disadvantages. Recording background measurements prolongs the system matrix acquisition and, moreover, the subsequent background subtraction introduces additional noise for larger frequency indices. Furthermore, SNR measures, which are based on empty scanner measurements ([1,2]), tend to be sensitive to harmonics of the excitation frequency. This results in small SNR values (sometimes even below the noise level) at frequency indices corresponding to harmonics of the excitation frequency. Thus, in the filtered system matrix components frequencies are suppressed, which might be useful for reconstruction. In this manuscript we propose an alternative method to remove the background from the measured system matrix by utilizing a mixing factor based filter in the DCT (discrete cosine transform) domain and a novel SNR measure, which is not biased by empty scanner measurements.

II. Material and Methods

II.I. Mixing Factor based Filtering

For a fixed frequency index k, the spatial distribution of the corresponding row-vector of a measured 2D system matrix exhibits a strong correlation to tensor products of Chebyshev polynomials [3]. The relation between the number of wave hills and the frequency index k is given by

$$k = m_x(N_D + 1) + N_D m_y, \qquad (2)$$

with mixing factors $m_x, m_y \in \mathbb{Z}$ and $N_D \in \mathbb{N}$ linking the excitation frequencies according to $N_D/(N_D + 1) = f_y/f_x$. Frequency domain filtering has been introduced in [3,4]. However, both procedures described there do not account for either the structure of the particle signal or the structure of the background in the corresponding domain. In order to overcome this deficiency, we define a filtered version of the measured system matrix by

$$S_{filt} = \Psi_{DCT}^* (B_{MF}^r \odot (\Psi_{DCT} S)), \qquad (3)$$

with $\odot$ denoting the Hadamard product. Here, the unitary operator Ψ_{DCT} represents the 2D DCT-II transform and B_{MF}^r denotes a frequency selection based on mixing factors belonging to frequency index k, cf. (2). To be precise, the filter B_{MF}^r is binary, consisting of a $r \times r$ rectangle of 1's, which is, e.g., for the x-receive coil, centered at $(m_x + 2, m_y + 1)$ in the DCT domain. This is motivated by the fact that the number of wave hills strongly correlates to the discrete frequency of the cosine basis function of the DCT; thus the filter is a hypothesis for DCT-domain-subsets relevant for the particle signal. We suppose, therefore, that non-static as well as static background effects are reduced to a minimum, as opposed to the methods from [3,4]. Here thresholding does not discriminate large coefficients corresponding to the particle signal from those belonging to the background. The choice of r depends on the discretization of the FOV and is empirically chosen to be 2 in the following.

II.II. A Mixing Factor Based SNR

For frequency selection in the DCT-domain we have to define an analogue for the SNR mentioned in Section I, relying on empty scanner measurements, which are not available anymore. We propose the following measure: With $\Gamma_{MF}^r = B_{MF}^r \odot \Psi_{DCT} S$, define SNR_{MF}^r by

$$SNR_{MF}^r = \frac{\|\Gamma_{MF}^r\|_2}{\|\Psi_{DCT} S - \Gamma_{MF}^r\|_2}. \qquad (4)$$

With this measure, the signal-to-noise-ratio should be large whenever the particle signal is well localized within the region defined by B_{MF}^r, where r should be chosen appropriately. In addition, the remaining DCT coefficients also characterize static and non-static components of the background in few significant low frequency coefficients.

III. Results

Two system matrices, provided in [5], are filtered as previously described. A comparison between background correction by subtraction and by filtering of a frequency component at a harmonic of the excitation frequency is shown in Fig. 1.

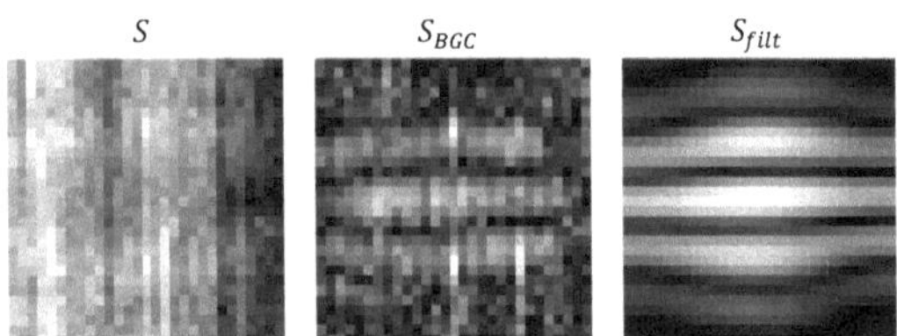

Figure 1: *Absolute values of a measured, background subtracted and filtered 2D system matrix component.*

The background subtraction does improve the measured frequency component, whereas the filter approach is capable of fully recovering the particle signal. The filtering approaches from [1,3] perform accurately, only when the background is properly removed. In the following,

reconstruction results based on background subtraction (S_{BGC}), are compared with those based on S_{filt}, using two different phantoms. Both reconstructions were performed with a single Karcmarz iteration, a regularization parameter $\lambda = 10^{-10}$ and a lower cutoff frequency of 70 kHz. For the S_{BGC} case, the standard SNR measure is used, the reconstruction with S_{filt} is performed both with standard SNR and SNR_{MF}^r. The results are shown in Fig. 2.

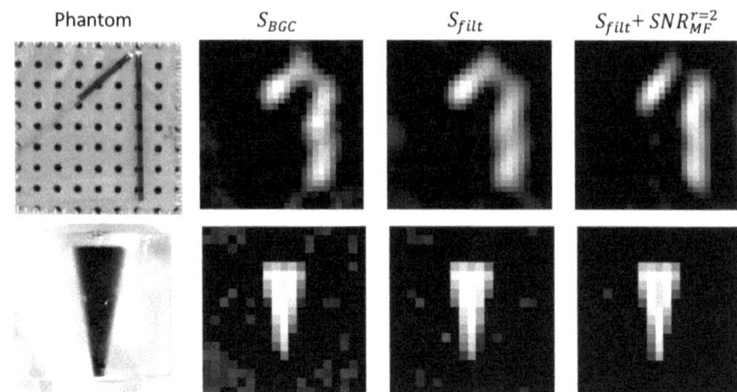

Figure 2: *Reconstruction results based on background corrected and filtered SM's (r = 2).*

The chosen threshold values are 2.0 for both SNR and SNR_{MF}^r in the upper row and 1.8 in the lower row. In all cases u_{BGC} is used.

IV. Discussion and Conclusion

The results in Fig. 2 show, that a filtered system matrix in combination with the new proposed SNR measure leads to improved reconstruction results. In particular, we refer to the rightmost image in the upper row, relying on (4). Moreover, noise artifacts are reduced to a minimum (Fig 2, lower phantom), in accordance with the results shown in Fig. 1.

In conclusion, the proposed method may eventually perform a background-particle separation without an empty scanner measurement, thereby reducing experimental efforts considerably. Reconstruction quality can be further improved by using the mixing factor based SNR_{MF}^r-measure, which is not biased by empty scanner measurements.

ACKNOWLEDGEMENTS
We gratefully acknowledge the financial support of the Federal Ministry of Education and Research (BMBF grant number 05M16WFA).

REFERENCES
[1] K. Them *et al.* Sensitivity Enhancement in Magnetic Particle Imaging by Background Subtraction. In *IEEE Trans. Med. Imaging*, 35(3):893, 2016. doi: 10.1109/TMI.2015.2501462.
[2] T. Knopp *et al.* Weighted Iterative Reconstruction for Magnetic Particle Imaging. In *Phys. Med. Biol.*, 55(6):1577, 2010. doi: 10.1088/0031-9155/55/6/003.
[3] L. Schmiester *et al.* Direct Image Reconstruction of Lissajous-Type Magnetic Particle Imaging Data Using Chebyshev-Based Matrix Compression. In *IEEE Trans. Comput. Imaging*, 3(4):671, 2016. doi: 10.1109/TCI.2017.2706058.
[4] A. Weber *et al.* Reconstruction Enhancement by Denoising the Magnetic Particle Imaging System Matrix Using Frequency Domain Filter. In *IEEE Trans. Magn.*, 51(2):1, 2015. doi: 10.1109/TMAG.2014.2332612.
[5] T. Knopp *et al.* MDF: Magnetic Particle Imaging Data Format. 2016. arXiv:1602.06072.

Poster Session 01

Interpretation of Cartesian Data based on a Simulated Human-Sized MPI Brain Imager

P. Szwargulski[a,b*], M. Graeser[a,b], F. Thieben[a,b], N. Gdaniec[a,b], F. Werner[a,b], M. Boberg[a,b], F. Griese[a,b], M. Möddel[a,b] , and T. Knopp[a,b]

[a] Section for Biomedical Imaging, University Medical Center Hamburg-Eppendorf, Hamburg, Germany
[b] Institute for Biomedical Imaging, Hamburg University of Technology, Hamburg, Germany
* Corresponding author, email: p.szwargulski@uke.de

Abstract: Recently the first proof of concept for a human scaled MPI scanner for brain applications was presented. It features a new imaging concept with a mechanically moveable selection field and uses a dynamic Cartesian imaging sequence. In this work, different kinds of data processing and image reconstruction approaches for Cartesian sequences are compared.

I. Introduction

The first human-scaled magnetic particle imaging (MPI) scanner for applications in the head [1] was designed to be capable for imaging volumes in the scale of a human brain. The scanner was developed as a field free point (FFP) scanner with a fast (~25 kHz) one-dimensional drive field and a slow (~2 Hz) orthogonal focus field enabling imaging of one imaging plane in about 0.5 s. The acquired data can be interpreted and reconstructed in different ways using a system matrix based reconstruction. One way is the interpretation of the Cartesian dataset as a single sequence with a period length determined by the slow focus field. An alternative is the interpretation as a stack of one-dimensional scans arranged in a multi-patch dataset [2]. For both, the state of the art single frame iterative Kaczmarz reconstruction can be used. If the individual scans of the multi-patch dataset are reconstructed independently a post-processing of the reconstructed images [3] is necessary. But the multi-patch dataset can also be reconstructed jointly solving a single system of equations [4]. In this work, different types of data interpretation and reconstruction methods are presented and compared based on simulated MPI data. Further, the influence of averaging multiple line scans to reduce the amount of data is investigated.

II. Material and Methods

II.I. Imaging Sequence

The design of the scanner includes a selection field that is capable of generating an FFP with a gradient strength of about $0.2\ \mathrm{Tm^{-1}\mu_0^{-1}}$ in the strongest direction. The current design is equipped with a one-dimensional drive field coil that is capable to move the FFP sinusoidally along the x-axis with a frequency of $f_x \approx 25$ kHz. The excitation field amplitude is set to be $6\ \mathrm{mT\mu_0^{-1}}$ to stay below the estimated limit for nerve stimulation in the head [1]. To extend the imaging sequence from 1D to 2D, the selection field coils generate additional dynamic focus fields. The focus field moves the FFP along a sinusoidal trajectory in the y-direction with a frequency $f_y \approx 2$ Hz. The field amplitude was ~15 mT and the repetition time of the sequence was TR ≈ 0.5 s. This results in 13,000 single line scans within one repetition. Since the focus field was driven continuously, the mean shift between two line scans varies from no shift at the boundary up to 34 μm in the center. Using the given field strength the resulting field of view (FoV) is about $110 \times 140\ \mathrm{mm^2}$.

II.II. Continuous Cartesian Dataset

The naive way to interpret the data is to use the Fourier transformation over the entire sequence. This will result in a spectrum including 494,001 frequency components, since the spectral resolution is given as $\Delta f = 1/\mathrm{TR} \approx 2$ Hz. The position of the signal-carrying harmonic bands in the spectrum can be calculated by multiple of $m_x = f_x/\Delta f = 13{,}000$ and $m_y = f_y/\Delta f = 1$. For reconstruction of this dataset, the state of the art regularized Kaczmarz algorithm can be used. One drawback of this approach is that the data processing of those long data streams has a high computational effort and slows down the overall reconstruction process.

II.III. Averaged Cartesian Dataset

One way to reduce the amount of data is to average a subset of successive line scans and apply the Fourier transform on the resulting time series. Taking the average over 100 line scans will reduce the number of frequency components linearly to 4941. The factor to calculate the signal-carrying harmonic band will be reduced in the x-direction to $m_x = f_x/\Delta f = 130$. For reconstruction, the same state of the art method as for the non-averaged Cartesian dataset was used.

II.IV. Multi-Patch Dataset

As an alternative to the interpretation as a single sequence, the data can also be Fourier transformed line by line. This will result in the averaged case in 130 patches and in the non-averaged case in 13,000 patches. Each patch will include 39 frequency components. In these patches no frequency mixing can be detected, since only the pure harmonics of the drive field are stored. The multi-patch data can be reconstructed in the one hand patch-wise and combined to a single image in a post-processing step [3] or in the other hand jointly solving a single system of equations [4].

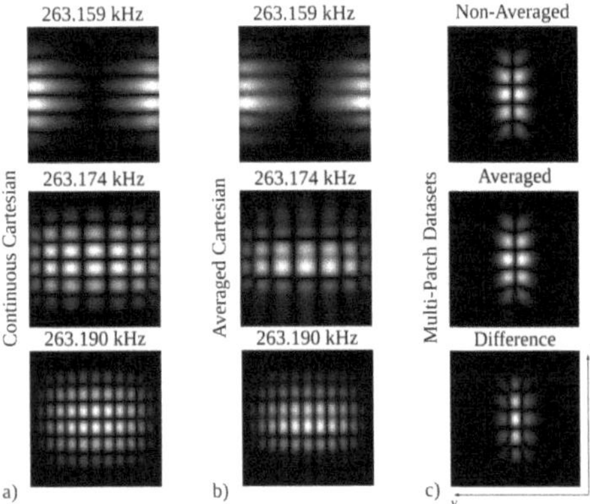

Figure 1: *In a) and b) three frequency components of the x-receive channel for the continuous and averaged Cartesian dataset are shown. All frequency components are included in the 10th harmonic band. In c) the 10th frequency components of the y-receive channel for the continuous and averaged multi-patch case are shown. Further, the absolute value of the difference between both is given.*

II.V. Simulation Environment

To analyze the different types of data interpretation and reconstruction methods a simulation study was performed. For this purpose, an ideal scanner configuration without noise including the field strengths and frequencies described in the section II.I was implemented. As base frequency 2 MHz were used. For simulation of the system matrices, 23 nm size particles without relaxation were used. For each case a system matrix on a 140×140 mm^2 FoV with 55×55 pixels was simulated. The data were resorted and combined to represent the averaged and the non-averaged case for both, the interpretation as a Cartesian dataset or as a multi-patch dataset. For testing the reconstruction, a software phantom including the letter "P" with a size of 76.4×49.5 mm^2 was designed and measurements were simulated solving the forward imaging equation with a high-resolution system matrix. The phantom is shown in Fig. 2. For reconstruction, a frequency selection was performed based on the mixing factors, excluding all frequencies below 75 kHz. The number of iterations was 50 and was kept constant for all cases. The relative regularization parameter was adapted to the size of the used system matrix to achieve the same effective regularization.

III. Results and Discussion

III.I. System Matrix Comparison

In Fig. 1 the system matrix components for the non-averaged and the averaged case for both, the Cartesian and the multi-patch data interpretation way are shown. As one can see, both Cartesian sequences include patterns that are structurally comparable. For the averaged case, an additional smearing of the patterns is visible. This could lead to a reduced achievable spatial resolution. It must be kept in mind, that averaging will lead to inconsistencies in the data, since the focus field shift between the blocks will be up to 3.4 mm. Inconsistencies in the data will result in signal leakage in frequency domain. Especially for higher averaging numbers this might be problematic. The smearing

can also be observed in the 10th harmonic of the y-receive channel of the multi-patch dataset, although it is less visible there. Therefore, additionally the difference image of both patterns is shown in Fig. 1.

III.II. Reconstruction Comparison

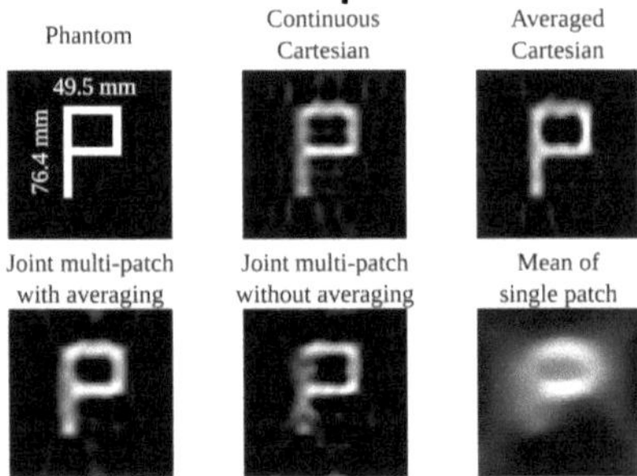

Figure 2: *Comparison of the reconstructed images using the different interpretation methods. For simulated data it can be seen that the averaged Cartesian and the averaged multi-patch interpretations lead to the best images.*

The reconstruction results are presented in Fig. 2. On the top left, the used software phantom is shown. On the bottom right the result for the post-processed single patch reconstruction is presented. Since for post-processing only the mean over all reconstructed images was chosen, the reconstructed image is blurred. To achieve better results an alternative post-processing method could be applied. The remaining reconstructed images include slight stripe artifacts at the bottom and on the top of the "P". This could be explained by the missing frequency components lower than 75 kHz. As one can see, the inconsistencies of the data engendered by the averaging has no negative influence on the image quality. For both cases, the Cartesian and the multi-patch approach, the averaging leads to a slight improvement in image quality. To investigate this effect in more depth, an analysis on the applicable number of averages will be necessary to find the admissible averaging limit. Further, the different data processing techniques and reconstruction methods need to be done on measured data of the MPI brain imager.

IV. Conclusions

As one can see, there are different ways to interpret the measured data of Cartesian MPI experiments leading to different reconstruction results. We have shown in a simulation study that a data reduction method using block averaging has no negative influence provided that the trajectory movement within an averaged block is small enough.

AUTHOR'S STATEMENT
Research funding: The authors thankfully acknowledge the financial support by the DFG (grant number KN 1108/2-1) and the BMBF (grant numbers 05M16GKA, 13XP5060B).

REFERENCES
[1] M. Graeser et al., arXiv:1810.07987
[2] F. Werner et al. Phys. Med. Biol.7;62(9):3407-3421.2017
[3] J. Rahmer et al. ISMRM.,19:629, 2011.
[4] T. Knopp et al. Phys. Med. Biol. 60 L15, 2015

Neural Network for Reconstruction of MPI Images

P. Koch[a]*, M. Maass[a], M. Bruhns[a], C. Droigk[a], T. J. Parbs[a], and A. Mertins[a]

[a] Institute for Signal Processing, University of Lübeck, Germany
** Corresponding author, email: koch@isip.uni-luebeck.de*

Abstract: In Magnetic Particle Imaging the reconstruction of the image given the voltage signal is not trivial. Since the system function cannot be measured in its entirety the reconstruction algorithms can only estimate the images. The standard reconstruction approaches usually rely on time consuming optimization concepts that involve the use of sophisticated priors. We studied the general possibility of learning the reconstruction with neural networks. The results reveal that the networks potentially can reconstruct the images while even learning priors. However, the structures used for harvesting the training data should be chosen wisely.

I. Introduction

In Magnetic Particle Imaging (MPI), voltage signals induced by superparamagnetic nanoparticles are acquired from which the particle distributions have to be reconstructed. One approach for reconstruction is based on the system matrix. Given the estimated system matrix, one common way to deal with the reconstruction is based on iterative algorithms like the Kaczmarz method [1]. Thus, the reconstruction of an image is usually an iterative optimization process that is often time consuming. The same holds when sophisticated priors are used for regularization. An alternative is to learn the inverse system in a data-driven fashion. For this purpose, machine learning techniques from the field of neural networks (NNs) can be adopted. First attempts to use neural networks for the particle distribution reconstruction have already been made [2,3]. However, both of these methods work in the frequency space, with only one-dimensional trajectory for the drive fields. Also, only dense NNs were used. In contrast, the method proposed here works with two-dimensional trajectory and operates in the time domain. Arguably, it appears promising to adopt so-called convolutional neural networks (CNNs). For example, in [4] CNNs were used for denoising and reconstruction of computed tomography images. Furthermore, CNNs have been adopted to reconstruct images of general inverse problems [5,6]. Due to the success of CNNs, we use this type of network for reconstruction of MPI images.

II. Material and Methods

II.I. Convolutional Neural Network

In this work, we propose a fairly small architecture (see Fig. 1). The network is similar to the one in [7] used for reconstruction of e.g. magnetic tomography images. The input of the network is the measured voltage signal as a vector. The first two layers of the network are dense layers. The size of the second dense layer defines the size of the reconstructed image. Subsequently, 2D convolution layers are deployed. The multiple feature maps produced by the first convolution

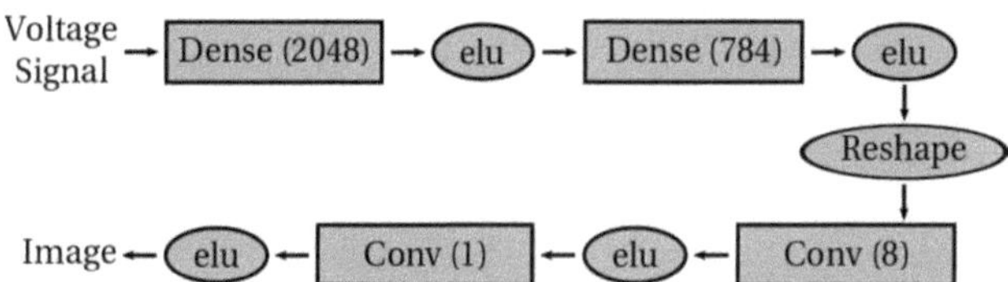

Figure 1: *Network architecture. Dense indicates a dense layer, where its size is specified in parenthesis. Conv denotes a 2D-convolution layer, where the number of 3x3 kernels is given in parenthesis. The reshape block represents the transition from a 1D signal to a 2D image (28x28 pixels).*

layer are fused to a single image by the single kernel of the second convolution layer. Thus, the output of the network is the reconstructed image. As activation function we used the exponential linear unit (elu)

$$f(\alpha, x) = \begin{cases} \alpha(e^x - 1), \text{for } x < 0 \\ x, \text{for } x \geq 0 \end{cases} \quad (1)$$

with $\alpha = 0.1$ for our experiments. This feed-forward network is trained in a supervised fashion. We tried two different loss functions: mean squared error (MSE) and mean absolute error (MAE) between the network's output and the ground truth. The loss is used to adapt the weights using the Adam optimizer.

II.II Test Setup

As a reference system, a linear minimum MSE (MMSE) estimator followed by a non-negativity constraint was used [8]. Given the observed signal u, an estimate $\hat{c}$ for the particle distribution c is calculated by $\hat{c} = \max(A \cdot (u - \bar{u}) + \bar{c}, 0)$, where

$$A = E\{(c - \bar{c})(u - \bar{u})^T\}E\{(u - \bar{u})(u - \bar{u})^T\}^{-1} \quad (2)$$

with the expectation operation $E\{\cdot\}$, $\bar{c} = E\{c\}$, and $\bar{u} = E\{u\}$. We conducted experiments on simulated data. For the creation of a dataset, the MNIST dataset [7] was used as particle distribution. It contains 70000 digital images of handwritten numbers between the digits zero and nine, where each image has a size of 28×28 pixels. The simulation of the voltage signal was based on the Langevin model of paramagnetism. The field of view (FOV) was defined to have size 20.4×20.4 mm^2, the frequency ratio for the Lissajous trajectory was $f_x/f_y = 31/32$, the particle size was 30 nm, and the body temperature of humans was assumed inside the simulation. To prevent inverse crime, the images were upscaled to 40×40 pixels. The voltage signals were corrupted with white Gaussian noise at a signal-to-noise ratio (SNR) of 20 dB. To cover the whole FOV, the dataset was augmented by three random rigid motions for each digit. In total, the dataset had 4×70000 voltage signals. All images showing a five form the test dataset (25252 samples) and the images of the other 9 digits were used for training the NNs.

III. Results

The approaches were compared with three error measures: MSE, MAE, and structural similarity (SSIM) index. For all measures, the average and standard deviation ($\pm$) over the whole test dataset were calculated (see Tab. 1). Both NNs outperform the linear MMSE estimator. The NN trained with MAE loss turned out to be superior to the one optimized under MSE loss with respect to the SSIM. Therefore, in Fig. 2, a few test images reconstructed by the NN with MAE loss are shown exemplarily. Even though the letter five was not included in the training data, it is quite accurately reconstructed. We used the trained model also for the reconstruction of vessel-like structures from their voltage signals (SNR of 20 dB). Examples can be found in Fig. 3. The reconstruction of this structures is reasonable but not as good as for the fives of the MNIST database (see Fig. 2).

IV. Discussion

The experiments verifies that for the reconstruction in MPI, nonlinear approaches that go beyond demanding $\hat{c} \geq 0$ are favorable. Furthermore, the nonlinear networks appear as a promising method for learning the inverse system. The results indicate that there is a significant difference between the structures of the vessel-like phantom and the MNIST numbers. It seems promising to present all different kinds of structures in the training dataset. However, the coarse structures as well as the background are reconstructed well. This shows the generalization ability of the network and indicates that the trained NN learned to invert the physical model. One drawback of the approach is the required amount of training data. In future research, we will focus on strategies to tackle the problem and apply the proposed technique to real data.

V. Conclusions

We proposed an end-to-end trained neural network capable of reconstructing MPI images from the voltage signal. The network can reconstruct structures that have never been presented during training. Since the networks outperform the linear MMSE estimator quite significantly, it becomes obvious that our nonlinear approach can learn and exploit the statistics of the data much better than a linear method.

Table 1: *Results for the networks and the MMSE estimator on the MNIST test data containing only the digit five.*

	MSE	MAE	SSIM index
NN (MSE loss)	0.0041 $\pm$ 0.0024	0.0232 $\pm$ 0.0086	0.9214 $\pm$ 0.0261
NN (MAE loss)	0.0042 $\pm$ 0.0024	0.0209 $\pm$ 0.0075	0.9510 $\pm$ 0.0246
Linear MMSE estimator	0.0087 $\pm$ 0.0038	0.0490 $\pm$ 0.0122	0.4803 $\pm$ 0.0895

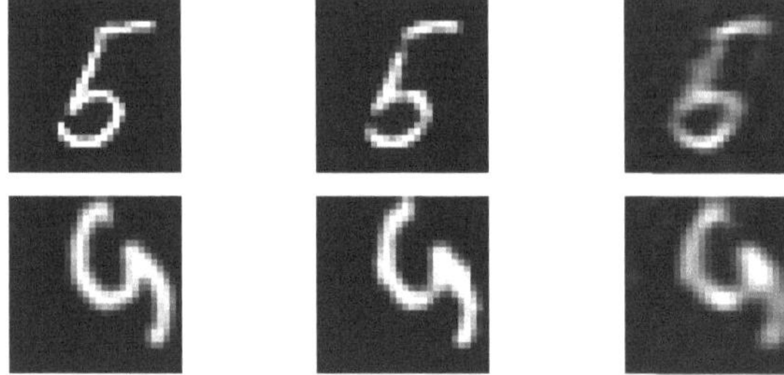

Figure 2: *Reconstructed MNIST images. First column: ground truth. Second column: reconstructions of NN trained with MAE loss. Third column: MMSE reconstructions.*

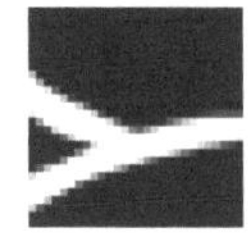
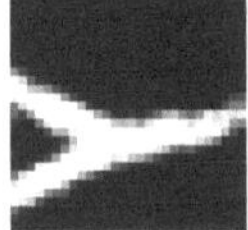
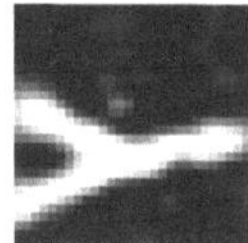

Figure 3: *Vessel images. From left to right; Ground truth, reconstruction of NN trained with MSE (MSE: 0.0110, MAE: 0.0411, SSIM index: 0.9081), and MMSE reconstruction (MSE: 0.0134, MAE: 0.0686, SSIM index: 0.5083).*

AUTHOR'S STATEMENT

This work was supported by the German Research Foundation under grant number ME 1170/7-1. Authors state no conflict of interest.

REFERENCES

[1] T. Knopp, J. Rahmer, T. F. Sattel, S. Biederer, J. Weizenecker, B. Gleich, J. Borgert, and T. M. Buzug. Weighted Iterative Reconstruction for Magnetic Particle Imaging. *Phys. Med. Biol.*, 55(6):1577-1589, 2010. doi: 10.1088/0031-9155/55/6/003.

[2] T. Hatsuda, T. Takagi, A. Matsuhisa, M. Arayama, H. Tsuchiya, S. Takahashi, and Y. Ishihara. Basic Study of Image Reconstruction Method using Neural Networks with Additional Learning of Magnetic Particle Imaging. *Int. J. Magn. Part. Imaging*, 2(2), 2016. doi: 10.18416/ijmpi.2016.1611002.

[3] B. G. Chae. Neural Network Image Reconstruction for Magnetic Particle Imaging. *ETRI J.*, 39(6):841-850, 2017. doi: 10.4218/etrij.2017-0094.

[4] E. Kang, J. Min, and J. C. Ye. A deep convolutional neural network using directional wavelets for low-dose X-ray CT reconstruction. *Med. Phys.*, 44(10):e360-e375, 2017. doi: 10.1002/mp.12344.

[5] K. H. Jin, M. T. McCann, E. Froustey, and M. Unser. Deep Convolutional Neural Network for Inverse Problems in Imaging. *IEEE Trans. Image Process.*, 26(9):4509-4522, 2017. doi: 10.1109/TIP.2017.2713099.

[6] B. Zhu, J. Z. Liu, S. F. Cauley, B. R. Rosen, and M. S. Rosen. Image reconstruction by domain-transform manifold learning. *Nature*, 555(7697):487-492. doi: 10.1038/nature25988.

[7] Y. LeCun, L. Bottou, Y. Bengio, and P. Haffner. Gradient-Based Learning Applied to Document Recognition. *Proc. IEEE*, 86(11):2278-2324, 1998. doi: 10.1109/5.726791.

[8] J. M. Mendel. *Lessons in Estimation Theory for Signal Processing, Communications, and Control*. Prentice Hall, 1995.

Determining the Relation between Iron Mass and Spatial Resolution for a Human-Sized Magnetic Particle Brain Imager

F. Thieben[a,b,*], M. Graeser[a,b], M. Boberg[a,b], P. Szwargulski[a,b], M. Moeddel[a,b], T. Knopp[a,b]

[a] *Section for Biomedical Imaging, University Medical Center Hamburg-Eppendorf, Hamburg, Germany*
[b] *Institute for Biomedical Imaging, Hamburg University of Technology, Hamburg, Germany*
* *Corresponding author, email: f.thieben@uke.de*

Abstract: The determination of brain perfusion is an important issue for the diagnosis of vascular diseases. Since the total iron dose is limited, the ability to measure and resolve low iron concentrations is of great interest. In this work, we investigated the relation between decreasing iron mass and spatial resolution for a human-sized MPI brain imager. We find the full-width at half maximum of a small delta sample to be a good initial measure for the spatial resolution. In our experiments, the achievable resolution showed only slight decrease over one decade of iron mass.

I. Introduction

The imaging modality magnetic particle imaging (MPI) determines the spatial distribution of superparamagnetic iron-oxide nano-particles [1]. One targeted application for MPI is perfusion imaging of stroke, which was proven to be feasible in mice by Ludewig et al. [2]. Depending on the size of the stroke a reasonable spatial resolution is necessary. In [3] a volume of 42 ml was modelled as this is above a typical stroke volume within the middle cerebral artery-territory [4]. Thus, a MPI system with a spatial resolution of 10 mm could resolve these strokes. Experimental system specifications for spatial resolution are usually done with high iron mass. Knopp et al. simulated the spatial resolution depending on the particle size and took the signal to noise ratio (SNR) of the measured signal into account [5]. In clinical imaging one typically works with low iron concentrations as the tracer has to be injected systemically. Thus the relation between iron mass and spatial resolution is of great interest. In this work, the spatial resolution was investigated systematically using two common methods. On the one hand using the full-width at half maximum (FWHM) of a small delta sample and on the other hand using two separated samples at a defined distance. The results of the two methods were compared for the first time in the context of MPI. All measurements were done with a human-sized MPI brain imager [3].

II. Material and Methods

II.I. Phantom Design

A resolution phantom (RP) was designed which allows two samples to be positioned at edge-to-edge distances from 5 mm to 25 mm in 1 mm steps and 25 mm to 45 mm in 5 mm steps along the x- and y-direction of our MPI system. A series of cubic delta samples with an edge length of 6.3 mm containing 250 µl Perimag (lot 05617 102-05, micromod, Germany) with decreasing iron mass was used for all measurements [2 mg, 500 µg, 125 µg, and 31.25 µg].

II.II. Resolution experiments

The measurements were performed using the human-sized brain imaging device presented in [3]. The drive field amplitude was set to 6 mT at a frequency of 25.699 kHz in x-direction. For 2D imaging an additional sinusoidal dynamic selection field was applied in y-direction with a repetition time of 0.5 s. The gradient strength in the field free point (FFP) varies between 0.16 T/m and 0.21 T/m in y-direction and is twice as large as in x-direction. For the signal detection two independent receive coils in x- and y-direction were used. A system matrix (SM) based approach was used to reconstruct the images. The SM was measured using a 250 µl delta sample containing undiluted Perimag (8.5 mg/ml) on a 28 × 28 grid covering a field of view (FOV) of 140 mm × 140 mm in x- and y-direction. The resulting pixel size was 5 mm. In the first experiment, each sample with a certain iron mass was placed in the center of the FOV for imaging. For reconstruction, the iterative regularized Kaczmarz algorithm was used with a fixed number of iterations. The number of frequency components was kept constant for all reconstructions. In a next step, the FWHM was determined from the interpolated signal. In an optimization algorithm, the relative regularization parameter λ was chosen to minimize the FWHM whilst maintaining a high image SNR. Since this excludes single pixel artifacts a condition was added to obtain a signal to artifact ratio in the image greater than two, i.e. the maximum in the region of interest (ROI) divided by the maximum outside this ROI. In the second experiment, two samples with the same iron mass were mounted on the RP at the premeasured FWHM distance and imaged in x- and y-direction. Similar to the previous experiment λ was chosen to optimize the spatial resolution. We define two samples to be resolvable if the signal intensity in image domain drops down under half of the maximum value in the middle between the two samples. We find this approach to be more conservative than the approach in [3]. If the samples at measured distance could not be resolved, the distance was increased by 1 mm, until it could be resolved. Otherwise the distance was decreased in 1 mm steps until they could no longer be resolved. Exemplary images of the two evaluation methods are shown in Fig. 2.

III. Results

In Fig. 1 the relative regularization parameter λ in dependence of the iron mass is presented. For the FWHM experiments as well as for the spatial resolution experiments the optimized λ increased with decreasing iron mass. In the spatial resolution measurements, three of four choices for λ were lower than the ones for the FWHM measurements. This was due to the fact that there were two samples in the FOV. Hence the total iron mass increased and thereby λ could be reduced.

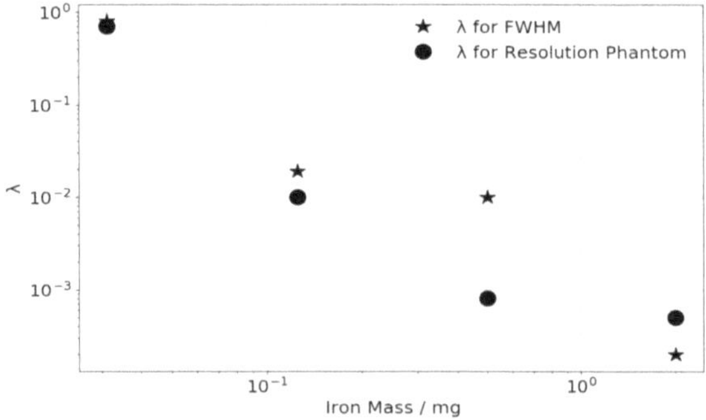

Figure 1: *Applied regularization parameter λ depending on the iron mass. The stars mark the used λ for the FWHM measurements of a delta sample. Dots mark the applied λ for the measurements with the spatial resolution phantom.*

The calculated FWHM of the measured iron mass are illustrated in Fig. 2. The FWHM for the x-direction remained below 7 mm until 125 µg. In y-direction, an increase could be observed with a resolution below 11.6 mm at 125 µg.

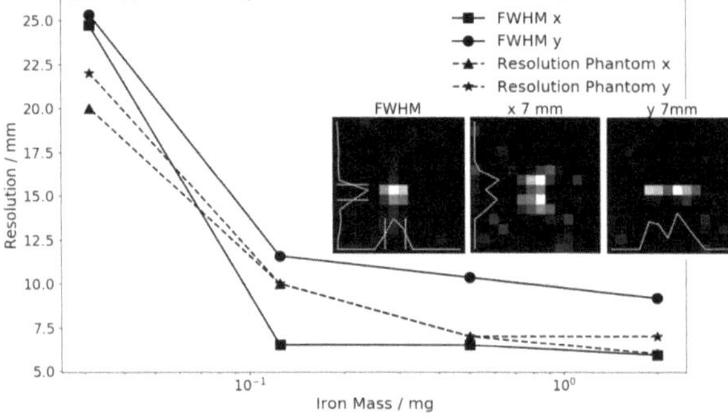

Figure 2: *Results of the resolution phantom with a certain iron mass in x- and y-direction are shown and connected as dotted lines. The FWHM for a delta samples are presented and connected as solid lines for both directions as well. Exemplary the reconstructed images for the 500 µg samples are given. In each image, additionally the profile lines throughout the center of the reconstructed image are illustrated.*

The spatial resolution of the RP is shown as well and is within the range of the FWHM measurements. The samples placed on the RP in an edge-to-edge distance of 10 mm could be resolved with an iron mass of 125 µg in x- and y-direction. For higher iron mass the spatial resolution was close to the SM pixel size of 5 mm. The better spatial resolution at 31.25 µg with the RP could be linked to the increased total iron mass. Starting at 2 mg, all experiments follow the same trend where the spatial resolution decreases slightly in the first decade with decreasing iron mass.

IV. Discussion

With the excitation in x-direction and the receive channels in x- and y-direction one would predict a higher resolution in x-direction. However, due to the higher gradient strength of the selection field in y-direction the MPI system shows a uniform spatial resolution. The measured spatial resolution showed only a slight decrease over one decade of iron mass and was close to the system specified spatial resolution of 5 mm in x-direction and 6 mm in y-direction evaluated in [3]. The FWHM in y-direction is wider than in x-direction, which we attribute to the position of the samples, which were placed in the middle between two SM positions in y-direction. Thus the signal was partitioned between two pixels. The steep resolution slope at iron mass below 125 µg can be attributed to the loss of frequency components for such low iron mass. Further investigations have to be done regarding the size of the used samples, which were bigger than the SM pixel size.

V. Conclusions

Within this work, we demonstrated that the presented imager achieves a uniform spatial resolution of 10 mm in x- and y-direction with decreasing iron mass down to 125 µg. We find the FWHM of a single sample to be a good indicator for the spatial resolution in MPI, but no replacement for a dedicated resolution phantom study.

Author's statement
Research funding: German Research Foundation (DFG, grant number KN 1108/2-1) and the Federal Ministry of Education and Research (BMBF, grant numbers 05M16GKA, 13XP5060B). Conflict of interest: Authors state no conflict of interest. Informed consent: Informed consent has been obtained from all individuals included in this study.

REFERENCES
[1] B. Gleich and J. Weizenecker. Tomographic imaging using the nonlinear response of magnetic particles. *Nature*, 435(7046):1217-1217, 2005. doi: 10.1038/nature03808.
[2] P. Ludewig et al. Magnetic particle imaging for real-time perfusion imaging in acute stroke. *ACS nano* 11.10:10480-10488, 2017. doi: 10.1021/acsnano.7b05784.
[3] M. Graeser et al. Human-sized Magnetic Particle Imaging for Brain Applications. 2018. *arXiv:*1810.07987 [physics.med-ph]
[4] C. Sperber and H.-O. Karnath. Tomography of acute stroke in a sample of 439 right brain damaged patients. *NeuroImage: Clinical*, 10:124-28, 2016. doi: 10.1016/j.nicl.2015.11.012
[5] T. Knopp et al. Prediction of the spatial resolution of magnetic particle imaging using the modulation transfer function of the imaging process. *IEEE transactions on medical imaging* 30.6:1284-1292, 2011 doi: 10.1109/TMI.2011.2113188.

Rapid PCI: An Alternative X-space Based Image Reconstruction for Rapid Scanning Trajectories

S. Kurt[a,b*], M. Utkur[a,b], Y. Muslu[a,b], and E. U. Saritas[a,b,c]

[a] *Department of Electrical and Electronics Engineering, Bilkent University, Ankara, Turkey*
[b] *National Magnetic Resonance Research Center (UMRAM), Bilkent University, Ankara, Turkey*
[c] *Neuroscience Program, Sabuncu Brain Research Center, Bilkent University, Ankara, Turkey*
[*] *Corresponding author, email: kurt@ee.bilkent.edu.tr*

Abstract: Magnetic Particle Imaging (MPI) has limited pFOV size due to drive field safety limits. Therefore, wider FOVs can be imaged by numerous overlapping pFOVs. However, processing each pFOV separately and combining them to form an image requires additional processing steps that can cause a sensitivity against noise, nanoparticle relaxation, and interference for the regular x-space reconstruction. In this work, we offer an alternative x-space based image reconstruction method which does not require pFOV processing. The proposed method promises improved image quality and a robustness against non-ideal signal conditions.

I. Introduction

In Magnetic Particle Imaging (MPI), there are two main methods for image reconstruction: system function reconstruction [1-3] and x-space reconstruction [4,5]. Regular x-space reconstruction requires partial field-of-view (pFOV) processing steps: speed compensation of the received signal, gridding to the nonequidistant field free point (FFP) positions followed by regridding to Cartesian space, and a DC recovery algorithm [6]. We have recently proposed an alternative x-space based image reconstruction that does not require these processing steps [7]. The preliminary experimental results of this technique called pFOV Center Imaging (PCI) utilized a trajectory where the pFOV center was moved to discrete positions. Here, we extend our technique to rapid scanning trajectories that continuously move the pFOV center. We demonstrate with experiments that rapid PCI is more robust against relaxation and interference artifacts.

II. Material and Methods

II.I. Theory

The proposed pFOV Center Imaging (PCI) utilizes the signal samples at the centers of the pFOVs. The reason behind this is the fact that the FFP speed is identical at the centers of all pFOVs, giving a chance to simplify the reconstruction process.

The first step of the technique is forming a "raw PCI image", $\hat{\rho}_{rpci}(x)$, by *directly* assigning the time-domain signal values corresponding to *equidistant* pFOV centers to corresponding pixels of $\hat{\rho}_{rpci}(x)$. We have previously shown that $\hat{\rho}_{rpci}(x)$ can be expressed in terms of ideal MPI image, $\hat{\rho}(x)$, as follows [7]:

$$\hat{\rho}_{rpci}(x) = \alpha \left(\hat{\rho}(x) * h_{pci}(x) \right) \tag{1}$$

where

$$h_{pci}(x) = \delta(x) - \frac{4}{\pi W} \sqrt{1 - \left(\frac{2x}{W}\right)^2} \tag{2}$$

Here, α is a constant related to the speed of the FFP at the pFOV center and W is the total extent of each pFOV. $h_{pci}(x)$ depends only on W, therefore it is a fully known kernel (independent of nanoparticle type). Thus, the ideal MPI image $\hat{\rho}(x)$ can be recovered via deconvolution of $\hat{\rho}_{rpci}(x)$ with the known kernel $h_{pci}(x)$.

For deconvolution process, we used a regularized deconvolution with a Laplacian operator (*deconvreg* function in MATLAB). Regular x-space reconstruction was also implemented for comparison purposes.

II.II. Imaging Experiments

Imaging experiments were performed on our in-house MPI scanner (Fig. 1a-b) with (-4.8, 2.4, 2.4) T/m selection field gradients in (x, y, z) directions [8]. A 10 mT drive field was applied at 9.7 kHz along the z-direction. Instead of a focus field, we used a robotic arm to slowly move the phantom in the scanner. The drive field and the robotic arm motion was applied simultaneously and continuously throughout the imaging experiment. The robotic motion along the z-direction had a constant speed of 0.0292 m/s, corresponding to a 0.07 T/s slew rate. This results in a scan time of 1.9 sec to cover a 5.5-cm length line in z-direction. For the x-direction, the arm moved to 9 discrete positions. The total FOV was 5.5x0.7 cm^2 in z-x plane, with a total scan time of 17.1 sec. The imaging phantom was prepared using Perimag (Micromod, GmbH, Germany) with 30 mmol Fe/L concentration. Two 3-mm diameter vials containing Perimag SPIOs were prepared with a separation of 9 mm (see Fig. 1c).

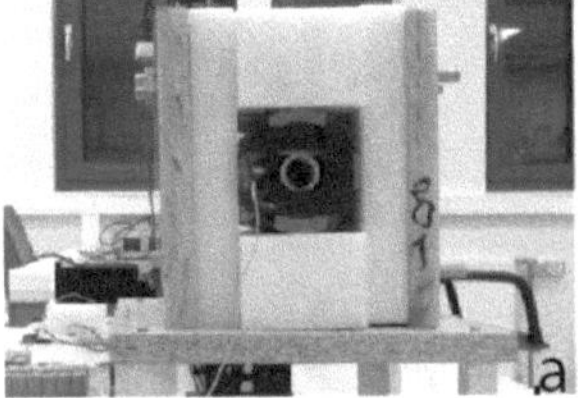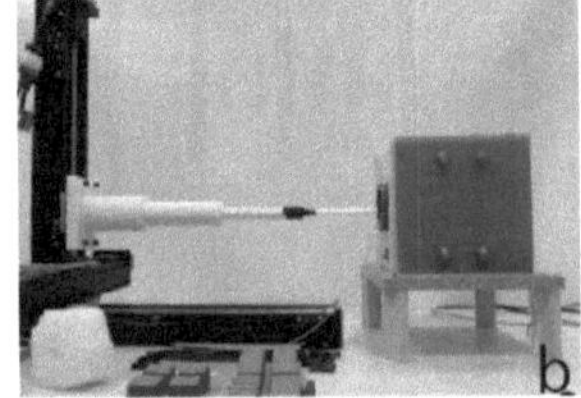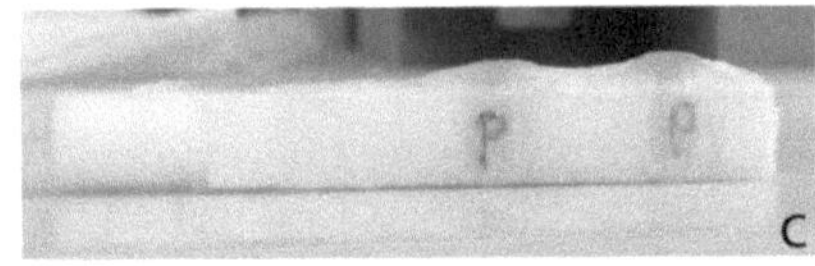

Figure 1: In-house MPI Scanner. (a) Front view. (b) Side view. (c) Phantom used in the imaging experiment: Perimag nanoparticles with 30 mmol Fe/L concentration in two 3-mm vials separated by 9-mm distance.

III. Results

Fig. 2 shows imaging experiment results for the rapid scanning trajectory. The regular x-space reconstructed image (Fig. 2b) displays artifacts that stem from pFOV processing steps. Speed compensation at the edges of the pFOVs requires signal to be divided by small numbers, which cause an amplification of both noise and interferences. Moreover, the delay in signal caused by relaxation further skews the speed-compensated pFOV images along the scanning direction. As a result, the pFOV boundaries manifest as periodic vertical stripes in the final reconstructed image. In addition, the image intensity increases along the scanning direction, causing a pile up of image intensity on the left side of the image (see red arrow in Fig. 2b). In contrast, the proposed PCI technique does not need pFOV processing, and therefore does not exhibit the aforementioned artifacts. As seen from Fig. 2c, the resulting image has significantly improved quality with respect to regular x-space reconstructed image.

Imaging Phantom with 2 Vials

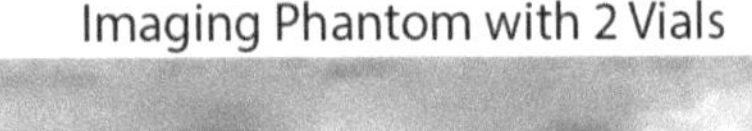

Regular X-space Reconstruction

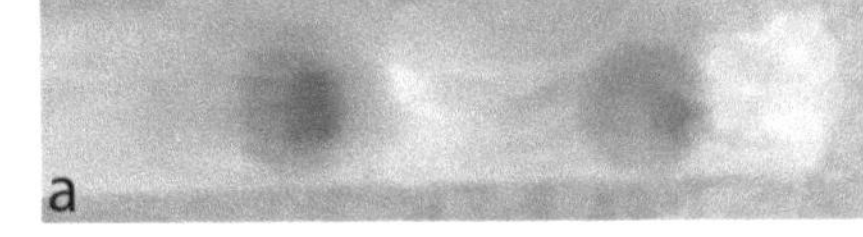

Proposed PCI Reconstruction

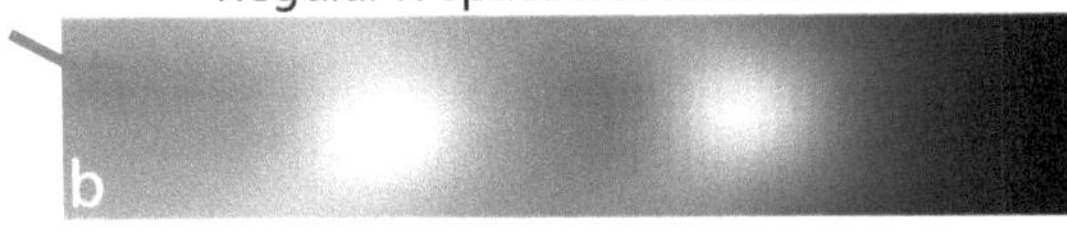

Figure 2: Imaging experiment results. (a) Top view of the imaging phantom with 2 vials. (b) Regular x-space reconstructed image. (c) Proposed PCI reconstructed image.

IV. Discussion

For PCI to be applicable, pFOV centers should be closely spaced. This makes the trajectories that have high overlap between pFOVs suitable for PCI. This condition is not a limitation but a realistic scenario for trajectories. Due to drive field safety limits, pFOV sizes cannot be more than ~1 cm for human torso imaging. Together with the limits on the slew-rate, that will lead to trajectories present large pFOV overlaps. Processing each pFOV independently gives a complexity to regular x-space reconstruction. Therefore, using the realistic high overlaps as an advantage, bypassing the pFOV processing steps reduces the complexity of reconstruction significantly.

The continuous trajectory used in this work decreases the scan time considerably compared to a trajectory that moves pFOV center to discrete positions (17.1 sec vs. 3 min 34 sec). Importantly, the performance of the proposed reconstruction is not adversely affected by this acceleration, as it preserves image quality for the rapid trajectory.

V. Conclusions

We extended our previously proposed an alternative x-space based reconstruction technique (PCI) for rapid scanning trajectories that are the real aims of the proposed method. It is shown that for trajectories that include simultaneous excitation and movement of FFP, proposed method is a good alternative for image reconstruction in MPI.

AUTHOR'S STATEMENT
Research funding: This work was supported by the Scientific and Technological Research Council of Turkey (TUBITAK 115E677). Conflict of interest: Authors state no conflict of interest.

REFERENCES
[1] B. Gleich and J. Weizenecker. Tomographic imaging using the nonlinear response of magnetic particles. *Nature*, 435(7046):1214-1217, 2005. doi: 10.1038/nature03808.
[2] J. Weizenecker, *et al*. A simulation study on the resolution and sensitivity of magnetic particle imaging. *Phys Med Biol,* 52(21):6363-6374, 2007. doi: 10.1088/0031-9155/52/21/001.
[3] J. Rahmer, *et al*. Signal Encoding in magnetic particle imaging: properties of the system function. *BCM Medical Imaging,* 9:4, 2009. doi: 10.1186/1471-2342-9-4.
[4] P. W. Goodwill and S.M. Conolly. The X-space formulation of the magnetic particle imaging process: 1-D signal, resolution, bandwidth, SNR, SAR, and magnetostimulation. *IEEE Trans Med Imaging,* 29(11):1851-1859, 2010. doi: 10.1109/TMI.2010.2052284.
[5] P. W. Goodwill and S.M. Conolly. Multidimensional X-Space Magnetic Particle Imaging. *IEEE Trans Med Imaging,* 30(9):1581-1590, 2011. doi: 10.1109/TMI.2011.2125982.
[6] K. Lu, *et al*. Linearity and Shift Invariance for Quantitative Magnetic Particle Imaging. *IEEE Trans Med Imaging,* 32(9):1565–1575, 2013. doi: 10.1109/TMI.2013.2257177.
[7] S. Kurt, *et al*. An Alternative X-space Based Image Reconstruction without Partial FOV Processing. *Proc of the 8th International Workshop on Magnetic Particle Imaging,* Hamburg, Germany, p.43-44, 2018.
[8] M. Utkur, *et al*. A 4.8 T/m Magnetic Particle Imaging Scanner Design and Construction. *21st National Biomedical Engineering Meeting,* Istanbul, Turkey, 2017. doi: 10.1109/BIYOMUT.2017.8479214.

A Super-Resolution Network for MPI

A. Ö. Arol[a,b*], A. A. Ozaslan[a,b], Semih Kurt[a,b], T. Çukur[a,b,c], and E. U. Saritas[a,b,c]

[a] *Department of Electrical and Electronics Engineering, Bilkent University, Ankara, Turkey*
[b] *National Magnetic Resonance Research Center (UMRAM), Bilkent University, Ankara, Turkey*
[c] *Neuroscience Program, Sabuncu Brain Research Center, Bilkent University, Ankara, Turkey*
* *Corresponding author, email: arol@ee.bilkent.edu.tr*

Abstract: In this study, we use a learning-based approach to implement a single image super-resolution (SR) network for improving the image quality in x-space-based magnetic particle imaging (MPI). Our method directly learns an end-to-end mapping between gridding-reconstructed blurred x-space images and the underlying nanoparticle distributions. Through numerical simulations, we show that the spatial blurring in x-space reconstruction can be significantly reduced with the proposed SR network.

I. Introduction

Two main image reconstruction methods have been proposed for magnetic particle imaging (MPI) [1]. The first method, system function reconstruction (SFR), needs extensive calibration scans where a voxel-sized sample is placed individually at each point in the field-of-view (FOV) and scanned. The main limitation of SFR is the duration of the calibration scan. Although there are some procedures for reducing the calibration time, calibration scan needs to be repeated every time a scan parameter (e.g., FOV or voxel size) is changed [2,3]. The alternative approach is x-space reconstruction, in which the signal is first speed compensated and then directly mapped to the instantaneous position of the scanned point. This approach does not require any calibration measurements; however, it produces blurry images that reflect convolution of magnetic nanoparticle (MNP) distribution with a point spread function (PSF) [4,5].

Here, we introduce a convolutional neural network (CNN) model to improve image quality in x-space reconstruction. The proposed model is inspired by the success of single-image super-resolution (SR) networks in various computer vision problems [6]. The proposed single-image SR network utilizes gridded x-space MPI images as low-resolution input images. In addition, this method can handle moderate changes in the scanning parameters and requires fewer calibration scans.

II. Material and Methods

II.I. Neural Network Architecture

Single-image SR is a classical problem in computer vision that aims to recover a high-resolution image from its low-resolution counterpart. Due to lack of input information at high spatial frequencies, SR is an ill-posed problem with infinitely many solutions. To overcome this problem, many learning-based approaches have been developed, utilizing machine-learning algorithms to capture the relation between low- and high-resolution versions of an image based on training data.

A class of single-image SR networks take bicubic interpolated images as inputs and then attempt to remove the blur that results from interpolation [6]. Here, we adopt this technique to MPI. First, a blurry image is reconstructed and gridded from the observed signal on the receive coil using an x-space-based automated gridding algorithm that we have previously developed [5]. SR network takes gridded MPI image as input, and reduces blurring to more accurately estimate the MNP distribution.

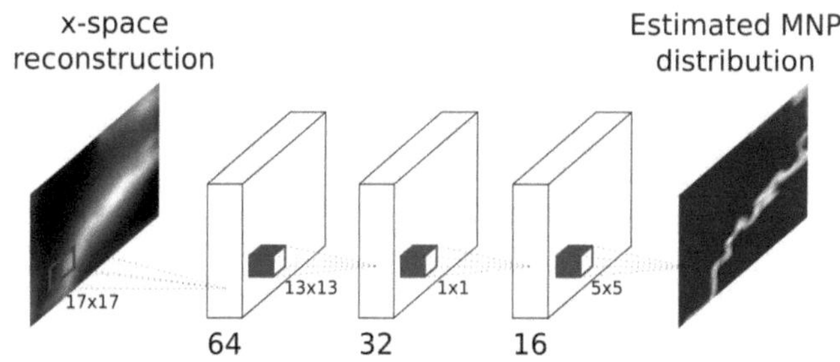

Figure 1: *The super resolution (SR) network architecture proposed in this work, which is based on convolutional neural network (CNN) blocks. The input to the SR network is the gridded x-space MPI image. Filter sizes and number of channels are denoted.*

We implemented the SR network for MPI based on convolutional layers, as illustrated in Fig. 1. Four convolutional layers were used and rectified linear units were employed between hidden layers as activation functions. The ith layer can be expressed as the following operation:

$$F_i(X_{i-1}) = X_i = max(0, W_i * X_{i-1} + B_i). \quad (1)$$

where W_i and B_i represent the filters and biases respectively. X_i is the result of ith layer and '$*$' denotes the convolution operation. Sizes of filters are denoted in Fig. 1. Mean square error (MSE) was used as the loss function to train the network.

This network learns the end-to-end mapping between x-space reconstructed blurry image and the underlying nanoparticle distribution.

II.II Numerical Experiments

To evaluate the proposed network, here we performed simulations based on an MPI system with 2cm×2cm FOV. MNPs with 25 nm diameter (with Langevin response) were placed on 280×280 grid in this FOV. Magnetic field gradients of (3, 3, -6) T/m/μ_0 were generated along (x, y, z) directions. For scanning the FOV, we used the Lissajous trajectory with frequencies 24.75 kHz and 25 kHz. The images were reconstructed using an x-space-based gridding algorithm that we have previously proposed, which automatically tunes the reconstruction parameters from the scanning trajectory [5].

To train the network, we generated a dataset of 12,000 realistic MPI images. We used 10,000 images as training set and 2,000 images as validation set. When generating this dataset, we utilized an approach similar to the coded calibration scenes (CSS) that we have recently proposed [7], where each MNP on the grid is connected to the next, as shown in Figure 2. Next, we trained the SR network using the resulting gridded MPI images as the input and the underlying MNP distributions as the output. The CCS method was previously proposed to reduce the calibration time for SFR-based MPI. Similarly, it has the potential to reduce the number of input-output pairs needed for the training dataset.

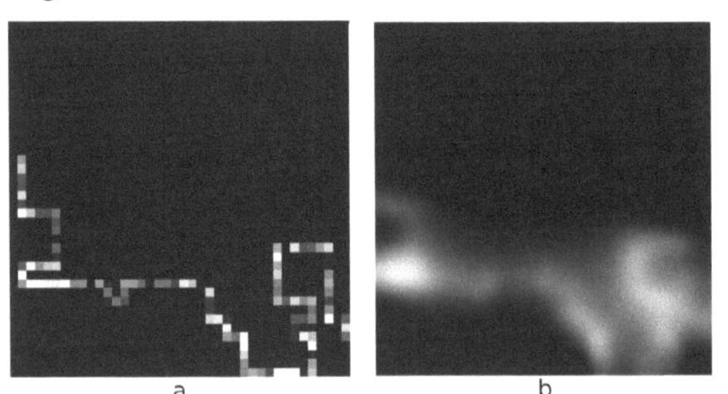

Figure 2: *A sample training dataset pair. The network is trained using (a) the connected MNP distributions as the output and (b) gridding reconstructed x-space images as the input.*

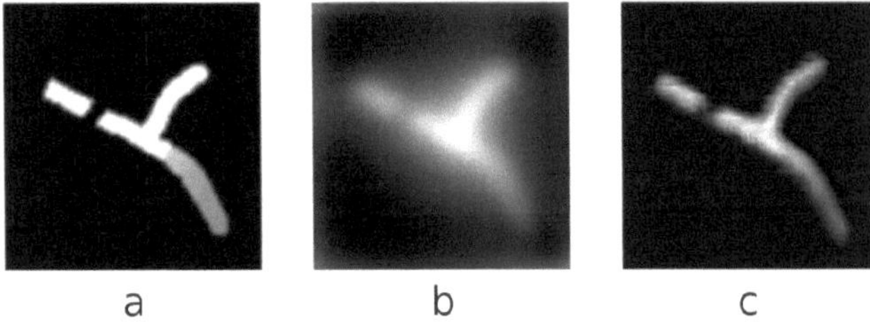

Figure 3: *A sample result from the proposed network. (a) MNP distribution, (b) gridding reconstructed x-space image, and (c) the output of the proposed SR network.*

III. Results & Discussion

Figure 3 shows a phantom, the corresponding gridding reconstructed x-space image (i.e., the input to the SR network), and the image obtained by using the proposed SR network. Note that for the given grid size of 280×280, SFR approach would require 78,400 calibration scans to acquire the full system matrix. Here, only 10,000 images were used to train the SR network. While the SFR approach requires repeating the calibration procedure when there is a change in scanning parameters and trajectories. Preliminary simulations suggest that the proposed SR network can handle moderate changes in scanning parameters (results not shown). In addition, it has the potential to be trajectory independent as it uses the gridded x-space image as input, as opposed to using the time-domain or frequency-domain MPI signal that would directly depend on the trajectory.

V. Conclusions

In this work, we proposed a new learning-based approach using CNNs to alleviate the blurring in x-space reconstructed MPI images. The proposed method requires fewer calibration scans when compared to the calibration measurements needed for a full system matrix. It also has the potential to handle different scanning parameters and trajectories, without the need for additional training.

AUTHOR'S STATEMENT
Research funding: The author state no funding involved. Conflict of interest: Authors state no conflict of interest.

REFERENCES
[1] B. Gleich and J. Weizenecker. Tomographic imaging using the nonlinear response of magnetic particles. Nature, 435(7046):1217-1217, 2005. doi: 10.1038/nature03808.
[2]. P. Goodwill and S. Conolly. Multidimensional X-Space Magnetic Particle Imaging. *IEEE Transactions on Medical Imaging*, 30 (9): 1581-1590, 2011. doi: 10.1109/TMI.2011.2125982.
[3]. J. Weizenecker, B. Gleich, J. Rahmer, H. Dahnke and J. Borgert, "Three-dimensional real-time in vivo magnetic particle imaging", Physics in Medicine and Biology, vol. 54, no. 5, pp. L1-L10, 2009.
[4] P. W. Goodwill and S. M. Conolly, "The X-Space Formulation of the Magnetic Particle Imaging Process: 1-D Signal, Resolution, Bandwidth, SNR, SAR, and Magnetostimulation," IEEE Transactions on Medical Imaging, vol. 29, no. 11, pp. 1851–1859, Nov. 2010.
[5] AA Ozaslan, A Alacaoglu, OB Demirel, T Cukur, EU Saritas. "A Generalized Reconstruction Technique for Non-Cartesian X-Space MPI", Proc of the 8th International Workshop on Magnetic Particle Imaging, Hamburg, Germany, p. 133-134, March 2018.
[6]. C. Dong, C. Loy, K. He and X. Tang, "Image Super-Resolution Using Deep Convolutional Networks", IEEE Transactions on Pattern Analysis and Machine Intelligence, vol. 38, no. 2, pp. 295-307, 2016.
[7] S Ilbey, CB Top, EU Saritas, HE Gven. "Fast System Calibration for MPI Using a Rotating Coded Calibration Scene", Proc of the 8th International Workshop on Magnetic Particle Imaging, Hamburg, Germany, p. 63-64, March 2018.

First MPS MObile Universal Surface Explorer

P. Vogel [a*], **M.A. Rückert** [a], **and V.C. Behr** [a]

[a] *Experimental Physics 5 (Biophysics), University of Würzburg, Würzburg, Germany*
[*] *Corresponding author, email: Patrick.Vogel@physik.uni-wuerzburg.de*

Abstract: Magnetic Particle Spectroscopy (MPS) is a useful modality to extract specific parameters from superparamagnetic iron-oxide nanoparticle (SPIONs) samples. To guarantee access to many research facilities and groups, a mobile handheld MPS device is presented offering a simple and intuitive handling, a robust and application-oriented design as well as inexpensive hardware.

I. Introduction

Magnetic Particle Imaging (MPI) is a tomographic method for three-dimensional localization of super-paramagnetic iron oxide nanoparticles (SPIONs) based on the nonlinear response to time-varying magnetic fields [1].

In addition to further developments in hardware and reconstruction methods for MPI, a better understanding of the tracer itself is essential. Magnetic particle spectroscopy (MPS) can be utilized to study the dynamic and behavior of SPIONs in time-varying magnetic fields [2], and to extract SPION-specific parameters, such as the Néel- or Brown-relaxation time, which can be used to enhance the quality of reconstruction results in MPI devices [3].

At the moment, most MPS devices are custom built and use different frequencies, magnetic field strengths and post processing steps. Because of the current lack of standardization, the comparison of data from different groups is limited. In addition, only few facilities and researchers have access to MPS devices. Furthermore, most MPS devices are not suited for easy, fast and flexible measurements in different environments or samples, such as PCR samples for SPION testing or petri dishes for cell labeling.

The MPS MOUSE (MObile Universal Surface Explorer) is a handheld device that will provide MPS access to many researchers through its ease of use, robust design and mobility as well as its flexibility.

II. Material and Methods

MPS devices consist of a transmit coil for generating a strong alternating magnetic field, a receive coil, an amplifier and an evaluation unit. Presently available MPS devices provide high sensitivity, but are very costly, not mobile and their handling requires special training. In addition, for many applications there are only reduced requirements for MPS devices:

1. Simple and intuitive handling

2. Robust and application-oriented design

3. Mobility and use of inexpensive hardware

II.I. MPS MOUSE hardware

For magnetic field generation, a transmit (tx) and receive (rx) system was developed, which can be used for multiple applications offering different sensitive areas simultaneously. Thus, several field of views (FOV) can be used for different measurements, e.g. for PCR samples (FOV I) and/or petri-dishes (FOV II). The tx-rx system consists of a planar transmit coil and several receive coils assembled in a gradiometer design (see Fig. 1).

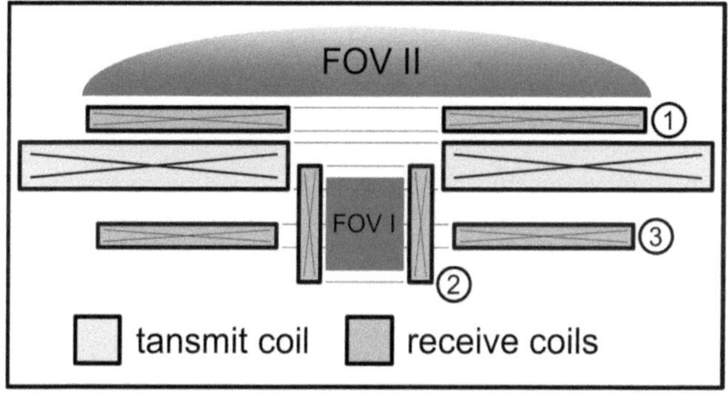

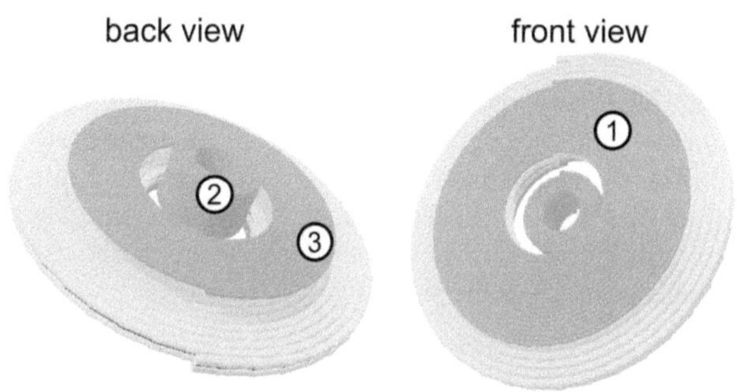

Figure 1: ***Top:*** *Sketch of transmit and receive coils. The receive coils are assembled in a gradiometer design to enable different FOVs for PCR sample (FOV I) and/or petri-dish measurements (FOV II).* ***Bottom:*** *3D rendering of the coils.*

A novel pulse amplifier approach based on a resonant circuit design is used to produce a short-term strong magnetic field, which is manageable with only a few electrical components. By using high performance batteries and special pump circuits, the transmit chain is able to generate magnetic fields up to 50 mT and more at the top of the scanner. This reduces spatial and energetic requirements and the cost of the complete system.

For control and data acquisition, a microcontroller (PSoC 5LP, Cypress, USA) is used, which can be controlled via Bluetooth by a mobile computer [4]. The host software is implemented in RAD Studio 10.3 (Embarcadero, USA) offering cross-platform compatibility resulting in a high flexibility. The software features several measurement modes as well as customized access to the processed data optimized for users, from novices to experts.

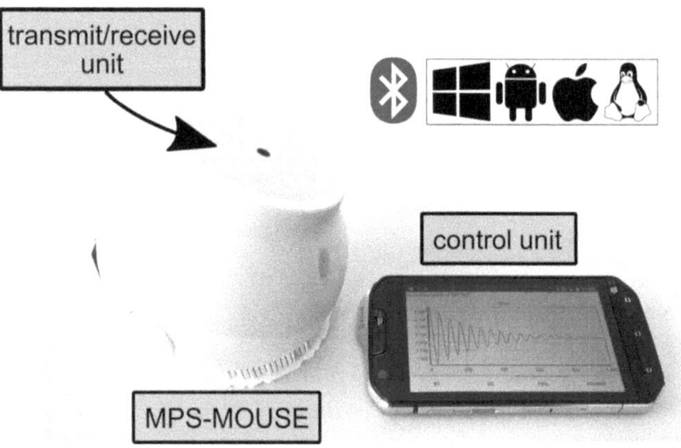

Figure 2: *Image of the MPS-MOUSE prototype. The system is designed to be used as handheld device or benchtop device for flexible measurements. Any (mobile) computer can serve as control unit.*

For a higher sensitivity, an active cancellation technique is used to suppress residual excitation signals. This enables functionality with the on-board 12 bit analog-digital-converter (ADC) of the microcontroller.

III. Results

In Fig. 3 an initial experiment with the MPS-MOUSE prototype is shown demonstrating the processed signal without (left) and with (right) 30 µl undiluted Resovist® (Bayer, Germany) positioned in FOV I (see Fig. 1). The magnetic field strength is 29.5 mT at a frequency of 20.3 kHz, the acquisition time is 1 ms at a sampling rate of 2 MS/s. The yellow magenta graph shows the time signal (with active cancellation) and the yellow graph shows the absolute spectrum of the signal.

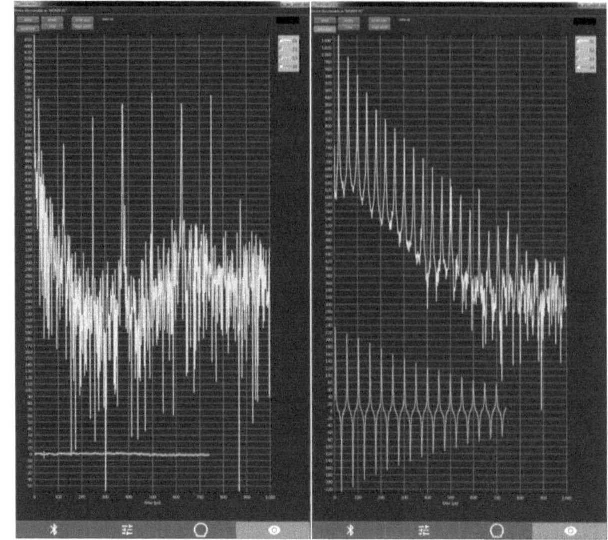

Figure 3: *Signal of a first experiment using the MPS MOUSE without (left) and with (right) Resovist®. Screenshots directly taken from the mobile application The magenta graph shows the time signal and the yellow graph indicates the spectrum.*

IV. Conclusions

The first prototype of the MPS mouse serves as a reference model to validate functionality (pulse operation for magnetic field generation, data acquisition, data transfer, evaluation routines, etc.), robustness and stability. The material cost of the device is far below current commercially available MPS devices, granting many research facilities access to this technology.

ACKNOWLEDGEMENTS

This work is funded by DFG (German Research Council) (VO 2288/2-1).

AUTHOR'S STATEMENT

Authors state no conflict of interest.

REFERENCES

[1] B. Gleich and J. Weizenecker. Tomographic imaging using the nonlinear response of magnetic particles. *Nature*, 435(7046):1217-1217, 2005. doi: 10.1038/nature03808.
[2] S. Biederer, et al., Magnetization response spectroscopy of superparamagnetic nanoparticles for magnetic particle imaging, *J. Phys. D.*, 42, 1-7, 2009.
[3] T. Knopp, et al., Magnetic Particle Imaging: From Proof of Principle to Preclinical Applications, *Physics in Medicine & Biology*, vol. 62(14):R124. 2017.
[4] M.A. Rückert, et al., WOTAN – loW cOst ulTra smAll formfactor coNsole for MPI, *Proc. on IWMPI #8*, P36, Hamburg, 2018.

Combined Active and Passive Cancellation of Receive Chain Direct Feedthrough

J. Beuke[a*], K. Brandt[a], A. Malhotra[a], A. Behrends[a], T. Friedrich[a], K. Gräfe[a], P. Rostalski[b] and T. M. Buzug[a]

[a] *Institute of Medical Engineering, University of Lübeck, Lübeck, Germany*
[b] *Institute for Electrical Engineering in Medicine, University of Lübeck, Lübeck, Germany*
* *Corresponding author, email: {beuke,buzug}@imt.uni-luebeck.de*

Abstract: Magnetic Particle Imaging (MPI) is a novel imaging modality, which can visualize magnetic nanoparticles using various magnetic fields. For signal acquisition it is necessary to remove the direct feedthrough into the receive chain prior to digitization. In this article a combination of a passive cancellation circuit with a gradiometric receive coil and an active cancellation with an injection transformer is shown. An attenuation of 97 dB could be achieved while maintaining the fundamental frequency of the particle signal, potentially improving image quality, both in terms of spatial resolution as well as signal to noise ratio.

I. Introduction

Magnetic Particle Imaging (MPI) uses magnetic fields to measure the distribution of superparamagnetic iron oxide nanoparticles (SPIONs) exploiting their nonlinear magnetization curve. It features a high temporal resolution which can partly be attributed to the simultaneous excitation and receiving [1]. This poses the problem of the direct feedthrough of the excitation signal into the receive chain. Since the excitation signal is several orders of magnitude stronger than the desired particle signal, a dampening of the undesired feedthrough must be achieved. Otherwise, the analogue-to-digital converter (ADC) used for digitizing the signal is unable to resolve the particle signal due to its limited dynamic range [2].

The use of analogue band-stop filters is a common solution to this problem. The fundamental frequency is attenuated while the higher harmonics from the particles can pass the filter mainly unaltered. The filter does not only affect the feedthrough but also the first harmonic of the particle signal, which poses a challenge for reconstruction [3]. A solution to this is the cancellation approach, where an inverted feedthrough signal is used to only cancel out the undesired signal and leave the particle signal unchanged. This can be realized for instance by replicating the field generator and connecting the receive coils reversely [2]. Another approach is a gradiometer coil which uses windings of opposing direction in order to generate the inverted signal. This will be explained further in section II.II. This work extends the passive cancellation using a gradiometer coil with an active cancellation, where the inverse signal is created using a digital-to-analogue converter (DAC). This will be explained further in section II.III. A similar approach has been used for removing power amplifier harmonics from the send chain [4] and for enabling multi-frequency MPI [5].

II. Material and Methods

II.I. Scanner

The MPI scanner used for this study is a field free line (FFL) scanner based on Halbach cylinders. It features a gradient of 5 T/m at a bore size of 4 cm. With a single excitation solenoid generating a field with 20 mT amplitude at 25 kHz in combination with a rotation of the gantry, a native 2D acquisition is possible. Using a movable sample holder enables 3D imaging [6].

II.II. Passive Cancellation

A gradiometer consists of two parts. The receive part is placed close to the field of view (FOV) and senses the magnetization of the SPIONs while a cancellation part further away from the FOV is connected in series but with opposing winding direction. The excitation field ideally induces the same voltage in both parts which cancel each other. The particle signal mainly couples into the receive part and therefore is not cancelled [2].

Due to the limited length of the excitation coil, the field is not homogeneous. Since the dampening depends on a close match of amplitude and phase of the opposing signals, it is favorable to be able to adapt the cancellation part's positions to the field of the excitation coil. For this reason, a gradiometer coil with movable cancellation parts has been simulated in COMSOL Multiphysics (5.3a, COMSOL Group, Sweden) and built using litz wire with a diameter of 0.5 mm and a 3D printed coil support. Moving the outer coil parts can be done using strings. The resulting coil is shown in fig. 2.

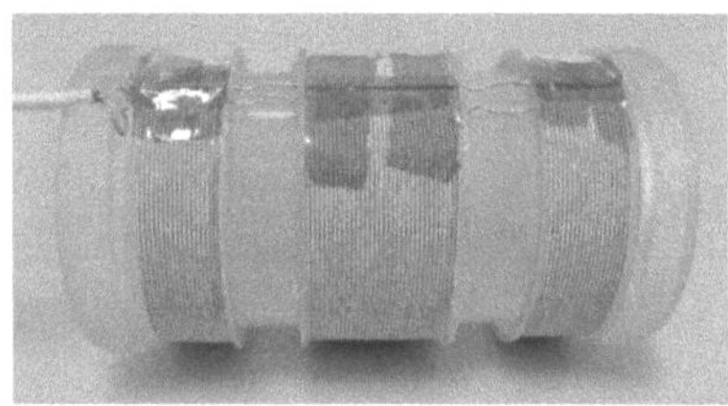

Figure 2: *Gradiometric receive coil used for passive cancellation. The receive part has a length of 2 cm and the cancellation part a length of 1 cm each. The inner diameter is 4 cm.*

II.III. Active Cancellation

The principal idea of active cancellation is to calculate the inverse signal for the cancellation digitally and output it via a DAC. For matching the signal amplitudes and separating the grounds, a transformer can be used. Here, the active cancellation is done by using a 1:1 toroidal air core injection transformer (Fig. 3) which has its secondary windings in series with the receive coil. The signal generation is performed with a Red Pitaya (Red Pitaya d.d., Slovenia) using a custom software [7]. The dampening signal can be adjusted in phase and amplitude to match the receive signal. The residual signal is then amplified using a commercial low noise amplifier (LNA) (SR560, Stanford Research Systems, Inc., California) and measured with an oscilloscope (HDO6104-MS, Teledyne LeCroy, New York). The gain of the LNA is determined with a network analyzer (E5601B, Agilent Technologies, California).

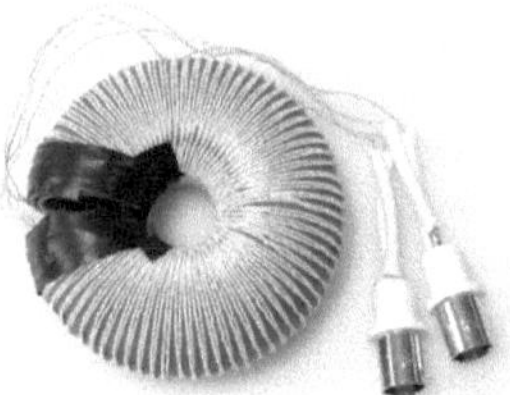

Figure 3: *Toroidal injection transformer used for active cancellation.*

II.IV. Active cancellation tuning process

The signal generation can be tuned using a MATLAB (MATLAB 2018b, The MathWorks, Inc., Natick, Massachusetts) programming interface. For the measurements, the LNA was first set to a gain of 1. Subsequently, the amplitude and phase of the dampening signal, a sinusoid of 25 kHz, were tuned manually, minimizing the residual signals amplitude. The gain of the LNA was increased during the tuning process to be able to clearly depict the residual signal above the noise level.

III. Results

After tuning, the gradiometer coil provides an attenuation of the induced voltage by 58 dB. The active cancellation gives further 39 dB, but a distortion of the residual signal can be observed. The distortion is changing over time.

IV. Discussion

The achieved attenuation of 97 dB brings the approach in the range of systems with analogue filters. It allows for a more flexible approach in dealing with the feedthrough, since e.g. temperature drifts can be compensated electronically. The observed distortion is attributed to the low impedance of the transformer primary windings. This can easily be mitigated using a larger air core transformer or a specifically chosen ferrite core and should prevent a possible influence on the imaging results.

V. Conclusions

It was shown that a combination of active and passive cancellation can achieve an MPI system design without a need for analogue filters. This decreases the size requirements while keeping the fundamental frequency of the particle signal unchanged and adding flexibility. A further improvement to the system would be the integration of the active cancellation with a noise matching transformer in order to maximize the SNR. Since the DAC oversamples the dampening signal, a low pass filter for removing quantization noise could be added. In the next step, an automatic tuning process integrated with the acquisition of an empty measurement will be developed. This process is planned to work with a fixed gain LNA. Therefore, the field strength is increased in small steps to avoid saturation of the LNA while phase and amplitude of the dampening signal are optimized. This enables an easy use in the imaging process and is expected to result in images of a higher quality.

ACKNOWLEDGEMENTS

The authors thankfully acknowledge the financial support by the German Research Foundation (DFG, grant number BU 1436/9-1) and the Federal Ministry of Education and Research (BMBF, grant number 13GW0069A).

AUTHOR'S STATEMENT
The authors state no conflict of interest.

REFERENCES

[1] B. Gleich and J. Weizenecker. Tomographic imaging using the nonlinear response of magnetic particles. *Nature*, 435(7046):1217-1217, 2005. doi: 10.1038/nature03808.

[2] M. Gräser, T. Knopp, M. Grüttner, T. F. Sattel and T. M. Buzug. *Analog receive signal processing for magnetic particle imaging.* Medical Physics 40.4 (2013), S. 042303. doi: 10.1118/1.4794482.

[3] K. Lu, P. W. Goodwill,E. U. Saritas, B. Zheng, and S. M.Conolly. Linearity and shift invariance for quantitative magnetic particle imaging. *IEEE Transactions on Medical Imaging 32*(9) (2013), 1565-75. doi: 10.1109/TMI.2013.2257177

[4] B. Zheng, W. Yang, T. Massey, P. W. Goodwill and S. M. Conolly. High-power active interference suppression in magnetic particle imaging. 2013 International Workshop on Magnetic Particle Imaging (IWMPI). doi: 10.1109/iwmpi.2013.6528381.

[5] D. Pantke, M. Straub and V. Schulz. Passive and Active Compensation of Drive Field Feed-Through for Multi-Frequency MPI. 2018 International Workshop on Magnetic Particle Imaging (IWMPI).

[6] M. Weber, J. Beuke, A. von Gladiss, K. Gräfe, P. Vogel, V. C. Behr and T. M. Buzug. Novel Field Geometry featuring a Field Free Line for Magnetic Particle Imaging, *IJMPI* 4(2) (2018). doi: 10.18416/IJMPI.2018.1811004

[7] https://github.com/tknopp/RedPitayaDAQServer, commit a371802, Nov 12, 2018

Verification of the Linear System Response of a Single-Sided MPI Device

Y. Blancke Soares[a]*, K. Gräfe[a], A. von Gladiss[a], C. Debbeler[a], K. Lüdtke-Buzug[a] and T. M. Buzug[a]*

[a] *Institute of Medical Engineering, University of Lübeck, Lübeck, Germany*
* *Corresponding author, email: {soares, buzug}@imt.uni-luebeck.de*

Abstract: A single-sided MPI scanning device allows for an unlimited object size. In this work, we present the results of a dilution series measurement to analyze the linearity of the system response of a single-sided MPI scanner topology in reconstructed images. Two-dimensional phantom measurements were performed using different dilutions of Resovist. For reconstruction, a Kaczmarz algorithm and a Tikhonov regularization with a static regularization parameter were used. We are able to confirm the linearity of the single-sided device as the signal in reconstructed images decreases linearly with increasing dilution proportion.

I. Introduction

In 2005, Weizenecker and Gleich [1] presented MPI for the first time. Two years later the idea of a single-sided scanning device was published to overcome restricting factors like the size of the measured object due to the scanner configuration [2]. Since then, the development of the single-sided setup has made great progress regarding the scanner geometry and scanner extensions for three-dimensional measuring [3, 4]. The development has reached a point where the system needs to be technically evaluated. Especially, the linearity of the system has to be verified, which is important for ensuring the quantification of MPI measurement results [5, 6].

In this work, we present the results of dilution series measurements to analyze the system response in terms of the linearity of the single-sided MPI scanner topology.

II. Material and Methods

II.I. Scanner Configuration

The single-sided scanning device consists of four sending coils, two circular and two D-shaped, which serve to generate three drive fields and one selection field. A receive coil for each field direction is implemented to receive the particle response.

For excitation, a base frequency of 2.5 MHz is used, which is divided by the frequency dividers $f_{d_x} = 99$ and $f_{d_y} = 96$ leading to the respective frequencies $f_x = 25.25$ kHz and $f_y = 26.04$ kHz for a two dimensional measurement. Since the signals in y- and z-direction are redundant in this study, measurement time was reduced by omitting the excitation in z-direction [4]. The repetition time T_R, which is the time needed for measuring one frame, can be calculated with

$$T_R = \frac{lcm(f_{d_{x,y,z}})}{f_0},\tag{1}$$

where lcm represents the least common multiple. In this case, the repetition time is 1.3 ms.

II. II. Phantom and Measurements

For the recording of a system matrix, the particle concentration of a point sample of 8 µl undiluted Resovist (Bayer-Schering, Berlin, Germany) with an iron content of 28 µg/µl is measured at each 8 x 16 positions in the 16 x 32 mm² FOV, recording 200 measurements per frame for averaging. After subtracting an empty system matrix, frequencies are selected by setting an SNR threshold of 3.65, which is evaluated by visual observation of the plotted system matrix SNR. For the measurements, we used a perspex-made phantom with five holes in four rows, each hole having a capacity of 10 µl, as shown in Fig. 1 (left). On the right side of Fig. 1 is a sketch of the phantom. The tracer was filled into the indicated position as it is closest to the scanner and the axis of rotation.

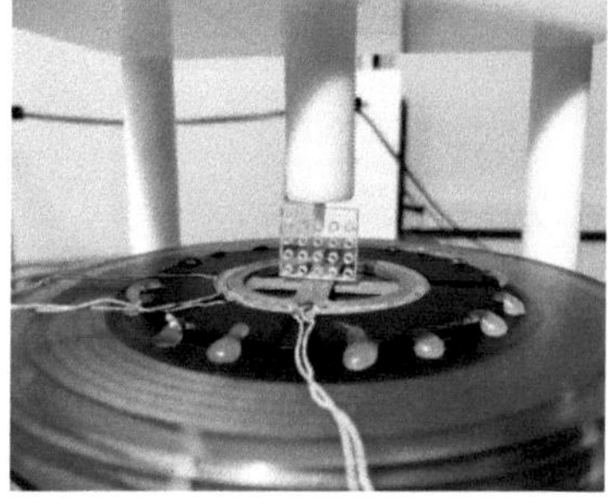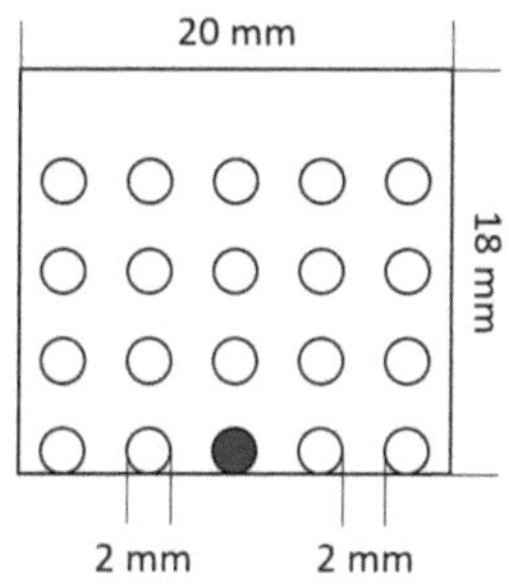

Figure 1: *(left) Fixed perspex phantom for the sensitivity study in the holder, consisting of 20 holes with a capacity of 10 µl each. (right) Sketch of the used phantom with specified dimensions and the position of the tracer indicated.*

Before reconstruction, the sample measurement is background corrected by subtracting an empty measurement. In addition, a measurement of undiluted Resovist is performed, which is used to normalize and compare the reconstructed dilution measurement signals.

Subsequently, 10 µl are measured with 90% Resovist and 10% distilled water, followed by dilutions up to 90% distilled water in 10% increments. Each dilution was measured ten times to quantify the measurement inaccuracies.

II.III. Reconstruction

The calibration-based reconstruction uses the acquisition of a system matrix S by measuring a cube-shaped sample at each position in the FOV. The linear equation

$$\hat{S}c = \hat{u}, \tag{2}$$

has to be solved, which is an ill-posed problem. $\hat{S}$ represents a system matrix, in which certain frequency components are selected based on an SNR above a selected threshold. $\hat{u}$ is the induced voltage, and c the concentration of the tracer. (2) is solved with an iterative Kaczmarz algorithm with 500 iteration steps. In addition, a Tikhonov-regularization with a constant regularization factor is used to stabilize the results. By using a static regularization parameter, measurement results become comparable to each other.

III. Results

A selection of reconstructed images for each dilution is shown in Fig. 2. The values of the pixels representing the position of the tracer were averaged for determining the signal intensities.

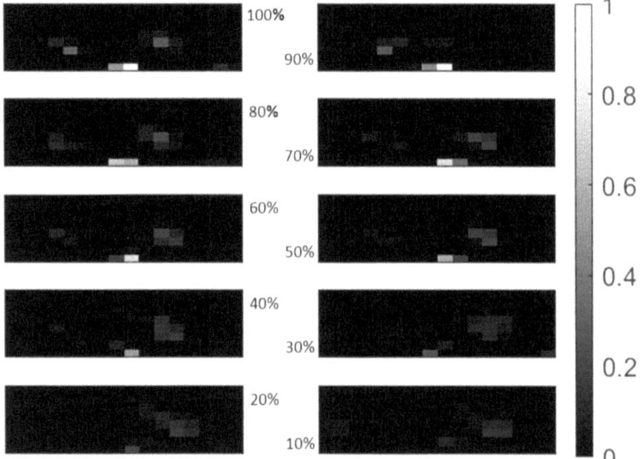

Figure 2: Reconstructed images of the phantom at different dilution steps. The intensity values at the corresponding pixels, indicated by the colorbar, are normalized to the maximum value of undiluted Resovist.

Fig. 3 shows a plot in which each group contains the normalized signals from ten measurements of the respective dilution. A linear increase in the signal curve can be observed with decreasing proportion of distilled water in the dilution. The regression line shows the linear increase of the measured signal from 40% Resovist in the dilution corresponding to an iron content of about 112 µg iron to 100% undiluted Resovist. The remaining values are excluded because of the high noise level.

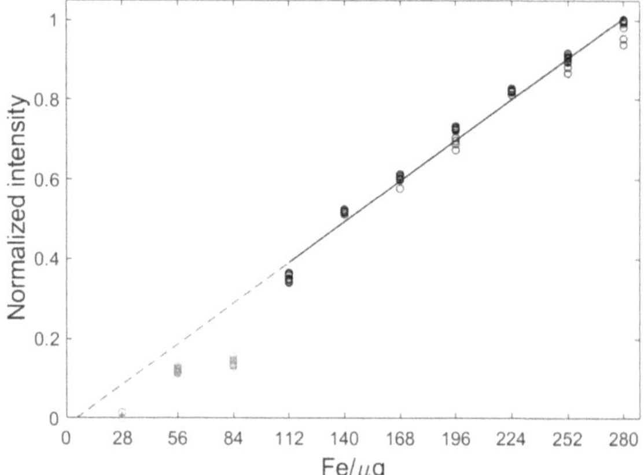

Figure 3: Reconstructed signal of the corresponding phantom positions at each dilution step normalized to the maximum signal of the reconstructed undiluted Resovist measurement respectively.

IV. Discussion

The reconstruction results show a linear behavior of the system down to 40% Resovist in the dilution corresponding to the calculated iron content of about 112 µg. The signal decreases linearly with increasing proportion of distilled water. The detection limit of the system is reached at 20% Resovist in the dilution corresponding to the calculated amount of about 56 µg iron in magnetite. No signal was measured at 10% Resovist in the dilution. In order to achieve a higher sensitivity of the system, one possible approach is to vary the amount of measurements for averaging or to perform hardware adjustments.

V. Conclusions

The dilution study has demonstrated a linear behavior of measurement results of the single-sided MPI scanner. Due to the characteristic behavior of Resovist, as described in [7], additional tracers can be used to support the presented results. Further sensitivity improvements can be made. This is a prerequisite for quantifiability of MPI.

ACKNOWLEDGEMENTS

The authors thank the DFG (BU 1436/9-1) and the German Federal Ministry of Education and Research (01DL17010A and 13GW0230B) for financial support.

REFERENCES

[1] B. Gleich and J. Weizenecker. Tomographic imaging using the nonlinear response of magnetic particles. *Nature*, 435(7046):1217-1217, 2005. doi: 10.1038/nature03808.

[2] T. F. Sattel et al. Single-sided device for magnetic particle imaging. *J. Phys. D*, 42(2):022001, 2009. doi: 10.1088/0022-3727/42/2/022001.

[3] K. Gräfe et al.. 2D Images Recorded with a Single-Sided Magnetic Particle Imaging Scanner. *IEEE Trans. Med. Imag.*, 35(4):1056-1065, 2016. doi: 10.1109/TMI.2015.2507187.

[4] K. Gräfe et al. First Phantom Measurements with a 3D Single-Sided MPI Scanner. *IWMPI*, 201-202, 2018.

[5] K. Bente et al. Sensitivity study for an MPI FFL scanner. *IWMPI*, 2015. doi: 10.1109/IWMPI.2015.7107070.

[6] O. Kosch et al. Preparing system functions for quantitative MPI. *IJMPI*, 3(2), 2017. doi: 10.18416/ijmpi.2017.1706002.

[7] N. Löwa et al. Concentration dependent MPI tracer performance. *IJMPI*, 2(1), 2016. doi: 10.18416/ijmpi.2016.1601001.

Towards resolution phantoms for multi-centric comparison of instrumentation

O. Kosch[a*], M. Graeser[b,c], J. Wells[a], P. Radon[a], H. Paysen[a], T. Knopp[b,c] and F. Wiekhorst[a]

[a] *Department 8.2 Biosignals, Physikalisch-Technische Bundesanstalt, Berlin, Germany*
[b] *Institute for Biomedical Imaging, Technical University Hamburg, Hamburg, Germany*
[c] *Section for Biomedical Imaging, University Medical Center Hamburg-Eppendorf, Hamburg, Germany*
[*] *Corresponding author, email: olaf.kosch@ptb.de*

Abstract: The achievable resolution of different magnetic particle imaging (MPI) for scanner instrumentations is a highly-requested trait. Based on different long-term stable phantoms we developed a benchmark to determine and compare the MPI resolution of different MPI instrumentations. Here, we show first results of a comparison of standard and improved MPI hardware architectures operated at Charité Berlin and University Medical Center Hamburg-Eppendorf with regard to the benefit in image resolution.

I. Introduction

The MPI technology is still under development, and demands further improvements of the instrumentation, especially to increase the signal to noise ratio (SNR). This requires measurements of phantoms with magnetic nanoparticle (MNP) as imaging tracer in a long-term stable, defined state, to determine advantages of technical changes. To this end, we have developed phantoms containing freeze-dried MNP tracer material [1]. Here, we demonstrate results acquired at two MPI scanners at Charité Berlin and University Medical Center Hamburg-Eppendorf using these phantoms. We compared the results on different MPI hardware instrumentations to compare and assess the image resolution and the capability of the devices for quantification.

II. Material and Methods

II.I. Phantoms

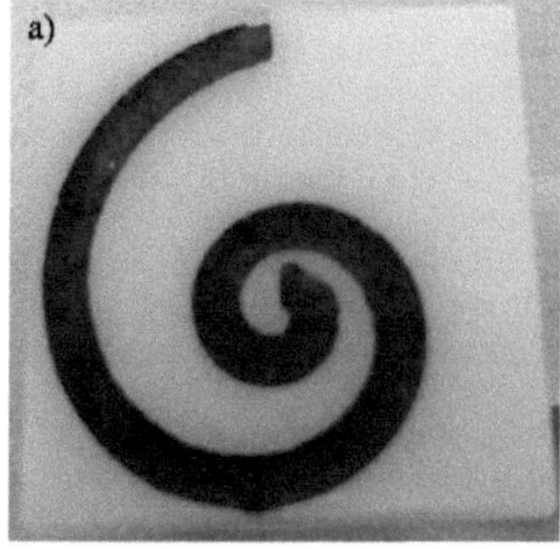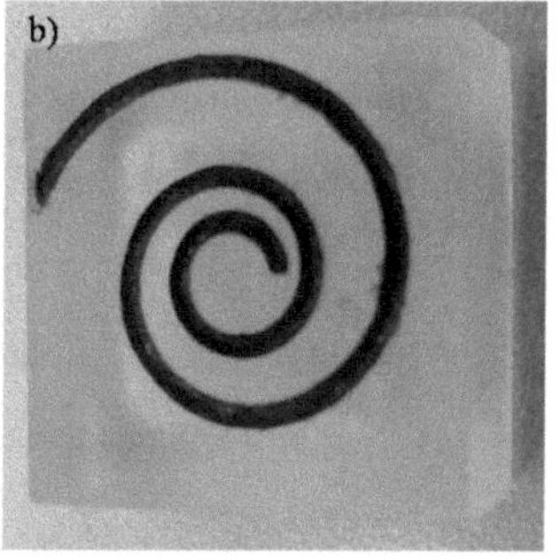

Figure 1: *Phantoms with exponential growing spiral layout with a) 2 mm channel and b) 1 mm channel width, filled with freeze-dried perimag.*

Two 3D-printed phantoms were designed to analyze the achievable image resolution [1]. They contain a channel with quadratic cross section (either with a width of 2 mm or 1 mm)

forming an exponential growing spiral. Fig. 1a) shows a photograph of the 2-mm phantom filled with 200 µL of perimag (micromod, Rostock, Germany) freeze-dried in mannitol and Fig. 1b) the 1-mm phantom filled with 72.6 µL both at original iron concentration of $c(Fe) = 152.2$ mmol/L. Since MNPs in liquid suspension may show signal changes over time [2], especially when subjected to magnetic excitation fields we chose immobilized MNPs to avoid this issue. The achievable resolution of the reconstructed images is determined by the visually minimal resolvable gap between the segments of the neighboring channel. Fig. 2 depicts the schematically gap distances of the two phantoms.

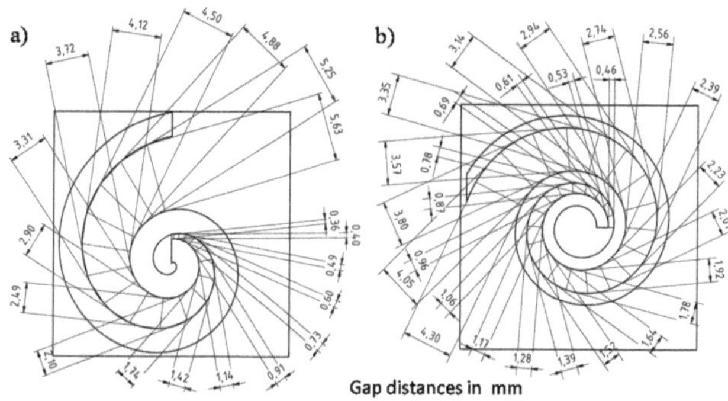

Figure 2: *Gap distances in a) the 2-mm phantom and b) the 1-mm phantom.*

II.II. MPI measurement and reconstruction

The MPI measurements were performed using the two preclinical MPI systems (Bruker MPI 25/20 FF) installed at Charité University Hospital Berlin and University Medical Center Hamburg-Eppendorf using drive field amplitudes of 12 mT in all directions, selection gradient fields of 1.25 T/m in x- and y-direction, and 2.5 T/m in z-direction. Additionally, both scanner systems are equipped with a separate receive coil. The one in Berlin [3] has a inner coil diameter of 72 mm and the one in Hamburg [4] 46.68 mm. The system functions (SF) were measured in both devices using a reference volume of 13.5 µL ($3x3x1.5$ mm^3) freeze-dried perimag at original concentration at 33x33x33 voxel positions in a reconstruction volume of $26.4x26.4x13.2$ mm^3.

All 3D reconstructions were performed under the same conditions (Kaczmarz-algorithm with 20 iterations and a regularization factor $\lambda_r=10^{-5}$). The 2-mm phantom was reconstructed using the measurement data of the original x-channel (standard coil) with an SNR threshold of 4 and the 1-mm phantom was reconstructed incorporating the data of the different separate receive coils of the devices applying an SNR-threshold of 6.

III. Results

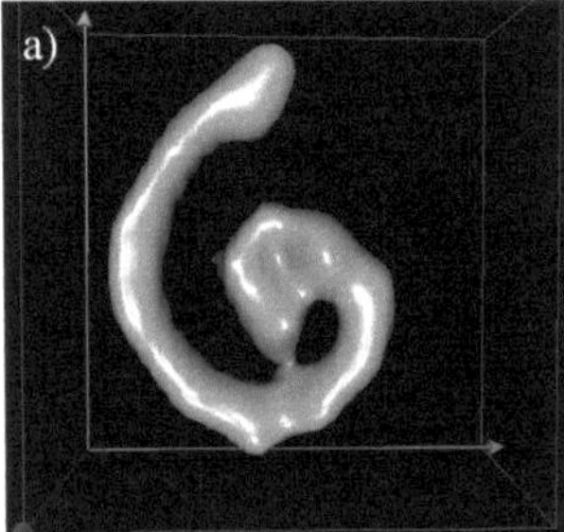
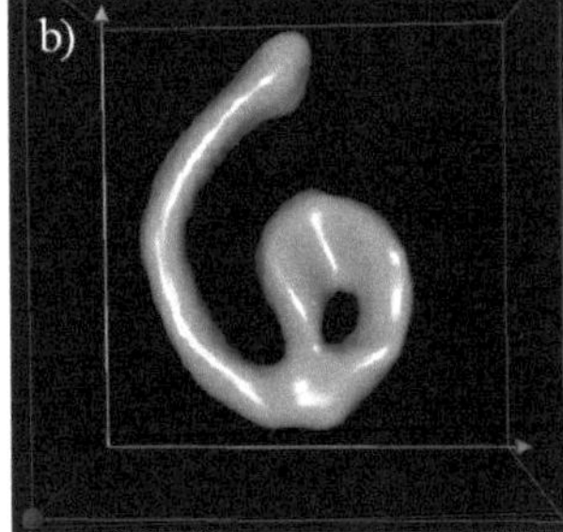

Figure 3: *Reconstructed volumes of the 2-mm phantom using the original x-coil at the MPI-scanner a) in Berlin and b) in Hamburg.*

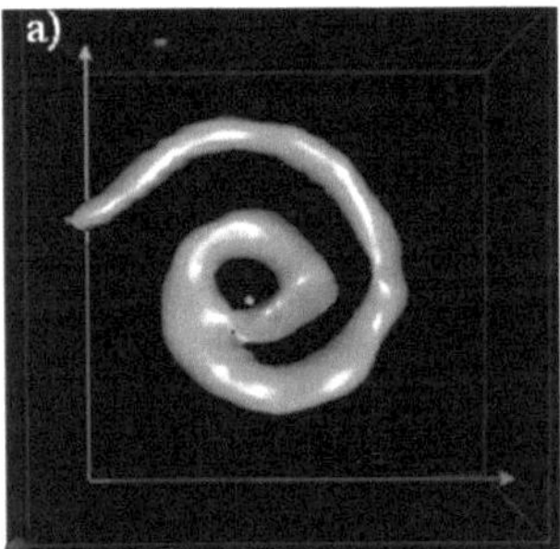
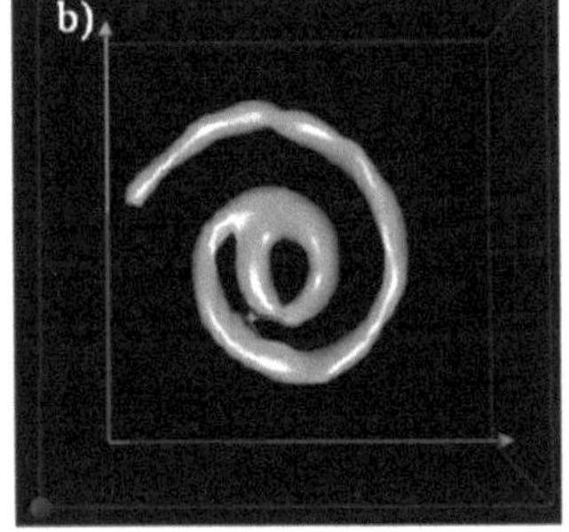

Figure 4: *Reconstructed volumes of the 1-mm phantom applying the separate receive coil a) in Berlin and b) in Hamburg.*

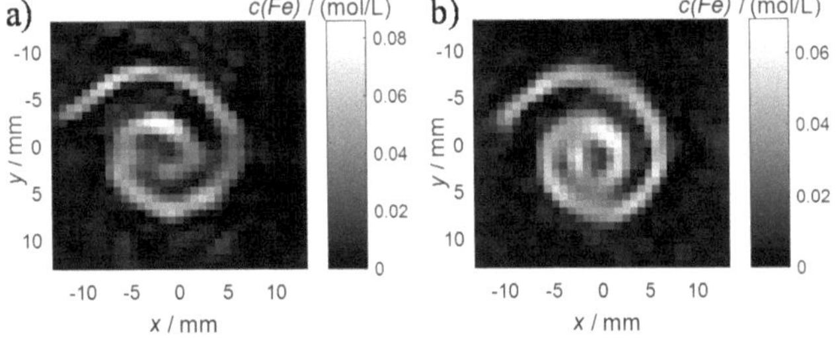

Figure 5: *Projection of the maxima of the reconstruction results in z-direction to the xy-plane applying the separate receive coil in a) Berlin and b) in Hamburg.*

For the measured data of the standard coil Fig. 3 shows the reconstructed volume of the 2-mm phantom using a threshold of 0.2 of the respective maximum value both yielding about

the same spatial resolution of about 2.2 mm for both sites (compared to Fig. 2a). Fig. 4 shows the reconstructed volumes of the 1-mm phantom using the separated receive coils of the two devices. At this a threshold of 0.2 was used in Fig. 4a) and 0.35 in Fig. 4b) for the 46-mm separate receive coil and a resolution limit of 1.5 mm for the 72-mm coil in Berlin and 1.0 mm for the 46-mm coil in Hamburg was achieved. Fig. 5 depicts the reconstructed quantitative images of the 1-mm phantom.

IV. Discussion

The 46-mm separate receive coil has a significant higher sensitivity and a higher spatial resolution compared to the 72-mm coil mainly related to the smaller diameter [1]. However, in the quantitative image the 46-mm coil leads to a wider distribution of the channel. This might be due to a small overmodulation, even by a reduced amplification. To address this, more measurements of phantoms at lower iron concentrations are required.

V. Conclusions

We applied a standard instrumentation to image the 2-mm phantom by MPI in Berlin and Hamburg and determined the same resolution. The implementation of the separate receive coils leads to an increased sensitivity and in this manner to a better image resolution. Our results show the potential of long-term stable resolution phantoms for MPI image quality comparison purposes. This allows to assess and compare the performance of identical hardware components operated at different sites as well as the evaluation of improvements by newly developed instrumentations. In the next steps we will develop more resolution phantoms with e.g. lower MNP content to enable the full characterization of instrumentations in a bigger sensitivity range, like the 46-mm coil.

ACKNOWLEDGEMENTS

This work was supported by the Deutsche Forschungsgemeinschaft research program "quantMPI" (DFG grant TR408/9-1) and "Matrix in Vision", (DFG SFB 1340/1 2018, projects A02) and "AMPI: Magnetic particle imaging: Development and evaluation of novel methodology for the assessment of the aorta in vivo in a small animal model of aortic aneurysms ", SHA 1506/2-1 and the DFG core facility for the measurement of ultra-low magnetic fields.

REFERENCES

[1] O. Kosch, H. Paysen, J. Wells, F. Ptach, J. Franke, L. Wöckel, S. Dutz, F. Wiekhorst, P. Evaluation of a separate-receive coil by magnetic particle imaging of a solid phantom, *J. Magn. Magn. Mater.* 471 (2019) 444–449. doi:10.1016/j.jmmm.2018.09.114.

[2] J. Wells, O. Kazakova, O. Posth, U. Steinhoff, S. Petronis, L. Bogart, P. Southern, Q.A. Pankhurst, C. Johansson, Standardisation of magnetic nanoparticles in liquid suspension, *J. Phys. D. Appl. Phys.* (2017). doi:10.1088/1361-6463/aa7fa5.

[3] H. Paysen, J. Wells, O. Kosch, U. Steinhoff, J. Franke, L. Trahms, T. Schaeffter, F. Wiekhorst, Improved sensitivity and limit-of-detection using a receive-only coil in magnetic particle imaging, *Phys. Med. Biol.* (2018). doi:10.1088/1361-6560/aacb87.

[4] M. Graeser, T. Knopp, P. Szwargulski, T. Friedrich, A. Von Gladiss, M. Kaul, K.M. Krishnan, H. Ittrich, G. Adam, T.M. Buzug, Towards Picogram Detection of Superparamagnetic Iron-Oxide Particles Using a Gradiometric Receive Coil, *Sci. Rep. 7* (2017). doi:10.1038/s41598-017-06992-5.

Towards particle independent calibration of magnetic particle spectrometers: Initial experiments

F. Fidler[a]*, K.-H. Hiller[a] and P.M. Jakob[a,b]

[a] *Magnetic Resonance and X-Ray Imaging MRB, Fraunhofer EZRT, Würzburg, Germany*
[b] *Experimental Physics V, University of Würzburg, Würzburg, Germany*
* *Corresponding author, email: florian.fidler@iis.fraunhofer.de*

Abstract: In this work, a macroscopic manufactured probe was rated on the calibration of magnetic particle spectrometers that mimics a particle with a non-linear behavior. Its suitability for magnetic particle spectrometers was tested in a first initial experiment. The suggested probe consists of a small coil with crossed diodes in parallel. The coil defines the coupling to the spectrometer and the non-linear behavior to the transmit field is given by the non-linear characteristic of the diodes. This system can be miniaturized and all of the necessary properties can be evaluated outside the scanner.

I. Introduction

Magnetic particle spectrometers and imagers offer the possibility of quantitative measurements. The measured voltages are related directly to the concentration and the particle properties. Unfortunately the signal detection chain in most cases consist of inductive elements, filters and amplifiers which complicates the quantitative evaluation of the acquired signal in terms of magnetic moment and its nonlinear behavior to applied magnetic field.

There are some strategies on the market for calibrating spectrometers, like small probes generating a well-known signal on a certain frequency to measure the amplitude and phase behavior of the detection system [1]. These probes are connected to external mostly synchronized equipment [2]. For comparison of different scanners, identically manufactured particles are used [3]. For general adjustment of the amplitude and phase paramagnetic substances like Dysprosium can be used in those cases where the transmit signal is also part of the detected signal [4].

These methods suffer from the lack of an exactly known particle system that can be used for calibration. Calibration with small probes is time consuming and hard to implement in magnetic particle imagers where strong time varying gradients are present. Paramagnetic substances deliver valuable information but do not allow the measuring of frequency response of the system. In most cases where a particle system is used for calibration, this calibration is repeated for all used particles, resulting for example in the possibility to quantify iron content in magnetic particle spectrometers [5].

In this work a macroscopic manufactured probe is used, that mimics a particle sample with non-linear behavior, but due to its well-known components it can be described exactly based on independent measurement outside the spectrometer. Its suitability for magnetic particle spectrometers is evaluated in a first initial experiment. The suggested probe consists of a small coil with crossed diodes in parallel. The coil defines the coupling to the spectrometer and the non-linear behavior to the transmit field is given by the non-linear characteristic of the diodes. This system can be miniaturized and all of the necessary properties can be evaluated outside the scanner.

II. Material and Methods

The proposed probe built for the initial testing is shown in Fig. 1. The coil is a solenoid with 25 windings of 0.2mm copper and a diameter of 4 mm. It is mounted on a PVC rod and connected via crossed diodes inside the coil volume. The diodes are standard surface mounted device diodes (RB481Y). This ensured a highly nonlinear behavior at low field strength, since the barrier voltage of those diodes is low in comparison to silicon diodes. This probe fits into a 6 mm glass tube. The orientation of the coil is aligned with the excitation field from the used spectrometer. This kind of device is not limited to a specific field direction; the coil can also be designed with sensitivity to two or three field directions. The ideal coil configuration depends on the spectrometer design, a single, fixed field was investigated.

All measurements were performed in a commercial magnetic particle spectrometer, the MPS unit (Pure devices GmbH, Rimpar, Germany). For the initial test, the excitation field strength was set to 17 mT at a frequency of 20 kHz.

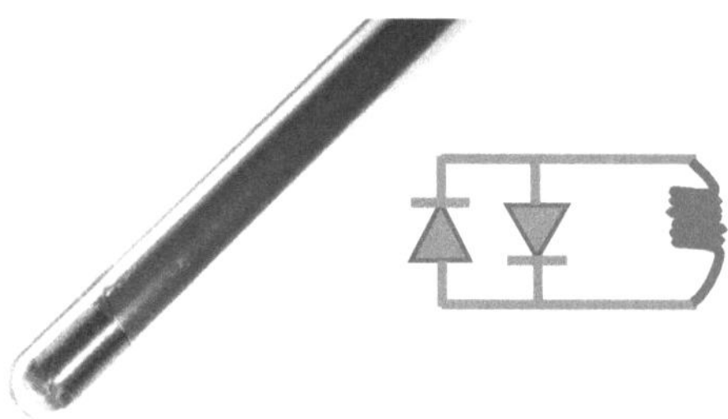

Figure 1: *The coil of the calibration probe has 25 windings and an inner diameter of 4 mm. Inside the coil it is connected via two crossed Diodes (see shematics).*

At this stage of testing, we were not able to do adequate independent characterization of the spectral behavior of the crossed diodes and unable to perform a complete calibration procedure based on this device.

III. Results

The proposed probe shows a strong nonlinear behavior as can be seen in Fig. 2.

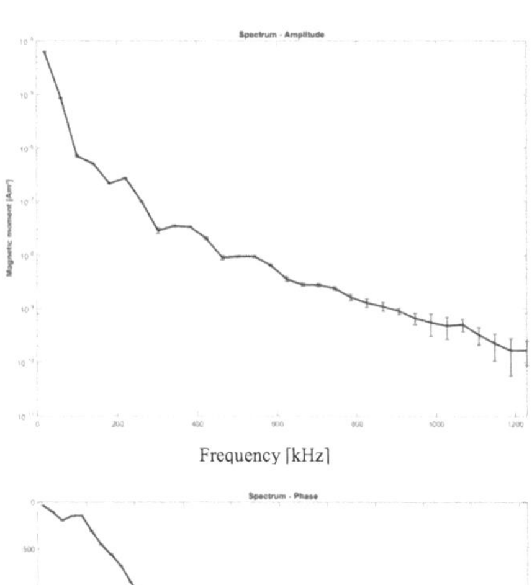

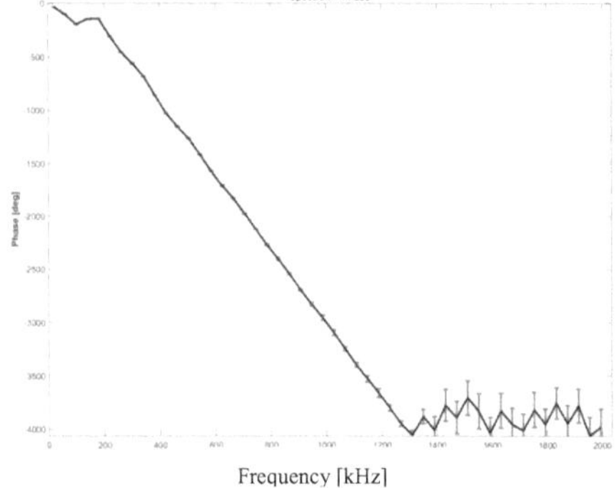

Figure 2: *The amplitude (top) and phase (bottom) of the odd harmonics is shown. Measurements were performed at an excitation frequency of 20 kHz and a field strength of 17 mT.*

Due to the additional induction of the probe itself, a large time shift can be seen, but does not affect the value of transfer function.

Beside the time shift, the general behavior of the acquired magnetization of the probe, it is comparable to typical particles. The magnetization is shown in Fig. 3.

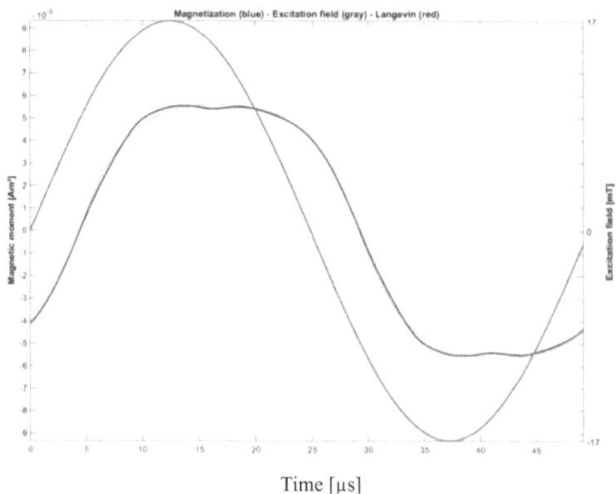

Time [µs]

Figure 3: *The excitation field (light grey) was 17 mT. The resulting magnetization (dark grey) shows time shifted particle like behavior. Additionally a Langevin model fit (thin line), including a fitted time shift, is shown.*

IV. Discussion

The results show a particle like behavior of the proposed probe. For a well-characterized probe, it should be possible to calculate a transfer function of the spectrometer from a single measurement without external equipment. This type of probes can be built for single or multiple directions of the magnetic field, depending on the problem. At this stage, due to the missing independent external characterization of the diodes, we were not able to show a complete calibration procedure bases on these types of probes. Still, implementing this setup in a magnetic particle imager is future work.

V. Conclusions

The results shown in this work are encouraging to consider macroscopic probes for a particle independent calibration process. This offers a quick and precise calibration procedure for magnetic particle spectrometers and maybe imagers.

AUTHOR'S STATEMENT
Research funding: The author state no funding involved. Conflict of interest: Authors state no conflict of interest. Informed consent: Informed consent has been obtained from all individuals included in this study. Ethical approval: The research related to human use complies with all the relevant national regulations, institutional policies and was performed in accordance with the tenets of the Helsinki Declaration, and has been approved by the authors' institutional review board or equivalent committee.

REFERENCES
[1] H. Paysen et al. Towards quantitative magnetic particle imaging: A comparison with magnetic particle spectroscopy. *AIP Advances*, 8, 056712, 2018. doi: 10.1063/1.5006391.
[2] M. Graeser et al. Two Dimensional magnetic particle spectrometry. *Phys. Med. Biol*, 62, 3378, 2017. doi: 10.1088/1361-6560/aa5bcd.
[3] P. Swargulski et al. Towards Standardized MPI Measurements. *Proc. IWMPI*, 2018.
[4] D.-X. Chen et al. Calibration of ac and dc magnetometers with a Dy2O3 standard. Rev. Sci. Instr., 82, 045112, 2011. doi: 10.1063/1.3581224.
[5] F. Weigl et al. Determination of the Total Circulating Blood Volume using Magnetic Particle Spectroscopy. *IJMPI*, 3(1):1217-1217, 2017. doi: 10.18416/ijmpi.2017.1703021.

Statistical Significance in Thrombus Characterization Using Magnetic Nanoparticle Spectroscopy of Brownian Rotation

J. B. Weaver[a,b,c*], H. Khurshid[d], C. V. Weaver[e], S. W. Gordon-Wylie[c], D. Ness[a,f], Y. Shi[b], D. A. Schartz[f], E. Demidenko[e], W. Wells[g] and C. J. Eskey[a]

[a] Department of Radiology, Dartmouth-Hitchcock Medical Center, Lebanon NH, USA
[b] Department of Physics, Dartmouth College, Hanover NH, USA
[c] Thayer School of Engineering, Dartmouth College, Hanover NH, USA
[d] Department of Applied Physics, University of Sharjah, Sharjah, UAE
[e] Section of Biostatistics and Epidemiology, Geisel School of Medicine at Dartmouth College, Lebanon, NH, USA
[f] Geisel School of Medicine, Hanover NH, USA
[g] Department of Pathology, Dartmouth-Hitchcock Medical Center, Lebanon NH, USA
* Corresponding author, email: john.b.weaver@hitchcock.org

Abstract: We are developing methods of characterizing blood clots in stroke to enable more effective personalized treatment. We present two developments in this effort: 1) Using magnetic spectroscopy of nanoparticle Brownian rotation of thrombin targeted nanoparticles to characterize the mechanical stability of the clot. 2) Identifying small numbers of nanoparticles on a clot. This required test single-sided, multivariate significance testing methods. We found that the clot organization and age can be characterized by thrombin targeted NPs and one-sided, multivariate statistical significance testing methods can be used to identify small numbers of magnetic nanoparticles (one nanogram on our systems).

I. Introduction

Stroke is a pernicious disease that kills many and is debilitating for many others. The economic costs and the costs in lives is very large. Ischemic strokes, where blood clots occlude an artery, are the most common. Treatment of ischemic stroke using endovascular procedures to physically remove the thrombus has been revolutionary in dramatically reducing both morbidity and mortality. There are several methods used including using suction to pull the thrombus into the catheter to be removed and using a stent like basket to scoop the thrombus into the catheter to be removed. These interventional procedures can eliminate permanent disability if performed relatively quickly following the blockage. However, these interventional procedures are not without problems. One of the most important is the thrombus breaking up while being removed forcing each fragment to be found and removed. We are using magnetic spectroscopy of nanoparticle Brownian rotation [1-5] to characterize the amount of thrombin presented on the surface of the thrombus and the thrombin present is reduced as the fibrin becomes more organized. We have found that the amount of thrombin on the surface of the clot can be characterized using thrombin targeted nanoparticles detected using magnetic spectroscopy of Brownian rotation.

The other component of this problem is understanding when significant amounts of NPs are present and when none. The problem is important if the clot fragments and we are forced to find each fragment. The question at that point is: Is there a clot fragment at that location or not? The question is difficult because the fragments can be small and the most likely clots to fragment are those with little thrombin on them to begin with. Other MPI methods have been used [8] to identify clots but they are not possible on a less expensive spectroscopic system such as those that we are trying to use at the point of care. The question is complicated because there are multiple frequencies so it is multivariate and we know more NPs should produce a larger signal so it is a one-sided significance test. There are no multivariate, one-sided significance tests; it is an area of current research. We introduced several possible tests and evaluated them on simulated spectra and on experimental spectra.

II. Material and Methods

II.I. Clot Characterization

We produced clots from animal blood using two methods: The first method is to interrupt clot formation at varying times to produce clots with varying fibrin organization [8]. The second method is to produce two types of clot: one "soft" that was thrombin rich and one "hard" that had less thrombin and more organized fibrin [9]. Both were formed from citrate stabilized pig blood. The hard clot was produced by introducing barium sulfate to induce the clotting cascade and the soft clot was formed by introducing thrombin directly. The clots were added to thrombin aptamer targeted nanoparticles (NPs). Magnetic spectra were gathered over time to estimate the binding. Both the relaxation time [5] and the relaxation adjusted number of NPs [6] were found over time for each clot.

II.II. Statistical Significance

We used five methods of testing statistical significance. The first is simple: use a one-sided t-test on the sum of the signal at all the frequencies, A-T. The second is a variance weighted z-test, V-Z. The third uses a single variable one-sided t-test to produce a p-value at each frequency and combine the p-values at each frequency using either Fisher's method, T-F, or Stouffer's method, T-S. Fisher's method and Stouffer's method were developed to perform meta-analyses. The final test is a multivariate t-test using one pooled variance, P-T.

We tested these methods in two ways: First, we used Monte Carlo like simulations to evaluate the power and bias of the tests. The results shown are for 8 frequencies and 4 repetitions with differences between the spectra ranging from zero to one noise standard deviation. Then the best of the tests were evaluated on experimental spectra taken with our current spectrometer [1,8]. Thirty spectra were taken on 250 nanograms of Micromod BNF Starch 100 nm NPs and another thirty spectra were taken on the 249 nanograms of NPs following the removal of 1 nanogram of NPs. The number of repeated spectra necessary to produce significance was evaluated.

III. Results and Discussion

It is important to confirm that multiple ways of producing clots yield the same spectroscopic results.

Both methods of producing clots produced the same results: The oldest, best organized clots had the fewest NPs bound and the relaxation time was reduced by the smallest amount. The youngest, least organized clots with the most thrombin had the most NPs bound and the change in relaxation time was greater. This confirms previously published results [8].

The larger relaxation changes for NPs bound to the thrombin rich clots probably reflect multiple bound sites for each NP.

All the proposed statistical significance tests can be useful in appropriate circumstances. When the variance in the noise at each frequency was the same, the pooled t-test was superior to all others. The T-S test was only slightly less powerful. The variance weighted z-test is not appropriate for small numbers of repetitions because of the artificial significance for small differences between spectra.

When the variance in the noise at each frequency was different, the T-S test was far superior to M-T.

For equal noise variance, seven repetitions were necessary on average to achieve significance for 1 nanogram difference for A-T, T-S and M-T tests. For unequal

variance, A-T and T-S tests achieved essentially the same power; 7 repetitions were required on average. The M-T required six. When the noise was unequal and higher, the T-S test required 12, the A-T test 22 and the M-T test 19 repetitions to achieve significance.

Table 1: Comparison of One-Sided, Multivariate Statistical Significance Tests.

		A-T	V-Z	T-F	T-S	M-T
Equal Variance	Integral Power	0.53	0.62	0.52	0.56	**0.58**
	Intercept	0.05	**0.09**	0.05	0.05	0.05
Unequal Variance	Integral Power	0.37	0.69	0.63	**0.64**	0.42

IV. Conclusions

Clots can be characterized using the number of NPs bound to them and their change in relaxation time.

The T-S test is a solid generally useful, simple one-sided, multivariate significance test that is appropriate for any variance pattern. However, the composite t-test using a pooled variance produced slightly more powerful results when the variance at each frequency was the same.

ACKNOWLEDGEMENTS
Funding from NIH/NIBIB under grant 1R21EB021456.

AUTHOR'S STATEMENT
There are no conflicts of interest.

REFERENCES
[1] Shi Y, Khurshid H, Ness DB, Weaver JB. Harmonic phase angles used for nanoparticle sensing. Physics in Medicine & Biology 2017, 62(20): 8102.
[2] Zhang X, Reeves DB, Perreard IM, Kett WC, Griswold KE, Gimi B, Weaver JB. Molecular sensing with magnetic nanoparticles using magnetic spectroscopy of nanoparticle Brownian motion. Biosensors and Bioelectronics 2013, 50(0): 441-446.
[3] Giustini AJ, Perreard I, Rauwerdink AM, Hoopes PJ, Weaver JB. Noninvasive assessment of magnetic nanoparticle–cancer cell interactions. Integrative Biology 2012, 4(10): 1283-1288.
[4] Rauwerdink AM, Weaver JB. Measurement of molecular binding using the Brownian motion of magnetic nanoparticle probes. Applied Physics Letters 2010, 96(3): 033702.
[5] Weaver JB, Kuehlert E. Measurements of Magnetic Nanoparticle Relaxation Times. Medical Physics 2012, 39(5): 2765-2770.
[6] John BW, Xiaojuan Z, Esra K, Seiko T-B, Daniel BR, Irina MP, Steven F. Quantification of magnetic nanoparticles with low frequency magnetic fields: compensating for relaxation effects. Nanotechnology 2013, 24(32): 325502.
[7] Starmans LW, Moonen RP, Aussems-Custers E, Daemen MJ, Strijkers GJ, Nicolay K, Grüll H. Evaluation of iron oxide nanoparticle micelles for magnetic particle imaging (MPI) of thrombosis. PLOS one 2015, 10(3): e0119257.
[8] Khurshid H, Shi Y, Berwin BL, Weaver JB. Evaluating blood clot progression using magnetic particle spectroscopy. Medical physics 2018, 45(7): 3258-3262.
[9] Chueh J-Y, Puri AS, Wakhloo AK, Gounis MJ. Risk of distal embolization with stent retriever thrombectomy and ADAPT. Journal of NeuroInterventional Surgery 2016, 8(2): 197-202.

A Schematic Kidney Phantom for Magnetic Particle Imaging

M. Schauerte*[a,b], P. Szwargulski[a,b], M. G. Kaul[c,], T. Knopp[a,b], M. Graeser*[a,b]

[a] Section for Biomedical Imaging, University Medical Center Hamburg-Eppendorf, Hamburg, Germany
[b] Institute for Biomedical Imaging, Hamburg University of Technology, Hamburg, Germany
[c] Department for Diagnostic and Interventional Radiology and Nuclear Medicine, University Medical Center Hamburg-Eppendorf, Hamburg, Germany
** Corresponding author, email: mats.schauerte@tuhh.de , ma.graeser@uke.de*

Abstract: The control of organ perfusion via medical imaging is an important diagnostic tool i.e. for the diagnosis of chronic kidney disease. In this work, a schematic phantom is constructed, which mimics the continuous branching of the vessels in the kidney as well as the perfusion of tissue, which cannot be spatially resolved. It is shown that in Magnetic Particle Imaging the visible drop in concentration of SPIOs can be correlated with the volume fraction of the tracer lumen and thus carries the information about the tissue perfusion.

I. Introduction

Chronic kidney disease is a severe condition with a global burden of over 200 million patients [1]. For diagnosis, information about the perfusion of the kidney is a useful parameter. This can be obtained by imaging the kidneys using ultrasound, CT, scintigraphy or MRI. All of these have their own advantages and disadvantages. Magnetic Particle Imaging (MPI) can combine a good spatial resolution, high temporal resolution, high sensitivity, and depth independent image quality [2]. In MPI the spatial distribution of superparamagnetic iron oxide nanoparticles (SPIOs), which serve as tracer, is imaged. Achievable resolutions range from 0.8 mm to 5 mm depending on the magnetic gradient strength, SPIO system and signal to noise ratio (SNR) [3]. If the phantom contains structures that are smaller than the achievable resolution, so-called partial volume effects occur.

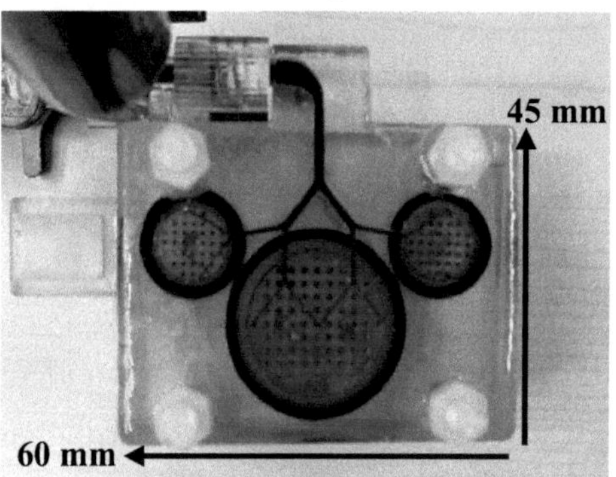

Figure 1: Implementation of the kidney phantom. The phantom consists of three layers. The upper and lower layers have further branching vein-like lumens, which flow into the middle layer. The fine perforation of the cylinders is well visible in the filled phantom. In the picture, the phantom was filled with black coffee for better demonstration.

Since the signal is linked to the absolute SPIO mass, the reconstruction spreads the signal intensity to the volume of the voxel, which underestimates the real local concentration.

In this work a 3D printed CAD phantom is constructed, which mimics the anatomy of a kidney with supplying vessels and a fine perforated area representing the capillaries within the kidney. In a static scenario the impact of fine capillary structures on the reconstructed concentration of SPIOs is examined. The calculated concentrations based on prior knowledge are compared to the reconstructed concentrations.

II. Material and Methods

The phantom is based on the anatomical data derived by digital subtraction angiography of a pig kidney. For the 3D printing process and the measurements, it was necessary to find a balance between anatomical precision and the ability to mathematically describe the phantom. Therefore, the shapes of the arterial and venous supplying vessels were designed as a steady and equiangular ramification over four levels. In addition, a separation of the arterial and venous system was desirable for future flow experiments. A capillary unit connects the supplying vessel structures. This unit consists of three cylindrical areas, perforated equidistantly by 1 mm holes in the large central cylinder and 0.75 mm holes in the small outer cylinders. In Fig. 1 one can see a picture of the phantom filled with black coffee to demonstrate the structure and the filling. Since the MPI system being used is not sufficient to resolve these fine structures, they are expected to appear as areas of constant concentration in the reconstructed image.

The phantom was printed using the Form 2 (FormLabs, Ltd.) stereolithographic desktop 3D-printer. A few limitations occurred regarding the minimal diameter of the supplying vessels, the capillary unit and the post-processing of the phantom. As preparation for the measurement the inside volume of the phantom is being calculated, and filled with the SPIOs (perimag, micromod, Germany) in a concentration of $c_0 = 0.236\,\mathrm{mg\,Fe\,ml^{-1}}$. The experiments were performed using a Bruker field free point MPI system. A 3D imaging sequence was applied with a drive field strength of 12 mT in all three directions and a selection field strength of G = diag(-0.6, -0.6, 1.2) Tm^{-1}.

To prove that the reconstructed image contains information on the lumen volume fraction of the capillary unit, the prior knowledge based on the CAD data is used to calculate the lumen ratio $\alpha = V_{cap} / V_{cyl}$ that is filled with tracer. The ratio of the capillary volume (V_{cap}) to the total cylinder volume (V_{cyl}) is then used to calculate the predicted concentration c_p of the image.

$$c_p = c_0 \cdot \alpha$$

The volume relation α of the areas of interest result in 0.1815 for the large and 0.155 for the small cylinder, respectively. The reconstruction of the image was done by using the iterative regularized kaczmarz algorithm in the frequency domain. In order to get the reconstructed value of c_0 an additional cubic tracer sample was used as reference measurement to address the nonlinear effects of the regularization on the reconstructed concentration. A correction factor between the applied concentration c_0 and the reconstructed concentration of a region of interest in the cubic sample, $c_{reco,cube}$, is calculated by $\beta = c_{reco,cube} / c_0$. This is done by calculating the mean of the intensities inside the region of interest within the reconstructed images. This correction factor was multiplied to the intensities of the reconstructed image and afterwards the corrected reconstructed concentration $\check{c}_{reco}$ was compared with the calculated concentration c_p.

$$\check{c}_{reco} = c_{reco} \cdot \beta$$

III. Results

In Fig. 2 the reconstructed images of the kidney phantom are shown. Most structures could be visualized in the reconstructed images. However, the small vessels with a diameter of 0.7 mm were contributing not enough signal, such that they were lost in the reconstructed images. The constant concentration expected in the perfusion areas showed fluctuations, which can be caused by the regularization.

Table 1: *Applied, reconstructed and corrected concentrations[mg Fe ml^{-1}] for the three cylinder regions and the relative error ϵ_r .*

	Small cylinder1	Small cylinder 2	Large cylinder
c_p	0.03657	0.03657	0.04283
c_{reco}	0.00256	0.00231	0.002969
$\check{c}_{reco}$	0.03750	0.03391	0.04358
ϵ_r	2.56 %	7.4%	1.8 %

As base for the calculation, the reconstructed concentration in each cylinder was averaged over a region of interest. After correction with $\beta = 14.679$, the relative error between calculated and reconstructed concentrations are between 2.56 % and 7.4 % for the small cylinders and 1.8 % for the large cylinder. As for the small cylinders, only 4 voxels in each plane are within the cylinder which can lead to errors as the model was not perfectly aligned with the system matrix grid due to its size and weight.

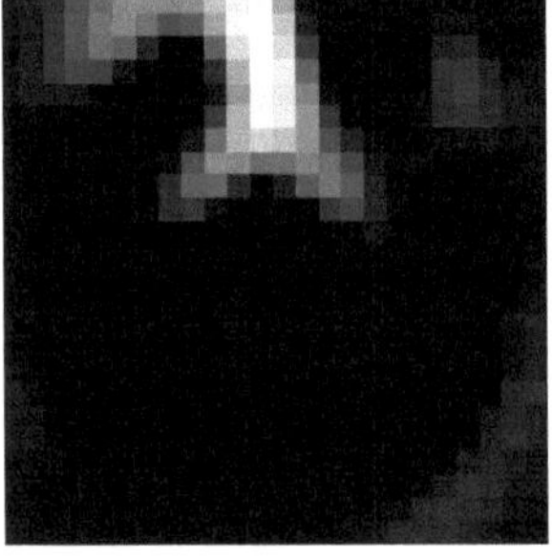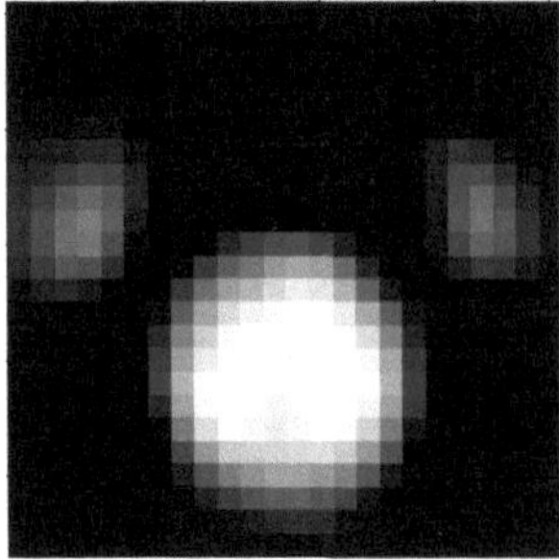

Figure 2: *Reconstructed images. Shown are two planes of the phantom. Left top plane containing the supply vessels. Right, center plane containing the capillary cylinders.*

IV. Discussion & Conclusion

The presented kidney phantom mimics the fine and coarse vessels of a real kidney. The fine structures in the central unit simulating the tissue were, as expected, impossible to resolve. The low relative difference between reconstructed and calculated concentration prove that the reconstructed image contains information about the lumen ratio of the phantom. It was necessary to use an additional reference sample to estimate the concentration insight the phantom. Therefore, the borders of the perforation area were disregarded, which contain variations in the signal strength. Due to the anatomy-like shape the phantom can be used for dynamic perfusion experiments. For this a steady flow though the phantom can be applied. After a tracer bolus is given, the time series can be used to calculate the perfusion of the tissue. In contrast to a real kidney the shape of the model is well known, the reconstruction and post processing of the data can be optimized to achieve good and reliable diagnostic data out of the measurements.

The measurements confirm that MPI contains information about the sub-resolution lumen ratio. For this it is necessary to correct the non-linear effects incorporated in the regularized reconstruction. The phantom showed to be reliable and a good base for perfusion imaging in MPI.

AUTHOR'S STATEMENT
Research funding: The project war funded by the German Research Fundation (KN 1108/2-1) and the German Federal Ministery of Education and Research (05M16GKA and 13XP5060B). Conflict of interest: Authors state no conflict of interest.

REFERENCES
[1] P.H Winocour, Diabetes and chronic kidney disease: an increasingly common multi☐morbid disease in need of a paradigm shift in care, *Diabetic Medicine*, 35(3), pp. 300-305, 2018, doi: 10.1111/dme.13564
[2] B. Gleich and J. Weizenecker. Tomographic imaging using the nonlinear response of magnetic particles. *Nature*, 435(7046):1217-1217, 2005. doi: 10.1038/nature03808.
[3] H. Bagheri et al. ,A mechanically driven magnetic particle imaging scanner Applied Physics Letters, 113, 183703, 2018 doi: 10.1063/1.5052646
[4] Knopp et al., Weighted iterative reconstruction for magnetic particle imaging, *Physics in medicine & biology* 55 (6), 1577 doi: 10.1088/0031-9155/55/6/003

Multi-modality Imaging of Prostate Cancer in Mice using Magnetic Particle Imaging, Magnetic Resonance Imaging and Near-infrared Imaging

Huijuan You[a,b]*, Wenting Shang[b,c], Hui Hui[b,c], Xin Yang[b,c], Jie Tian[b,c]* and Liang Wang[a]*

[a] *Department of Radiology, Tongji Hospital, Tongji Medical College, Huazhong University of Science and Technology, Wuhan, Hubei 430030, China*
[b] *Key Laboratory of Molecular Imaging, Institute of Automation, Chinese Academy ofSciences, Beijing, China*
[c] *Beijing Key Laboratory of Molecular Imaging, Institute of Automation, Beijing, 100190, China*
* *Corresponding author, Liang Wang; email: wang6@tjh.tjmu.edu.cn ; Jie Tian; email: jie.tian@ia.ac.cn*

Abstract: Prostate cancer is a common disease in males older than 50 years. Precision diagnosis of prostate cancer is challenging due to the low sensitivity using conventional imaging techniques i.e. CT and MRI. Here we design multi-modality probes which can target prostate cancer and detected it by using magnetic particle imaging, magnetic resonance imaging and near-infrared imaging. Our results showed that this multimodality imaging approach has potential to facilitate the clinical diagnosis by selecting the individualized therapy.

I. Introduction

Prostate cancer (PCa) is a common disease in males older than 50 years[1, 2]. With the discovery and application of more targeted receptors and metabolic intermediates in prostate cancer, the effective detection and evaluation the PCa will be greatly enhanced by molecular probes. Therefore, molecular imaging technology is playing an increasingly important role in the diagnosis of prostate cancer. As we know, fluorescence imaging (FLI) offers remarkably high sensitivity, but the tissue penetration depth is just around several millimeters[3, 4]. Magnetic resonance imaging (MRI) can provide high spatial resolution and excellent depth penetration, however, it has poor sensitivity[5]. Magnetic particle imaging (MPI) promises excellent depth penetration, positive contrast and almost no background from tissue[6, 7]. Hence, single modality imaging of most cancer is typically restricted by the sensitivity, depth and/or spatial resolution they can achieve, the diagnostic methods are difficult to achieve precise diagnosis of cancer. Therefore, it is indispensable to exploit the complementary information from multimodality imaging to obtain more tissue information that may be missed by a single one. The development of multi-modality nanoprobes enable substantial enhancement of imaging sensitivity, high depth of penetration, and high spatial resolution for imaging of the cancers[8]. Here, we synthesized multi-modality probes. And, we test the efficacy of the probes using the fluorescence imaging (FLI)[9], magnetic resonance imaging (MRI) and magnetic particle imaging (MPI)[6, 10].

II. Material and Methods

The multi-modality probes were synthesized with Indocyanine Green (ICG) bonded to Fe_3O_4 NPs. Firstly, the Fe_3O_4 NPs was carboxylated. Next, the ICG was sequentially bonded to the modified Fe_3O_4 NPs. The morphology and size of the Fe_3O_4-ICG NPs were observed by transmission electron microscopy (TEM) and dynamic light scattering (DLS), respectively. The in vitro FLI signal, MRI signal and MPI signal of the Fe_3O_4-ICG NPs were observed by optical molecular imaging system (IVIS®Spectrum, PerkinElmer, USA), MRI (1T, M3TM, AspectImaging, Isereal) and MPI (MOMENTUM, MagneticInsight, USA), respectively. The cytotoxicity of the Fe_3O_4-ICG NPs were detected by Cell Counting Kit-8 assay (CCK-8, Solarbio, USA). For in vivo imaging, BALb/c nude mice (male, 6-8 week) were using to establishe the orthotopic model of prostate cancer. After 8 weeks of tumor development, we injected the Fe_3O_4-ICG NPs in the tail vein and the FLI/MRI/MPI images were acquired using IVIS®Spectrum, M3TM and MOMENTUM, respectively.

III. Results

The TEM image revealed that Fe_3O_4-ICG NPs had a uniform morphology. The hydrodynamic diameter of the Fe_3O_4-ICG NPs was 20 ± 5nm based on DLS. The CCK-8 assay showed no obvious cytotoxicity was observed in these cells, indicating Fe_3O_4-ICG NPs had good biocompatibility. The in vitro FLI signal, MRI signal and MPI signal of the Fe_3O_4-ICG NPs were excellently observed by

IVIS®Spectrum, M3TM, and MOMENTUM, respectively. Together, these results indicated that the FLI/MRI/MPI probes were able to function efficiently in multi-modality imaging. The Fe_3O_4-ICG NPs could detect the BALb/c nude mice orthotopic prostate cancer. In vivo observation (24h) of orthotopic prostate cancer systemic administrated with Fe_3O_4-ICG using FLI, MRI and MPI, respectively. We observed the majority of the optical signal were in the orthotopic prostate cancer from the FLI (Fig.1A.). The FLI provided remarkably high sensitivity in the detection of prostate cancer. The MRI indicated marked signal reductions in orthotopic prostate cancer (Fig.1B.). Hence, the MRI imaging offered high spatial resolution and excellent depth penetration in the detection of prostate cancer. The MPI displayed distinct positive contrast and almost no background from tissue in orthotopic prostate cancer (Fig.1C.). These data confirmed that Fe_3O_4-ICG NPs can detect prostate cancer precisely.

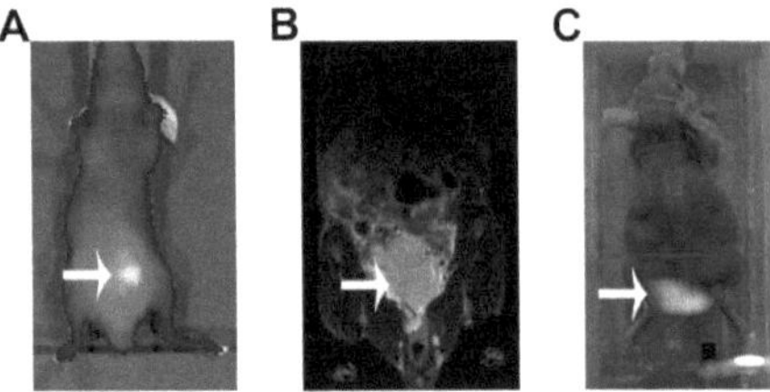

Figure 1: *FLI, MRI and MPI imaging results*

A. Fluorescence imaging (FLI). In vivo observation (24h) of orthotopic prostate cancer systemic administrated with Fe_3O_4-ICG using near-infrared imaging. B. Magnetic resonance imaging (MRI). In vivo observation (24h) of orthotopic prostate cancer systemic administrated with Fe_3O_4-ICG using magnetic resonance imaging. C. Magnetic particle imaging (MPI). In vivo detection (24h) of orthotopic prostate cancer systemic administrated with Fe_3O_4-ICG using Magnetic particle imaging.

IV. Discussion

Imaging has played a vital role in the diagnosis of PCa. All of the imaging modalities have their own advantages and intrinsic drawbacks, multi-modality probes enable integrate the advantages of more than one imaging modality to obtain complementary functions to improve the imaging sensitivity and specificity[11]. Here, we synthesized multi-modality probes Fe_3O_4-ICG NPs, which combined FLI, MRI and MPI imaging modalities together to obtain more tumor information. In this study, we conducted FLI, MRI and MPI experiments both in vitro and in vivo. We showed that the multi-modality probes Fe_3O_4-ICG NPs had high sensitivity and specificity in the nude mice bearing orthotopic prostate cancer. Timely detection of prostate cancer (including initial prostate cancer and biochemical recurrence of prostate cancer), accurate assessment of its staging and risk grading are the basis for rational selection of treatment options in clinically. The Fe_3O_4-ICG NPs can provide remarkably high sensitivity, high spatial resolution and excellent depth penetration in the detection of prostate cancer. Therefore, the multi-modality probes Fe_3O_4-ICG NPs can provide an effective method to locate the position of the prostate cancer and facilitate the clinical diagnosis by selecting the individualized therapy. There were still some limitations in this experiment. The Fe_3O_4-ICG NPs was not the probe that actively targeted tumors. The Fe_3O_4-ICG NPs reached tumor passively through the leaky vasculature surrounding the tumors by the Enhanced Permeability and Retention (EPR) effect. It depended passively on the EPR effects on targeting tumor regions. There are limitations in clinical applications. Maybe we can use targeted receptors in prostate cancer and make ligands grafted at the surface of nanoparticles[12]. These nanoparticles may actively target tumors by binding to the receptors overexpressed by prostate cancer.

V. Conclusions

In summary, we have successfully synthesized multi-modality probes Fe_3O_4-ICG and conducted FLI, MRI and MPI experiments both in vitro and in vivo. The Fe_3O_4-ICG NPs as a non-toxic muti-modality nanoparticle bases on FLI, MRI and MPI enable integrate the advantages of FLI, MRI and MPI imaging to obtain complementary functions to improve the imaging sensitivity and specificity. The Fe_3O_4-ICG NPs can provide remarkably high sensitivity, high spatial resolution and excellent depth penetration in the precisely detection of prostate cancer.

ACKNOWLEDGEMENTS
This paper is supported by National Key Research and Development Program of China No. 2017YFA0205200, 2016YFC0103803, National Natural Science Foundation of China under Grant No. 81227901, 81527805, 81671851, 61231004; Beijing Municipal Science & Technology Commission No. Z161100002616022; the R&D Project of the Chinese Academy of Sciences No. GJJSTD20170004.

AUTHOR'S STATEMENT
Conflict of interest: Authors state no conflict of interest.

REFERENCES
1. Magi-Galluzzi, C., Mod Pathol, 2018. 31(S1): p. S12-21.
2. Miller, K.D., et al., 2016. CA Cancer J Clin, 2016. 66(4): p. 271-89.
3. Hong, G., et al., Nat Med, 2012. 18(12): p. 1841-6.
4. Hong, G.S., A.L. Antaris, and H.J. Dai, Nature Biomedical Engineering, 2017. 1(1): p. 22.
5. Cheng, Z., et al., 2016. 2(1): p. 132-140.
6. Song, G., et al., Nano Lett, 2018. 18(1): p. 182-189.
7. Yu, E.Y., et al., Nano Lett, 2017. 17(3): p. 1648-1654.
8. James, M.L. and S.S. Gambhir, Physiol Rev, 2012. 92(2): p. 897-965.
9. Nguyen, Q.T. and R.Y. Tsien, Nat Rev Cancer, 2013. 13(9): p. 653-62.
10. Gleich, B. and J. Weizenecker, Nature, 2005. 435(7046): p. 1214-1217.
11. Gao, D. and Z. Yuan, Int J Biol Sci, 2017. 13(4): p. 401-412.
12. Danhier, F., O. Feron, and V. Preat, J Control Release, 2010. 148(2): p. 135-46.

System matrix dependent image quality of SPION infused polycaprolactone

H. Nilius[*a], **R. Siepmann**[a], **M. Orth**[b], **K. Mueller**[a], **F. Mueller**[a], **S. M. Dadfar**[c], **M. Darguzyte**[a], **V. Schulz**[a] **and S. D. Reinartz**[d]

[a] *Physics of Molecular Imaging Systems, RWTH Aachen University, Aachen, Germany*
[b] *Institut für Textiltechnik, RWTH Aachen University, Aachen, Germany*
[c] *Experimental Molecular Imaging, RWTH Aachen University, Aachen, Germany*
[d] *Department of Diagnostic and Interventional Radiology, Uniklinikum Aachen, Aachen, Germany*
[*] *corresponding author, email:* _henning.nilius@pmi.rwth-aachen.de_

Abstract: The most common cause of death worldwide is coronary artery disease (CAD) which is treated by percutaneous coronary intervention (PCI). Major disadvantages of PCI include harmful X-rays and an iodine contrast agent. MPI could overcome this disadvantage, but there are no MPI-visible stents available. Our approach to an MPI-visible stent is infusing polycaprolactone (PCL) with SPIONs. However, an appropriate sample has to be chosen for system matrix measurement. In this work we present different possibilities.

I. Introduction

CAD is the most common cause of death worldwide with 15,6% of all deaths in 2015 [1]. Patients with CAD have stenosis in the coronary arteries caused by arteriosclerotic plaques. Behind the stenosis the coronary blood flow is reduced and therefore, the oxygen demand of the myocardium cannot be fulfilled. The gold standard treatment for CAD is PCI. PCI uses X-rays and an iodine contrast agent to visualize the vessels and stents can be implanted. Major disadvantages of PCI include only a planar view, and higher risk for patients with reduced kidney function or hyperthyroidism, due to the iodine contrast agent. Furthermore, it exposes the patient and the practitioner to harmful ionizing radiation. MPI as a high sensitivity imaging technique based on magnetic fields rather than X-rays, can overcome these disadvantages [2]. Moreover, multi-color MPI and magnetic steering of devices add meaningful new possibilities especially for difficult interventions. However, new MPI-compatible devices have to be constructed, before it can become a viable alternative to PCI. While there are already some MPI-visible catheters, no specialized stents are available yet. Our work approaches the creation of such a stent by infusing the biodegradable polyester PCL with inhouse produced superparamagnetic nanoparticles (SPIONs). However, since the tracer is incorporated into a solid material, standard protocols for system matrix measurement did not deliver satisfying results. Here we present the progress of our work [3] and different ways to obtain a system matrix for incorporated SPIONs.

II. Material and Methods

II.I. Filament production

The filaments for this work were produced as presented in [2]. Five mixtures of a PCL granulate (PCL Capa 6506, Perstorp, Malmo, Sweden) and 0, 1, 2, 5 and 7 weight percent (wt%) of in-house produced air dried SPIONs, called "C2", were prepared [4]. Each of these mixtures were given into a. micro extruder (MC15, Xplore Instruments BV, Sittard, Netherlands) separately with an extruder temperature of 75° C and mixing speed of 5-6 RPM. The resulting extrusion force was 700 N. To produce thin filaments (see Fig. 1), the melt was winded with a winding speed of 50 m/min. The extruder was cleaned with pure PCL after each mixture until no visible sign of SPIONs remained.

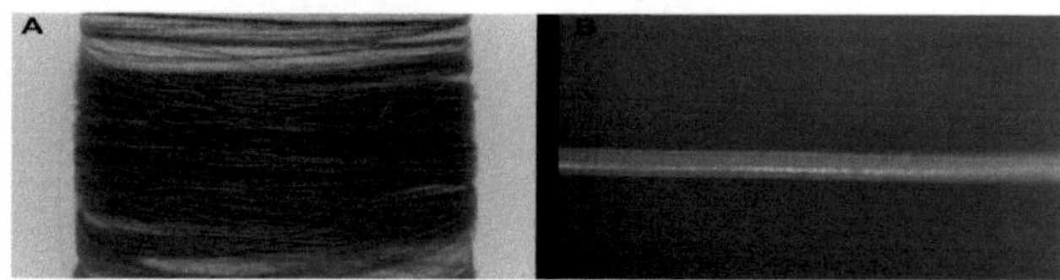

Figure 1: *A: PCL-filament with 2 wt% of SPIONs. The color of the filament changes from white for 0 wt% to black at 7 wt%. B: Microscopic image of 2 wt% filament. The monofilament has a smooth surface but shows thickness inhomogeneities.*

II.II. MPI measurements

An imaging phantom was created by forming an "E" out of the 7wt% yarn on an acrylic bloc. The long stroke of the phantom was 12 mm and the short strokes approx. 7 mm. Five different samples for system function measurement were prepared in small vials with a 1 mm³ chamber for the tracer: C2-SPION-powder, at 75°C melted 5 wt%-SPION-filaments, Synomag-D plain (Synomag-D plain, Micromod Partikeltechnik GmbH, Rostock, Germany), C2-particles in an aqueous solution at a. similar concentration to Synomag-D and 7 wt%-SPIONs-melt directly from the micro extruder. System matrices were than measured with 150 averages and a bandwidth of 1.25 MHz. The MPI image was made with a commercially-available MPI scanner (MPI PreClinical, Bruker Biospin, Ettlingen, Germany). The drive-field amplitudes were set to 14 mT in all directions with a gradient field of 2.5 T/m resulting in a field of view (FOV) of 22.4 x 22.4 x 11.2 mm in [x,y,z]-direction. We reconstructed the same measurement with all five system matrices. A Kaczmarz-algorithm with non-negative constraints was used and only frequency components of the system matrices with a SNR of over 4 were utilized. Then a maximum intensity projection (MIP) along the z-axis was calculated using MIPAV (Center for Information Technology, National Institutes of Health, Bethesda, United States of America).

III. Results

All filaments that were produced could be further processed. However, the frequency response showed mostly lower harmonics and a weaker signal strength compared to SPIONs at a similar concentration in an aqueous solution. The images reconstructed with the system matrix using C2-SPION powder showed a high signal intensity but were noisy. Also, the one using melted filaments showed a high intensity as well, but the shape of the imaging phantom was not distinguishable. The matrix with the 7wt%-SPION melt showed a similar resolution but a lower signal intensity. The system matrix measured with the Synomag-D showed the lowest signal strength and some artifacts at the corners of the FOV. However, the spatial resolution was higher than the system matrix using the powder. Liquid C2 showed a similar resolution to the Synomag-D-matrix but a higher signal strength. The reconstructed images are displayed in Fig. 2.

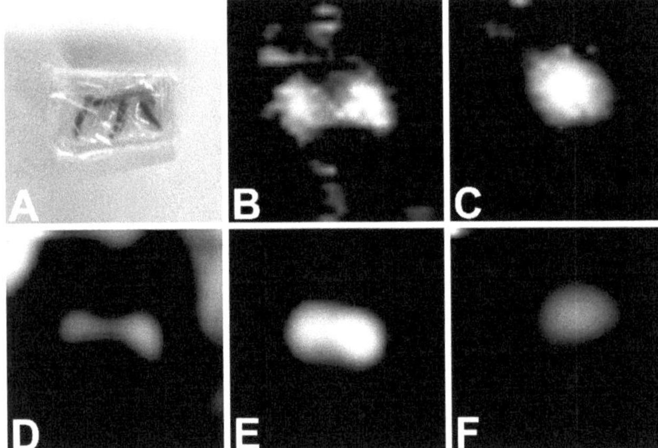

Figure 3: MIPs of the reconstructed images using system matrices with different samples (same window): A: imaging phantom, B: C2-Powder C: melted 5%wt-SPION filament, D: Synomag-D, E: liquid C2, F: 7wt%-SPION melt directly from the micro extruder

IV. Discussion

The filaments we produced could be further processed and showed a concentration dependent signal in the MPI [3]. Therefore, SPION infused PCL has the potential to be a suitable material for MPI visible stents or scaffolds. The frequency response of the filaments was shifted to the lower harmonics and the signal was weaker compared to SPIONs in water. One explanation is that the rotation of the SPIONs is hindered by the surrounding PCL. Therefore, the Brownian-relaxation is missing from the spectrum. The images reconstructed with the system matrix using melted filaments have a low resolution. A possible explanation could be that the concentration of SPIONs in the polyester is not high enough to measure a sufficient system matrix for reconstruction. Similar, the system matrix with the 7wt%-SPION-melt shows a low resolution as well. On the other hand, the concentration of the Synomag-D and the C2-solution was high enough resulting in a high resolution, but the signal intensity was lower than the powder sample. The images reconstructed with the C2-SPION powder system matrix had the highest signal intensity and the resolution was high enough to distinguish the form of the imaging phantom. Therefore, for a high resolution the samples should be in a liquid solution at a high concentration. For the highest sensitivity with acceptable resolution the powder should be used. The best spatial resolution we achieved was not high enough to distinguish the middle stroke of the "E". Nevertheless, it should be high enough to monitor stent degradation and structural damages to a stent.

V. Conclusions

MPI has the potential to be a meaningful alternative to PCI especially for difficult interventions and special patient groups. In this work, we showed that SPION infused PCL could be a viable material for MPI visible scaffolds. However, the right sample for the system matrix measurement has to be chosen. In this work we presented which sample is most suitable for which application. As next step we plan to create a stent out of SPION infused PCL and multi-color measurements.

ACKNOWLEDGEMENTS

We thank our colleagues from the department of "Physics of Molecular Imaging Systems" who provided knowledge and expertise that greatly assisted the research. Also, we like to thank the "Institute für Textiltechnik" for providing the equipment and expertise to create the filaments.

AUTHOR'S STATEMENT

Research funding: The author state no funding involved. Conflict of interest: Authors state no conflict of interest.

REFERENCES

[1] G. 2015 M. and C. of D. GBD 2015 Mortality and Causes of Death Collaborators, "Global, regional, and national life expectancy, all-cause mortality, and cause-specific mortality for 249 causes of death, 1980-2015: a systematic analysis for the Global Burden of Disease Study 2015.," *Lancet (London, England)*, vol. 388, no. 10053, pp. 1459–1544, Oct. 2016.

[2] B. Gleich and J. Weizenecker, "Tomographic imaging using the nonlinear response of magnetic particles," *Nature*, 2005.

[3] H. Nilius, R.Siepmann, M. Orth, M. Straub, S. M. Ali Dadfar, M. Darguzyt and V. Schulz: Towards the visualization of biohybrid implants with MPI: SPION infused PCL, *International Workshop on Magnetic Particle Imaging (8th IWMPI) 2018*

[4] S. M. Ali Dadfar, M. Darguzyte, D. Camozzi, J. Metselaar, S. Banala, N. Güvener, I. Slabu, U. Engelmann, M. Straub, V. Schulz, F. Kiessling and T. Lammers (Ongoing): Maximizing superparamagnetic iron oxide nanoparticles performance for MRI, MPI, and hyperthermia applications.

Evaluation of two iron oxide nanoparticle systems for their capabilities in MRI and MPI

Stefan Lyer [a,*], Maik Liebl [b], Harald Unterweger [a], Olaf Kosch [b], Rainer Tietze [a], Eveline Schreiber [a], Tobias Bäuerle [c], Michael Uder [c], Arnd Dörfler [d], Frank Wiekhorst [b], Christoph Alexiou [a]

[a] Universitätsklinikum Erlangen, ENT-Department, Section of Experimental Oncology and Nanomedicine (SEON), Else-Kröner-Fresenius Stiftung-Professorship, Erlangen, Germany
[b] Physikalisch-Technische Bundesanstalt, Berlin, Germany
[c] Universitätsklinikum Erlangen, Department of Radiology, Erlangen, Germany
[d] Universitätsklinikum Erlangen, Department of Neuroradiology, Erlangen, Germany
* Corresponding author, email: stefan.lyer@uk-erlangen.de

Abstract: Magnetic Particle Imaging (MPI) is a powerful new imaging technique for versatile purposes, which is dependent on magnetic nanoparticles as tracers [1]. The aim of the work shown here was to evaluate the possibilities of improving the MPI performance of two SPION systems by varying the synthesis parameters. Results: One system, SEON^{Dex} is very reproducibly size tunable but not suitable for MPI. SEON^{LA-HSA} is very sensitive against variations in its synthesis, but has a MPI performance in the range of Resovist®. By MPI we could image ex vivo the accumulation of SEON^{LA-HSA} in a rabbit spleen.

I. Introduction

Magnetic resonance and radiation based imaging techniques as well as ultrasound are important diagnostic methods in medicine. All three modalities have their advantages as well as their disadvantage and for all three modalities, contrast agents are available. These agents can improve the diagnostic value of the imaging by highlighting certain regions, in which an irregular state of the tissue or an organ or parts of them is located.

Magnetic Nanoparticles (MNPs) can be used as contrast agents in MRI. Unfortunately, MNPs did lose the race on the marked against Gadolinium based imaging agents, although very encouraging diagnostic value could be demonstrated e.g. by Harishinghani in 2003 for the detection of malignant lymph nodes in prostate cancer.

Despite of these setbacks a large number of scientists still is interested in MNPs because they have outstanding properties that go beyond imaging agents. MNPs can also be used as shuttles for drugs to improve their bioavailability and/or heating tissue as direct treatment.

Combining all these properties with a quantitative imaging modality like Magnetic Particle Imaging (MPI) offers a unique possibility: measuring or at least estimating the drug load in the tissue after the application by a medical device without taking biopsies or blood. Besides the technical development, there is only one additional prerequisite, which is to develop nanoparticles that are suitable of all this. We therefore started with two of our iron oxide nanoparticle systems that are quite far in development and might be good candidates for fulfilling the above-mentioned requirements.

The first nanoparticle system SEON^{DEX} has a crosslinked dextran coating and the second system has a double coating with lauric acid and albumin (SEON$^{LA-BSA \text{ and } -HSA}$). Both showed excellent biocompatibility *in vivo* and *in vitro*. In addition to that, we could demonstrate for the latter, a high efficiency in particle accumulation and drug deposition in a rabbit cancer and a rabbit atherosclerosis model. Beyond that, these nanoparticles can be heated for hyperthermia.

The aim of the project was to modify the synthesis parameter of both particle systems to optimize or improve their imaging properties for MPI.

II. Material and Methods

II.I. Nanoparticle systems used

Both nanoparticle systems are synthesized by wet precipitation of iron salts with ammonium hydroxide. The first is an *in situ* precipitation with dextran in the solution, which is later crosslinked by epichlorohydrin. The resulting nanoparticles have a size of 80 nm and a chain like structure. The second system is first precipitated at 80°C, followed by a first coating with lauric acid and a second coating with serum albumin resulting in nanoparticles forming nanoclusters with a size of ca. 65nm. For detailed description, see references [2, 3].

II.II. MPS- and MPI-Measurement

Magnetic particle spectroscopy (MPS) measurements of the SEON systems were performed using a commercial magnetic particle spectrometer (MPS-3 Bruker Biospin, Germany) as previously described in detail. For the MPS measurement, samples of 10 µL were placed in polymerase chain reaction tubes (Applied Biosystems, Darmstadt, Germany) into the pick-up coil system of the MPS. The magnetic response of the samples to an AC magnetic field of a frequency f_0 of 25 kHz and amplitude of B_{excit} of 25 mT was recorded for 10 s. MPI was performed with the preclinical MPI scanner (MPI 25/20 FF, Bruker/Philips, Germany) operated at Charité University Hospital, Berlin. A drive field strength B_{drive} of 12 mT in each direction at three slightly different frequencies around 25 kHz for generating 3D Lissajous trajectories was applied. The static selection field gradient ranged to 2 T/m. The field-of-view (FOV) defined by the system function covered 33 x 33 x 16.5 mm^3.

III. Results

III.I. SEON^{DEX}-Particles

We evaluated the following parameters: amount of dextran, amount of iron (at two different dextran amounts), NH$_3$-concentration, NH$_3$- drop speed, stirring speed and reaction temperature, respectively heating rate. The effects on the hydrodynamic particle size and volume susceptibility were very diverse. Whereas NH$_3$- drop speed, temperature and heating rate had no effect on the properties of the nanoparticles, an increase of dextran concentration led to a reduction of the hydrodynamic diameter. Finally, we demonstrated that an increase in the iron concentration led to a reproducible and systematic change in the particle size from 30 nm to 130 nm, accompanied by a proportional increase of the volume susceptibility. According to the Koenig-Kellar model, there is a relation between susceptibility and relaxation, so with the contrast properties of the magnetic material. To study this, five different SPION^{DEX} particles with different hydrodynamic diameters (30nm, 40nm, 50nm, 80nm and 130nm) were dispersed in an agarose gel. The results showed, that the T2* relaxivity was dependent on the size of the different nanoparticles and square dependent on their susceptibility.

The MPS amplitude of the third harmonic normalized to iron content A_3* followed the same scheme. Unfortunately, the values were too low for being suitable as MPI tracer.

III.I. SEON$^{LA-BSA \text{ and } -HSA}$-Particles

We varied following parameters during wet chemical processes: the amount of iron, the amount of lauric acid, the reaction time, the reaction temperature and the stirring speed. Unfortunately, variation of the parameters did not lead to a reproducible alteration of the particle size, but rather to an increased instability of the synthesis.

SEON$^{LA-BSA \text{ and } -HSA}$-nanoparticles, which in part were synthesized under dGMP-conditions, had similar A_3* values, in the range of Resovist® (A_3*=11.0 Am^2/kg(Fe)).

Since first tests showed, that it is possible to get MPI-images in phantoms, we wondered, if it is also possible to image these nanoparticles in organs, which accumulate nanoparticles. Imaging a rabbit liver is not possible with the current MPI-scanners due to their size. Therefore, we used the spleen of a rabbit that we treated with SEON^{LA-HSA} 24h before sacarification (Local Government of Lower

Franconia; 54.2532.1-54/12). After reconstruction, MPI could visualize excellently the shape of this spleen (Fig. 2A). The histological examination subsequently confirmed SPION-accumulation in the imaged spleen (Fig 2B).

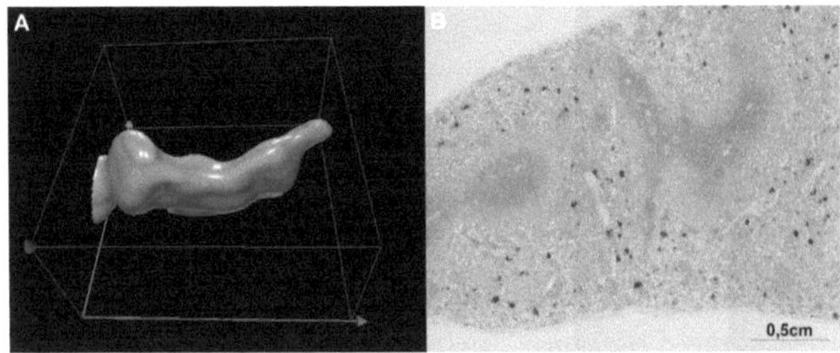

Figure 2: *A: MPI-image of a rabbit spleen with accumulated SEON^{LA-HSA}. B: Histological overview of a part of this spleen.*

IV. Conclusion

The particle system SEON^{DEX} can be modified via variations in the synthesis process, so that particle size and concomitantly the magnetic volume susceptibility can be altered in a reproducible way. It exhibits size-dependent relaxation times in MRI and is very biocompatible. Therefore, SEON^{DEX} has superb qualities to be used as a MRI contrast agent, but with current technical status, not as MPI tracer. Modifications in the synthesis of SEON$^{LA-BSA/-HSA}$ did not show a relation between synthesis parameters and reproducible size or susceptibility changes. The variation in the synthesis parameters of SEON$^{LA-BSA/-HSA}$ has therefore also no effect on the performance in MPS/MPI. The particle system SEON^{LA-HSA} shows good performance for MPS and has comparable values to Resovist®. In preliminary study, these particles were visualized in a rabbit spleen ex vivo and thus constitute a promising candidate for being an MPI tracer.

Our results demonstrate that SEON^{LA-HSA} enrichment in a target organ is feasible.

ACKNOWLEDGEMENTS

For technical assistance, we thank Mrs. Bianca Weigel and Mrs Julia Band For performing the MPS-measurements, we thank Mrs. Patricia Radon.

AUTHOR'S STATEMENT

Research funding: For financial support, we would like to thank the DFG (AL552/8-1) and (WI4230/1-3). Conflict of interest: The authors state no conflict of interest. Informed consent: Informed consent has been obtained from all individuals included in this study. Ethical approval: The research related to human use complies with all the relevant national regulations, institutional policies and was performed in accordance with the tenets of the Helsinki Declaration, and has been approved by the authors' institutional review board or equivalent committee.

REFERENCES

[1] B. Gleich and J. Weizenecker. Tomographic imaging using the nonlinear response of magnetic particles. *Nature*, 435(7046):1217-1217, 2005. doi: 10.1038/nature03808.

[2] H. Unterweger, et al.. Non-immunogenic dextran-coated superparamagnetic iron oxide nanoparticles: a biocompatible, size-tunable contrast agent for magnetic resonance imaging. Int J Nanomed 12 (2017) 5223-5238.

[3] J. Zaloga, et al.. Development of a lauric acid/albumin hybrid iron oxide nanoparticle system with improved biocompatibility. Int J Nanomed 9 (2014) 4847-4866.

Estimation of M-H curve of NMPs using optimization technique

S. M. Choi [a], J.C. Jung [a], and H.B. Hong [a*]

*[a] Intelligence and Robot system Research Group
ETRI, Daejeon, South Korea
* Corresponding author, email: hb8868@etri.re.kr*

Abstract: This paper describes a system that can draw magnetic characteristic curves without developing complex equations or new functions by introducing optimization theory to secure the magnetic characteristic curve. The method described in this paper optimizes the objective function (object function or cost function) by setting the objective parameter of the optimization and specifying the effective interval boundary value of the parameter. Finally, the M-H curve of the corresponding material was obtained by matching the MH curve measurement value of the material analyzed using the existing equipment such as MPMS.

I. Introduction

Nano-magnetic particles (NMPs) with non-linear magnetic properties such as superparamagnetic iron oxide are used in a variety of applications. NMPs need to be analyzed for magnetization behavior, one of the most basic properties of particles used for these applications. To date, several analytical methods have been developed for the analysis of NMPs. One of the most precise methods is a magnetometer using SQUIDs. These methods provide very precise and accurate analysis results. In many cases, however, the cost of equipment is expensive to maintain in a typical laboratory and the cost of operation is very high. In order to overcome this problem, this study introduces a study on the technique of securing the magnetic characteristic curves by using the optimization theory and a very simple coil system.

II. Material and Methods

The measurement system was prepared as shown in Fig 1. The excitation coil was manufactured by winding a 0.18 mm copper wire around a bobbin of peek material with an outer diameter of 10 mm (24 mm in length). Detection coils were prepared to be differential coils with 0.14 mm coils at 12 mm intervals in tubes (9 mm outer diameter 9 mm).

The current and signal acquisition of the coils were performed by a controller manufactured by UMLOGICs (Daejeon, Rep. Korea). In this experiment, an AC current of 45 KHz was applied to the coils. The NMPs used in the experiments were 50 nm size NMP purchased from Chemicell, Germany. In order to estimate the M-H curve, the measured values, known model functions and the parameters (Current, Frequency, Phase, Offset, Magnetic saturation, and Magnetic moment) are considered. The function model of magnetization (M) is a approximating the magnetization characteristics of SPIOs [1]. The values of the acquired data, $M(H(t))$ were optimized using (LM, Levenberg-Marquardt [2], and TRF, Trust Region Reflective [3] algorithm). Because LM algorithm sometimes diverge and won't work well without boundary condition. In fact, it could not limit the bound of parameters. On the other hand, 'TRF' shows better results with some limited bound, which is particularly suitable for large sparse problems with bounds. It is generally robust method. Finally, M is estimated for one or more loops, and M-H curves are generated using representative values of H and M values. All of the above tasks were done using python 3.6. Pseudo code is following.

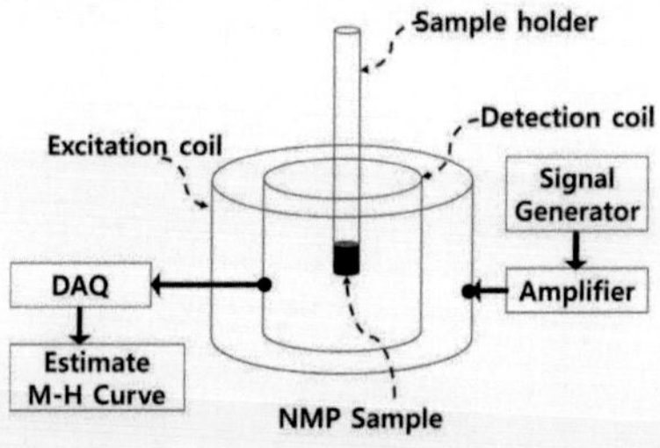

Figure 1: *Schematic drawing of the measurement system*

```
# Set parameters and their boundary

# Given parameter

amp = constant # amplitude of det. coil's signal at zeroing

freq = constant # frequency of signal on excitation coil

pi = 3.14

# Parameters to be estimated

offset, phase, Ms, m0 = 0 # unknown

params = [amp,freq,phase,offset,Ms,m0]
```

```
bounds = ([ amp *0.9999,freq*0.9999,-pi,-2,0,1e-2],
        [amp *1.0001,freq*1.0001,pi,2,5,3]) #[begin,end]


# Input data

measured = DAQ(detection coil) # means v= - DM/dt

x_data = Integral(filter(measured)) # means M(H(t))


# Define model function

define  model_func(t,amp,freq,phase,offset,Ms,m0) using
Langevin equation, where 't' is input, others are all
parameters

define getHt()=amp * cos(2*pi*freq*t - phase) + offset +
noise

# Estimate parameters using TRF optimization

params_estimated = optimize(model_func, x_data, bound)


# Reconstruct M-H curve

MHt_est =  model_func(t,params_estimated)

Ht_est = getHt(t,params_estimated)

plot(Ht_est,MHt_est)
```

III. Results+

Figure 2 shows the result of fitting the estimated curves to the actual measured curves. Since there is no function that can perfectly connect the value of the x-axis of the measured data with (such as Oe) and the estimated curve is expressed using the relative value. As shown in the Fig 2, the results of the M-H curve analyzed using the current optimization theory and the actual MPMS and the measured data are almost similar.

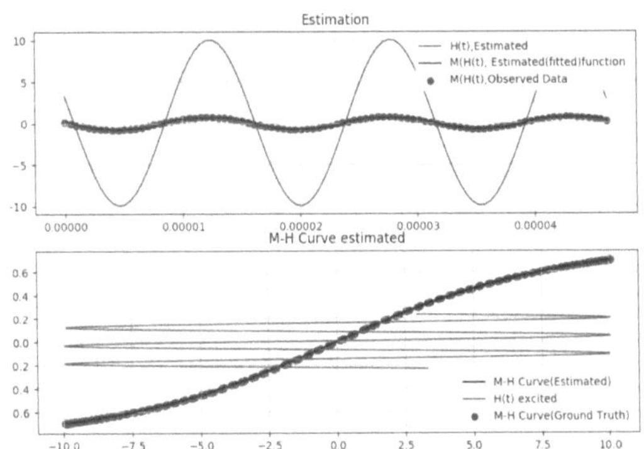

Figure 2:. *Results of the estimation and reconstructed M-H curve estimated with the ground truth*

IV. Discussion & Conclusion

In this paper, estimation of M-H curve theory has been represented based on a few numerical optimization algorithms. Until now, mathematical models have been used as a way to obtain such equipment without using expensive equipment. For example, Teliban proposed a method for creating M-H using a mathematical model based on the frequency mixing magnetic detection technique [4]. However, we propose a system, which can draw a magnetic characteristic curve without developing a complex formula or a new function by introducing optimization theory as a method to secure a magnetic characteristic curve. In this study, to overcome the some drawbacks of the conventional method of obtaining the magnetic characteristic curves algebraically by introducing equations into existing functions, the target parameters of the optimization was defined, and the effective interval boundary value of the corresponding parameters specified (Object function or cost function). In this study, we also have developed a calibration technique to match the MH curve measurement of the known material through conventional analytical instrument such as MPMS. The method proposed in this study may be the alternative in situations where it is difficult to use an expensive instrument or if it is necessary to screen these magnetic characteristics.

ACKNOWLEDGEMENTS
. This work was supported by Institute for Information & com- munications Technology Promotion (IITP) grant funded by the Korea government (MSIP) (No. B132-15-1001).

AUTHOR'S STATEMENT
Research funding: The author state no funding involved. Conflict of interest: Authors state no conflict of interest. Informed consent: Informed consent has been obtained from all individuals included in this study. Ethical approval: The research related to human use complies with all the relevant national regulations, institutional policies and was performed in accordance with the tenets of the Helsinki Declaration, and has been approved by the authors' institutional review board or equivalent committee.

REFERENCES
[1] B. Gleich and J. Weizenecker. Tomographic imaging using the nonlinear response of magnetic particles. *Nature*, 435(7046):1217-1217, 2005. doi: 10.1038/nature03808.
[2] Moré, Jorge J. "The Levenberg-Marquardt algorithm: implementation and theory." Numerical analysis. Springer, Berlin, Heidelberg, 1978. 105-116.
[3] Coleman, Thomas, Mary Ann Branch, and Andrew Grace. "Optimization toolbox." For Use with MATLAB. User's Guide for MATLAB 5, Version 2, Relaese II (1999).
[4] L. Teliban, et. al. *M(H)* shape reconstruction using magnetic spectroscopy. Journal of Magnetism and Magnetic Materials. 324:895-902, 2012. doi:10.1016/j.jmmm.2011.10.016

Effects of heating on tissue – safety limits and therapeutic aspects for MPI

Ulrike Grzyska[a], Franz Wegner[a] and Joerg Barkhausen[a]

[a] Department of Radiology and Nuclear Medicine, University Hospital Schleswig-Holstein, Lübeck, Germany
[*] Corresponding author, email: ulrike.grzyska@uksh.de

Abstract: Thermal effects of Magnetic particle imaging (MPI) can be used for targeted therapies but the application of heat to living systems is limited. In the range of 60-100°C hyperthermia results in immediate coagulation necrosis. However, even much lower temperatures show effects on cell viability or can be used to make cell tumor cells more sensitive to radiation- or chemotherapy. Therefore, the effects of temperature distribution on the cancer cells' viability, the heat resistance of various tumor cell types and potential applications of MPI warrant further investigation.

I. Introduction

The application of electromagnetic fields in medical imaging may result in tissue heating. On the one hand these thermal effects limit clinical applications but on the other hand they offer therapeutic options. For example, the use of MRI is limited in patients with pacemakers or defibrillators because the applied oscillating magnetic fields may cause heating of the devices. However, apart from the safety aspect heating offers a wide range of possible therapeutic applications. High Intensity Focused Ultrasound (HIFU) for example can be applied as an effective modality for thermal ablation of tumors.

Whereas the thermal effects of MRI are very well characterized, less is known about the limitations of heating of tissues and devices as well as the therapeutic options using MPI. A recent study investigated the heating of different stents in MPI [1]. It seems to be possible to perform MPI examination in patients with stents, as the majority of stents did not show significant temperature increases. However, *Duschka et al.* tested the heating of catheters and guidewires and detected material dependent heating characteristics of the devices [2]. But the authors concluded even though that it is not safely predictable whether a ferromagnetic material will show an increased temperature during the MPI examination or not.

With regard to therapeutic MPI applications *Salamon et al.* demonstrated the feasibility of thermal ablation in a liver tumor model by selective heating of a copper wire [3]. In a second study *Tay et al.* introduced a different approach: the applied magnetic nanoparticles (MNPs) were heated by means of the magnetic fields of an MPI-scanner [4] and in addition to the therapeutic effects the tissue temperature was monitored by means of the MPI signal of the MNPs [5].

To avoid harm to patients during hyperthermia a profound knowledge of biological effects caused by the application of heat is essential. In this work, we summarize some effects of heating on cells and tissues as reported in the literature. Furthermore, we compare heating applied by MPI to other modalities such as MRI and ultrasound.

II. Material and Methods

We performed a review of the most recent literature on this topic and analyzed the thermal effects induced by electromagnetic field as well as the therapeutic options of hyperthermia.

III. Results and Discussion

Any temperature change to higher temperatures is related to delivered energy. This energy causes thermal bio-effects ranging from moderate cell changes and antiproliferative effects to destruction of the cells followed by cell death and coagulation necrosis. In the last decade, several groups investigated the effect of high temperatures on different cell types. *Elengoe et al.* explored the heat sensitivity of human liver cells compared to breast cancer cells heating them up to 38°C, 40°C and 42°C for five different time intervals. The results clearly demonstrated that normal human liver cells are more heat resistant than tumor cells [6].

Another recent study showed that temperatures of up to 47°C for 1h using magnetic hyperthermia (MHT) induced by an alternating magnetic field (AMF) considerably dropped the viability of human bone cancer cells (osteosarcoma) to 54% [7]. Considering that exogenous heating produces cytotoxic effects, *Sanz et al.* showed that similar effects can even be found at lower temperatures starting with the loss of viability to 50% at 42.1°C [8]. They also showed that the occurrence of cytotoxic effects not only depends on the achieved temperature but also on the type of hyperthermia applied.

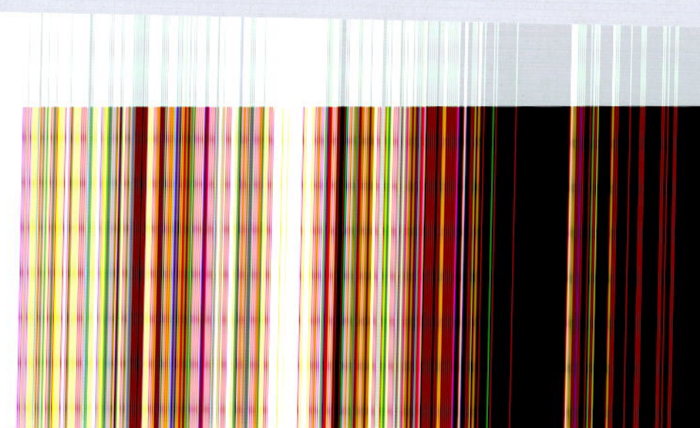

Table 1: Overview of the viability decrease in some selected studies showing the temperature needed to reduce the viability of human cancer cells by 50%.

Authors	Tested Cell Type	Temperature
Elengoe et al., 2013 (6)	Breast cancer cells	40°C (104°F) direct heat exposure for 4h
Herea et al., 2018 (7)	Osteosarcoma cells	49°C (120°F) with WHT for 1h in an AMF
Sanz et al., 2017 (8)	Neuroblastoma cells	42°C (108°F) for 30 min. with MHT

Abbreviations: AMF, alternating magnetic field; MHT, magnetic hyperthermia; WHT, water-based hyperthermia.

Although low temperatures of about 40 to 50°C have significant effects on tumor cells, immediate cell death and coagulation necrosis require temperatures of more than 60°C. First clinical studies applying high intensity focused ultrasound (HIFU) as a curative therapy approach in prostate cancer started in the 1990s. The advantage of this noninvasive treatment was the precise delivery of ultrasound energy to the tumor leading to targeted cell necrosis [9]. The most effective frequencies for therapeutic ultrasound range from 0.8 to 3.5 MHz. This waves lead to an interaction with biological tissue by oscillating the tissue and may rise its temperature up to 100°C, depending on the parameters and type of tissue being exposed. However, even at high temperatures the complete ablation remains challenging and therefore the treatment of malignant tumors has not found its way to clinical routine. However, excellent results can be obtained treating fibroids, a benign tumor of the uterus.

The effects of alternating magnetic fields on tumor cells can be enhanced by magnetic nanoparticles. *Rodríguez-Luccioni et al.* pointed out that the reduction of cell viability depends on the amount of iron oxide with the treated volume [10]. A recently introduced approach combines HIFU and MPI [11], because MPI enables to monitor the heating effect induced in the tissue by HIFU, as the nanoparticle signal changes due to temperature increase [5].

As mentioned above, cancer cells are more sensitive to heat than normal cells [6]. Compared to other techniques, magnetic hyperthermia in conjunction with magnetic nanoparticles provides several advantages including the combination of imaging, treatment and treatment monitoring as well as the possibility to treat tumors virtually anywhere in the human body. Therefore, MPI or MPI combined with HIFU can be considered an attractive approach for local hyperthermia and interventional, minimally invasive ablation of tumors.

IV. Conclusions

The use of hyperthermia in MPI as a treatment option for benign and malignant tumors is a promising technique. However, to prevail against the combined use of HIFU and MRI cost-effectives should be taken into account for all MPI developments in this field.

AUTHOR'S STATEMENT
Research funding: The author state no funding involved. Conflict of interest: Authors state no conflict of interest.

REFERENCES

[1] F. Wegner, T. Friedrich, N. Panagiotopoulos, S. Valmaa, J. P. Goltz, F. M. Vogt, M. A. Koch, T. M. Buzug, J. Barkhausen, and J. Haegele, "First heating measurements of endovascular stents in magnetic particle imaging," *Phys. Med. Biol.*, vol. 63, no. 4, 2018.

[2] R. L. Duschka, H. Wojtczyk, N. Panagiotopoulos, J. Haegele, G. Bringout, J. Rahmer, C. Bontus, T. M. Buzug, J. Borgert, J. Barkhausen, and F. M. Vogt, "Safety Measurements for Heating of Cardiovascular Interventions in Magnetic Particle Imaging (MPI) - First experiences," *J. Healthc. Eng.*, vol. 5, no. 1, pp. 79–94, 2014.

[3] J. Salamon, J. Dieckhoff, C. Jung, M. Möddel, M. G. Kaul, L. Späth, G. Adam, T. Knopp, and H. Ittrich, "Visualization of spatial and temporal temperature distributions in a liver tumor ablation model using Magnetic Particle Imaging," *IWMPI*, vol. Hamburg, pp. 187–188, 2018.

[4] Z. W. Tay, P. Chandrasekharan, A. Chiu-Lam, D. W. Hensley, R. Dhavalikar, X. Y. Zhou, E. Y. Yu, P. W. Goodwill, B. Zheng, C. Rinaldi, and S. M. Conolly, "Magnetic Particle Imaging-Guided Heating in Vivo Using Gradient Fields for Arbitrary Localization of Magnetic Hyperthermia Therapy," *ACS Nano*, vol. 12, no. 4, pp. 3699–3713, 2018.

[5] C. Stehning, B. Gleich, and J. Rahmer, "Simultaneous magnetic particle imaging (MPI) and temperature mapping using multi-color MPI," *Int. J. Magn. Part. Imaging*, vol. 2, no. 2, pp. 1–6, 2016.

[6] A. Elengoe and S. Hamdan, "Heat Sensitivity between Human Normal Liver (WRL-68) and Breast Cancer (MCF-7) Cell lines," *J. Biotechnol. Lett.*, vol. 4, no. 1, pp. 45–50, 2013.

[7] D.-D. Herea, C. Danceanu, E. Radu, L. Labusca, N. Lupu, and H. Chiriac, "Comparative effects of magnetic and water-based hyperthermia treatments on human osteosarcoma cells," *Int. J. Nanomedicine*, vol. 13, pp. 5743–5751, 2018.

[8] B. Sanz, M. P. Calatayud, T. E. Torres, M. L. Fanarraga, M. R. Ibarra, and G. F. Goya, "Magnetic hyperthermia enhances cell toxicity with respect to exogenous heating," *Biomaterials*, vol. 114, pp. 62–70, 2017.

[9] C. G. Chaussy and S. Thüroff, "High-Intensity Focused Ultrasound for the Treatment of Prostate Cancer: A Review," *J. Endourol.*, vol. 31, no. S1, 2017.

[10] H. L. Rodríguez-Luccioni, M. Latorre-Esteves, J. Méndez-Vega, O. Soto, A. R. Rodríguez, C. Rinaldi, and M. Torres-Lugo, "Enhanced reduction in cell viability by hyperthermia induced by magnetic nanoparticles.," *Int. J. Nanomedicine*, vol. 6, pp. 373–380, 2011.

[11] T. C. Kranemann, T. Ersepke, J. Franke, T. Friedrich, A. Neumann, T. Buzug, and G. Schmitz, "An MPI-Compatible HIFU Transducer: Experimental Evaluation of Interferences.," *IWMPI*, pp. 197–198, 2018.

Session 03: Reconstruction, Theory, and Nanoparticle Physics II

selection and drive fields yields a similarity measure to compare patches b and c:

$$\mu_{b,c}(\Omega) = \omega_0 \tilde{\mu}_{b,c}^{\text{SF}}(\Omega) + \sum_{k=1}^{K} \omega_k \, \nu_{b,c}^{k}(\Omega) \qquad (6)$$

with weights $\omega_k \in \mathbb{R}_0^+$ for $k = 0, \ldots, K$. With the weights one can balance the contribution of the individual fields to the global similarity measure.

II.III. Clustering

We used the clustering algorithm k-medoids to group patches into a desired number of clusters based on the cost matrix $\left(\mu_{b,c}(\Omega)\right)_{b,c \in I_C}$. The algorithm assigns each patch to a medoid $c \in I_C$ that leads to the smallest total costs. Each medoid stands for a selected system matrix and the number of medoids is given by the desired number of clusters.

III. Results

The measure and clustering was tested on a set of 15 system matrices measured at different FFP positions with the same gradient strength as it was used in [3]. The weights of the measure are chosen to be

$$\omega_0 = \frac{1}{4 \cdot \max_{r \in \Omega, c \in I_C} \left\| H_{\text{SF}}^c(T^{\xi_c}(r)) \right\|_2} \qquad (7)$$

$$\omega_k = \frac{1}{4 \cdot \max_{r \in \Omega, c \in I_C} \left\| p_{\text{DF}}^k(T^{\xi_c}(r)) \right\|_2}, \quad k = 1,2,3 \qquad (8)$$

which leads to a normalization of the contributing fields. The clustering and corresponding reconstructed images for preset numbers of 15, 9 and 1 system matrices are shown in Fig. 1. Using only 9 (60 %) of the system matrices selected by the clustering algorithm the reconstruction is visually similar to the reconstruction using all 15 system matrices. Particularly, it preserves the rectangular shape of the phantom much better than the efficient multi-patch reconstruction using only the central system matrix. Fig. 2 shows the structural similarity (SSIM) index of the reconstruction with 1 to 15 system matrices compared to the reconstruction where all system matrices are used. The larger the number of used system matrices, the better are the reconstruction results.

IV. Conclusions

The structure of the measure allows to weight and analyze differences in the selection and drive fields individually. It enables to select system matrices prior the calibration procedure which saves time during calibration and memory during reconstruction. As indicated by the progression of the SSIM index the reduction of system matrices in the reconstruction yields a slow increase of image artifacts. Note that the measure is not only applicable for image sequences

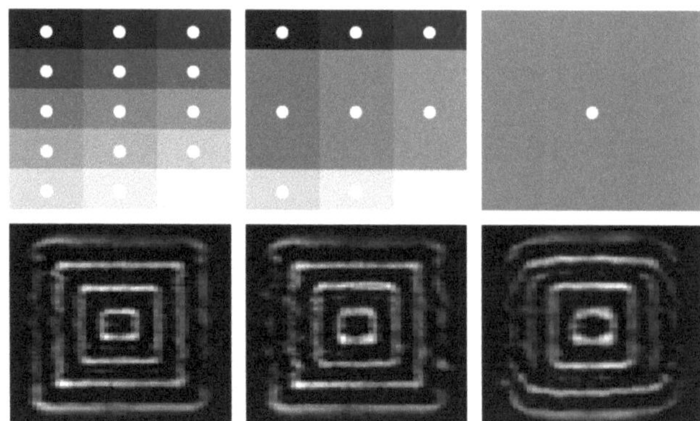

Figure 1: *Results for reusing different numbers of system functions for 15 patches. In the first row it is shown which system matrix (white dot) is used for which patch in the cluster (grey tone). Below the corresponding reconstruction results are shown. From left to right, the basic multi-patch approach, the general multi-patch approach, and the efficient multi-patch approach using a single system matrix are presented.*

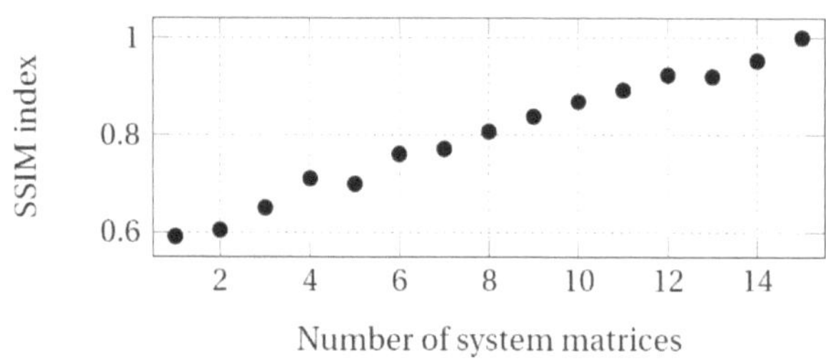

Figure 2: *The SSIM index quantifies the similarity of the optimal reconstruction using 15 system matrices with multi-patch reconstructions using 15 to 1 system matrices.*

with different FFP positions but also for those with various selection or drive field strengths.

AUTHOR'S STATEMENT

Research funding: The authors thankfully acknowledge the financial support by the German Research Foundation (DFG, grant number KN 1108/2-1) and the Federal Ministry of Education and Research (BMBF, grant number 05M16GKA). Conflict of interest: Authors state no conflict of interest. Informed consent: Informed consent has been obtained from all individuals included in this study.

REFERENCES

[1] M. Boberg, T. Knopp, and M. Möddel. Analysis and Comparison of Magnetic Fields in MPI using Spherical Harmonic Expansions. *Book of Abstracts IWMPI*, 2017.

[2] B. Gleich and J. Weizenecker. Tomographic imaging using the nonlinear response of magnetic particles. *Nature*, 435(7046):1214–1217, June 2005.

[3] P. Szwargulski, M. Möddel, N. Gdaniec, and T. Knopp. Efficient Joint Image Reconstruction of Multi-Patch Data reusing a Single System Matrix in Magnetic Particle Imaging. *IEEE Transactions on Medical Imaging*, 2018. ISSN 0278-0062. doi: 10.1109/TMI.2018.2875829.

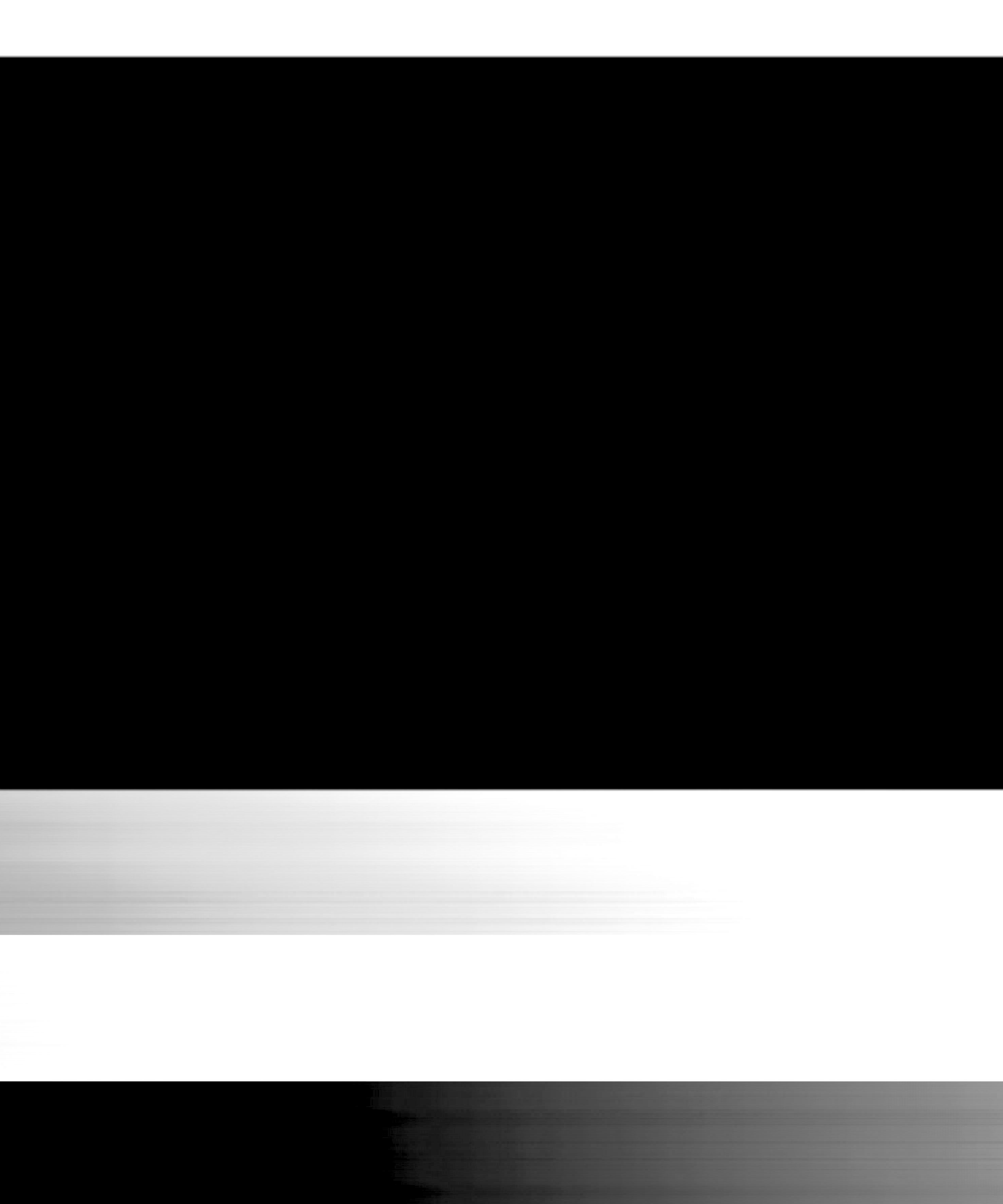

The signal from the entire line of scan after direct feedthrough filtering can be formulated as:

$$s_l(t) = \alpha \dot{x}_s(t)\hat{\rho}\big(x_s(t)\big) - \gamma \sin(\omega_0 t + \theta) \qquad (3)$$

$$x_s(t) = \frac{pFOV}{2}\cos(\omega_0 t) + \varphi t \qquad (4)$$

where φ is the focus field slew rate and $\gamma \sin(\omega_0 t + \theta)$ is the loss due to filtering. Here, we propose to sample $s_l(t)$ with a sampling period $T = \frac{2\pi}{\omega_0}$, i.e.,

$$s_l[n] = s_l(nT + \Delta t) = \beta\hat{\rho}(\Delta x + \varphi nT) - \hat{\gamma} \qquad (5)$$

Here, Δt is a potential timing offset in sampling, and Δx, β, and $\hat{\gamma}$ are constants. Note that after this sampling operation, the signal lost due to filtering is a DC term that is *constant for the entire line*. Assuming the FOV is wide enough, one end of the scanned line can be set to zero to determine $\hat{\gamma}$. Then, the ideal MPI image can be easily obtained as:

$$\hat{\rho}[n] = \frac{s_l[n] + \hat{\gamma}}{\beta} \qquad (6)$$

We refer to this method as "Harmonic Dispersion X-Space MPI (HD-X)", as it relies on the dispersion of information that is otherwise contained in the harmonics.

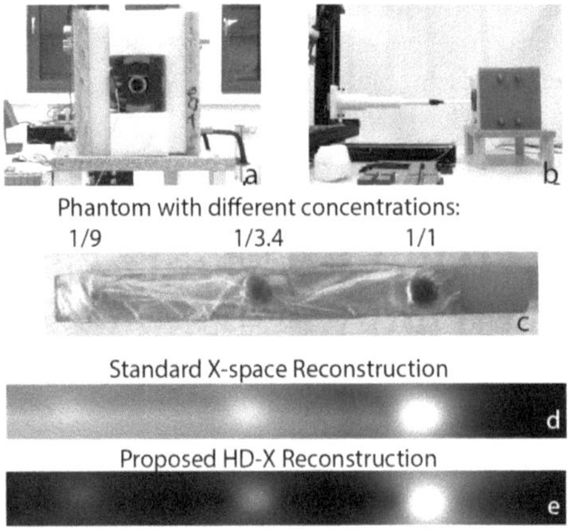

Figure 2: In-house FFP scanner and imaging experiment results. (a) Front and (b) side views of the scanner. (c) Phantom with 3 vials prepared by different concentrations of Perimag nanoparticles: 0.3/9, 0.3/3.4, 0.3 mol Fe/L. (d) Standard x-space reconstructed image. (e) Proposed HD-X reconstructed image.

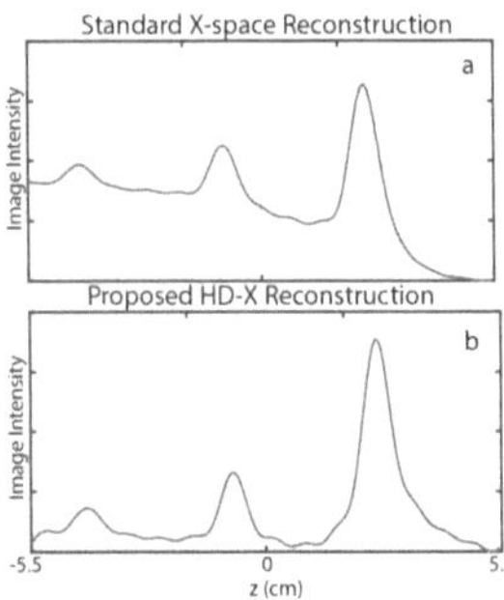

Figure 3: 1D cross-sections of the results in Fig. 2. (a) Standard x-space reconstruction. (b) The proposed HD-X reconstruction.

III. Material and Methods

Imaging experiments were performed on our in-house FFP scanner (Fig. 2a-b), with (-4.8, 2.4, 2.4) T/m selection field gradients, using 10 mT drive field at 9.7 kHz along the z-direction. To emulate the focus field, a robotic arm moved the phantom at a constant speed of 2.92 cm/s along the z-direction, corresponding to 0.07 T/s slew rate. The FOV was 11x0.7 cm^2 in z-x plane, covered in 9 lines in a total scan time of 34 sec. The imaging phantom contained 3 different concentrations (0.3, 0.3/3.4, 0.3/9 mol Fe/L) of Perimag nanoparticles (Micromod GmbH), prepared in 3-mm diameter vials separated at 2 cm distances (Fig. 2c).

IV. Results and Discussion

Figures 2 and 3 compare the proposed HD-X method with the standard x-space reconstruction. The standard x-space reconstruction suffers from a pile-up artifact in image intensity along the scanning direction due to the DC recovery algorithm failing in the presence of relaxation and interference effects. The proposed method, on the other hand, is robust to such effects and can successfully resolve even the vial with the lowest concentration (see Fig. 3b). These results demonstrate improved performance of the proposed technique for resolving low SNR regions.

Due to speed limitations of the robotic arm, the highest slew rate we could test was 0.07 T/s. Simulations suggest that the performance of the proposed method improves at higher slew rates, as the signal energy further disperses to the bands centered around the harmonics (results not shown). This is valid for slew rates extending up to 35 T/s, i.e., well beyond the 20 T/s human safety limit on slew rate.

V. Conclusions

In this work, a simplified approach to x-space reconstruction for linear trajectories is proposed. This technique relies on the dispersion of fundamental harmonic information to nearby bands, and it involves only filtering and sampling, without any pFOV processing. This simple approach proves to be robust against interference and relaxation effects.

AUTHOR'S STATEMENT

Research funding: This work was supported by the Scientific and Technological Research Council of Turkey (TUBITAK 115E677).

REFERENCES

[1] B. Gleich and J. Weizenecker. Tomographic imaging using the nonlinear response of magnetic particles. *Nature*, 435(7046):1214-1217, 2005. doi: 10.1038/nature03808.

[2] J. Rahmer, *et al.* Signal Encoding in magnetic particle imaging: properties of the system function. *BCM Medical Imaging*, 9:4, 2009. doi: 10.1186/1471-2342-9-4.

[3] P. W. Goodwill and S.M. Conolly. The X-space formulation of the magnetic particle imaging process: 1-D signal, resolution, bandwidth, SNR, SAR, and magnetostimulation. *IEEE Trans Med Imaging*, 29(11):1851-1859, 2010. doi: 10.1109/TMI.2010.2052284.

[4] P. W. Goodwill and S.M. Conolly. Multidimensional X-Space Magnetic Particle Imaging. *IEEE Trans Med Imaging*, 30 (9):1581-1590, 2011. doi: 10.1109/TMI.2011.2125982.

[5] K. Lu, *et al.* Linearity and Shift Invariance for Quantitative Magnetic Particle Imaging. *IEEE Trans Med Imaging*, 32 (9):1565–1575, 2013. doi: 10.1109/TMI.2013.2257177.

the actual jumps of the function c. If ψ is fixed correctly the resulting *Variably Scaled Discontinuous Kernel* (VSDK) Φ_ψ determines a discontinuous interpolant that is not affected by the Gibbs phenomenon. For the definition of the scaling function ψ the knowledge or a robust estimate of the edges of the distribution c is required. This can be obtained by edge detection methods such as the Canny edge detector or, in simpler cases, with a thresholding strategy from an initial reconstruction on the **LS** nodes.

III. Results

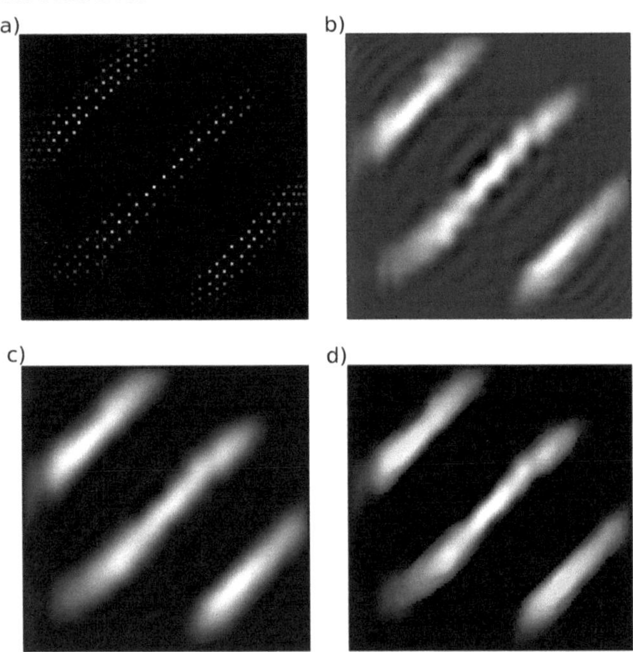

Figure 1: *a) Reduced reconstruction on the Lissajous nodes LS. b) Chebyshev interpolation on LS c) Classically filtered Chebyshev interpolation d) Interpolation using discontinuous kernel functions.*

We test the kernel-based interpolation method on a 2D MPI data set measured in [2] on a simple 3D phantom consisting of 3 parallel cuboids filled with Resovist©. The precise dimensions of the phantom and the conducted measurements are described in [2]. For the reconstruction, the system matrix information on a reduced number of 1249 Lissajous nodes **LS** in the acquisition plane was used. The particle concentration on the nodes **LS** displayed in Figure 1a) was computed by iteratively solving a linear system of equations with a weighted, reduced MPI system matrix and an additional Tikhonov regularization. To obtain the full reconstruction on the field of view Ω a Chebyshev interpolation based on the nodes **LS** was derived in [2]. As can be seen in Figure 1b), this Chebyshev interpolant displays some Gibbs artifacts close to the position of the discontinuities. In [3], classical and adaptive spectral filters were applied to reduce these artifacts. Such a spectral filtered polynomial approximant using a classical cosine filter is displayed in Figure 1c).

For this particular data set, we construct now an improved interpolant based on a discontinuous kernel. As a scaling function ψ we use the filtered Chebyshev reconstruction in Figure 1c) and apply a hard threshold at ⅕ of the maximal signal strength. In this way, a discontinuous scaling function ψ and a resulting discontinuous interpolation kernel Φ_ψ is obtained. The corresponding VSDK interpolant V(x) is shown in Figure 1d).

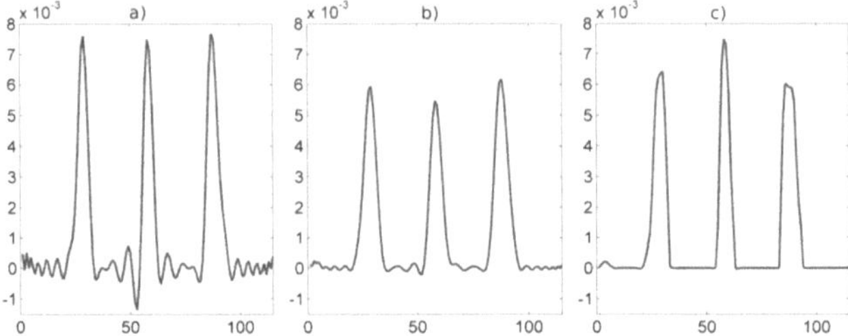

Figure 2: *Diagonals of the images in Figure 1: a) Chebyshev interpolation on LS b) Classically filtered Chebyshev approximation c) Interpolation using discontinuous kernel functions.*

IV. Discussion and Conclusions

The VSDK interpolant V(x) has some remarkable advantages compared to the other two displayed reconstructions displayed in Figure 1 b) and c). The Gibbs effect in Figure 1d) is now completely removed. This can in particular be seen in Figure 2 in which the distributions of the particles along the main diagonal of the images are illustrated. Further, compared to the filtered Chebyshev reconstruction given in Figure 1c), the VSDK reconstruction in Figure 1d) interpolates the original data exactly on the nodes **LS**. Finally, a slight blurring can be observed for the filtered reconstruction, whereas the edges in the VSDK reconstruction turn out to be sharper.

ACKNOWLEDGEMENTS

The authors gratefully acknowledge the support of RITA (Rete Italiana di Approssimazione) and of GeoEssential UE ERA-PLANET GA n. 689443.

REFERENCES

[1] T. Knopp, A.Weber. Sparse reconstruction of the magnetic particle imaging system Matrix. IEEE Trans. Med. Imaging. 32(8) (2013), 1473-80.
DOI: 10.1109/TMI.2013.2258029

[2] C. Kaethner, W. Erb, M. Ahlborg, P. Szwargulski, T. Knopp and T.M. Buzug. Non-Equispaced System Matrix Acquisition for Magnetic Particle Imaging based on Lissajous Node Points. IEEE Transactions on Medical Imaging 35, 11 (2016), 2476-2485. DOI: 10.1109/TMI.2016.2580458

[3] S. De Marchi, W. Erb and F. Marchetti. Spectral filtering for the reduction
of the Gibbs phenomenon for polynomial approximation methods on Lissajous curves with applications in MPI. Dolomites Res. Notes Approx. 10 (2017), 128-137. DOI: 10.14658/pupj-drna-2017-Special_Issue-13

[4] H. Wendland, Scattered Data Approximation. Cambridge University Press
(2004). DOI: 10.1017/CBO9780511617539

[5] M. Bozzini, L. Lenarduzzi, M. Rossini, R. Schaback. Interpolation with Variably Scaled Kernels. IMA J. Numer. Anal. 35 (2015), 199-219. DOI: 10.1093/imanum/drt071

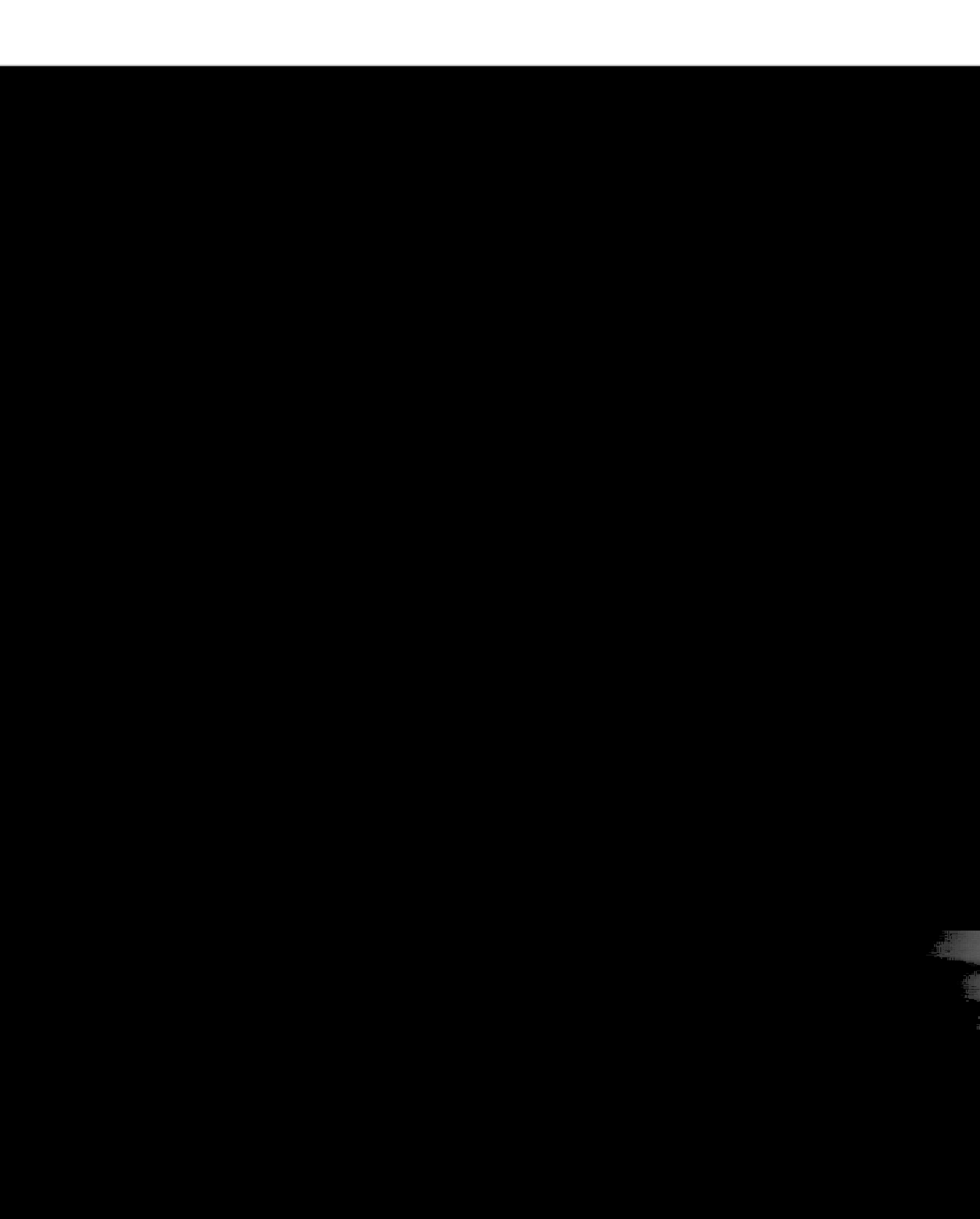

Different measurements have been performed on the particles such as AC susceptometry, magnetorelaxometry, vibrating sample magnetometry and magnetic particle spectroscopy also including parametric sweeps in temperature, frequency and/or viscosity [14]. From these measurements the following values have been obtained for SHP-25: $M_S = 366$ kA/m, $r_m = 10.5$ nm $\pm$ 4.2%, $r_h = 24.2$ nm $\pm$ 5.9% and $K_{uni} = 11.8$ kJ/m^3.

II.III. Details of comparison

To perform the comparison, the dynamic magnetic moment vs. magnetic field curves at field frequencies of 1 kHz and 25 kHz are studied using a field amplitude of 25 mT. These frequencies were chosen because of the fact that at 1 kHz the mechanical/Brownian motion is dominant whereas at 25 kHz the dynamics of the magnetization is dominant. As starting parameters for the simulation the measured values are used and then varied until the simulation results agree reasonable well (mean absolute error compared to the measurement smaller than 5%) with the observed behavior of the particles.

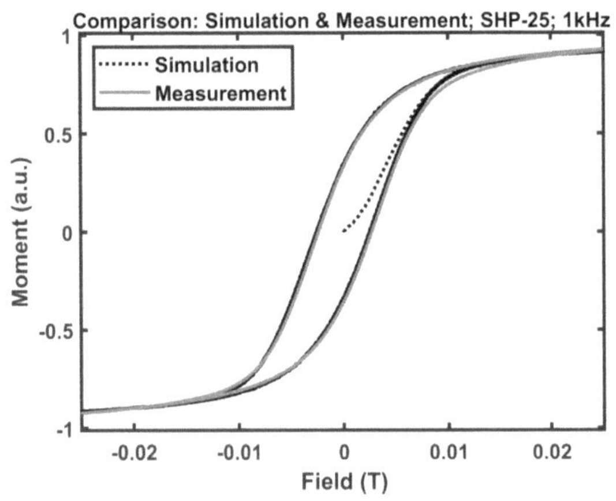

Figure 1: *Comparison of simulation and measurement for SHP-25 at 1 kHz after parameter variation. A good agreement between both is achieved. A slight difference is seen due to asymmetries in the measured signal which may be due to a very small phase error or offset field. This asymmetry would have gone unnoticed without the more symmetric simulation result.*

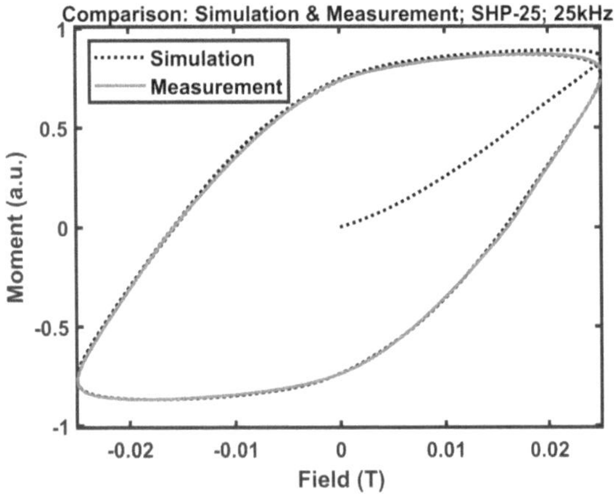

Figure 2: *Comparison of simulation and measurement for SHP-25 at 25 kHz after parameter variation. The same parameters as in Fig. 1 are used and also a good agreement is achieved.*

III. Results & Discussion

Fig. 1 and Fig 2 show the final results after successfully varying the simulation parameters. The parameters used for the displayed simulations are $M_S = 366$ kA/m, $r_m = 11.5$ nm $\pm$ 4.1%, $r_h = 20.0$ nm $\pm$ 6% and $K_{uni} = 16$ kJ/m^3 $\pm$ 40%. These values are very close to the experimental values. The increase (decrease) in r_m (r_h) was necessary to get the correct slope (coercivitiy) of the hysteresis in the 1 kHz measurement (Fig. 1) whereas the increase of K_{uni} and the broad width of K_{uni} are necessary to describe the hysteresis in the 25 kHz measurement (Fig. 2). The broad width of K_{uni} is reasonable due to the fact that the particles are nearly spherical and even a small variation in shape creates a massive variation in shape anisotropy [15]. The distributions of r_m and r_h are not of interest since only very broad distributions >10% lead to a visible change in behavior.

IV. Conclusions & Outlook

The work shows that simulations reproducing the measured behavior can be used to reliably extract particle parameters. Furthermore, due to the direct comparison between simulation and measurements, small errors in the experimental setup may be noticed giving hints on how to improve it. Having a properly validated method to simulate magnetic particles allows one to study parameter ranges which are not yet experimentally available and also allows one to predict the particles behavior under various different external conditions, such as different multidimensional field excitations, temperatures and/or viscosities. In the field of MPI, these simulation will allow one to perform different studies using parametric sweeps and infer on their influence on spatial resolution and/or temporal resolution under well-defined conditions without experimental uncertainties.

ACKNOWLEDGEMENTS

Funding by the Federal Ministry of Education and Research via the Project SAMBA-PATI (FKZ: 13GW0069A) and by the German Research Foundation (DFG) via SPP1681 (VI 892/1-1, LU 400/4-3) are gratefully acknowledged. Furthermore, this work was supported by the Laboratory for Emerging Nanometrology (LENA).

AUTHOR'S STATEMENT

No magnetic particles (simulated or measured) were harmed within the work of this paper.

REFERENCES

[1] C.A. Ross et al. J. Vac. Sci. Technol. B 17, 3168-3176 (1999)
[2] E. A. Périgo et al. Appl. Phys. Rev. 2, 041302 (2015)
[3] M. Arruebo et al. Nanoday 2, 22-32 (2007)
[4] B. Gleich & J. Weizenecker, Nature 435, 1217 (2005)
[5] S. Foner, Rev. Sci. Inst. 30, 548 (1959)
[6] S Biederer et al. J. Phys. D: Appl. Phys. 42, 205007 (2009)
[7] R.M. Ferguson et al. IEEE Trans. Magn. 49, 3441-3444 (2013)
[8] M. I. Shliomis & V. I. Stepanov. Adv. Chem. Phys. Vol. 87, 1 (1994)
[9] P. E. Kloeden & E. Platen. Numerical Solution of Stochastic Differential Equations, 2 ed. ,Springer (1995)
[10] Neumann et al. (2018), 8th Int. W. Magn. Part. Imag., 213.
[11] J. Weizenecker et al. Phys. Med. Biol. 57, 7317-7327 (2012)
[12] M Graeser et al. J. Phys. D: Appl. Phys. 49, 045007 (2016)
[13] S. A. Shah et al. Phys. Rev. B 92, 094438 (2015)
[14] F. Ludwig et al. J. Magn. Magn. Mater 360, 169-173 (2014).
[15] J.A. Osborn, Phys. Rev. 67, 351-357 (1945)

III. Results and Discussion

Figure 1 shows the hydrodynamic size dependence of third harmonic with respect to the MNPs of CMEADM and Et-CMDM series. In particular, we evaluated the third harmonic M_3 normalized by the fundamental harmonic M_1, M_3/M_1. d_H was proportional to d_C in the same series of the measured MNPs. In the CMEADM series, M_3/M_1 had a peak value around d_H= 54–64 nm. This is associated with the distribution of the multicore structure [6, 12]. The effective large core diameter in the multicore structure shows the high harmonic [5]. The effective size distributions of the measured samples showed that the multicore particles of the large effective core diameter were included in CMEADM-033 and -033-02 [12]. On the other hand, because the large core diameter increased the anisotropy energy barrier, M_3/M_1 was decreased.

On the other hand, M_3/M_1 in the Et-CMDM series was lower than that in the CMEADM series. It is characteristic that d_H in the Et-CMDM series were smaller than those in the CMEADM series despite their large d_C. This indicates that the large effective core diameter and small anisotropy in the multicore structure significantly enhanced the nonlinear property of the magnetization associated with the harmonic [12]. We also evaluated the dependence of the transition of the magnetic regime on the size and anisotropy of MNPs by the numerical simulation [13]. This gives the important insight for the development of MNPs for high harmonic because the non-linearity of the magnetization response is determined by the magnetic regimes.

IV. Conclusions

We evaluated the dependence of the harmonic on the d_C and d_H with respect to the different series of MNPs divided into small and large d_H. In the MNPs of the small d_H, the harmonic was lower than that in the MNPs of the large d_H despite their large d_C. The multicore structure was composed in the MNPs in large d_H. It is indicated that the effective core size dominantly affected the non-linear property of magnetization. Because d_H is associated with the effective core diameter of the multicore structure, the third harmonic was depended on d_H. However, the single-core structure is important for the biomedical application because the unexpected aggregation due to the change of the pH and the conjugation with proteins in blood is inhibited. In addition, the result in terms of the MNPs in the solid state will also be shown in the presentation.

ACKNOWLEDGEMENTS

This work was partially supported by the JSPS KAKENHI Grant Numbers: 15H05764, 17H03275, and 17K14693.

REFERENCES

[1] B. Gleich and J. Weizenecker. Tomographic imaging using the nonlinear response of magnetic particles. *Nature*, 435(7046):1217-1217, 2005. doi: 10.1038/nature03808.

[2] N. Panagiotopoulos, RL. Duschka, M. Ahlborg, G. Bringout, C. Debbeler, M. Graeser, C. Kaethner, K. Lüdtke-Buzug, H. Medimagh, J. Stelzner, TM. Buzug, J. Barkhausen, F. Vogt, J. Haegele. Magnetic particle imaging: current developments and future directions. *Int. J. Nanomed.* 2015, 10(1), 3097-3114, 2015. doi: 10.2147/IJN.S70488.

[3] D. Eberbeck, F. Wiekhorst, S. Wagner, and L. Trahms. How the size distribution of magnetic nanoparticles determines their magnetic particle imaging performance. *Appl. Phys. Lett.*, 98, 182502, 2011. doi: 10.1063/1.3586776.

[4] S.A. Shah, R.M. Ferguson, K.M. Krishnan. Slew-rate dependence of tracer magnetization response in magnetic particle imaging. *J. Appl. Phys.* 116, 163910, 2014. doi: 10.1063/1.4900605.

[5] T. Yoshida, N. B. Othman, K. Enpuku. Characterization of magnetically fractionated magnetic nanoparticles for magnetic particle imaging. *J. Appl. Phys.* 114, 173908, 2013. doi: 10.1063/1.4829484

[6] S. Ota, R. Takeda, T. Yamada, I. Kato, S. Nohara, and Y. Takemura. Effect of particle size and structure on harmonic intensity of blood-pooling multi-core magnetic nanoparticles for magnetic particle imaging. *Int. J. Magn. Part. Imaging*, 3(1):1703003, 2017. 10.18416/ijmpi.2017.1703003.

[7] N. Nitta, K. Tsuchiya, A. Sonoda, S. Ota, N. Ushio, M. Takahashi, K. Murata, and S. Nohara. Negatively charged superparamagnetic iron oxide nanoparticles: a new blood-pooling magnetic resonance contrast agent. *Jpn. J. Radiol*, 30(10):832—839, 2012. doi: 10.1007/s11604-012-0133-0.

[8] H. Gavilán, A. Kowalski, D. Heinke, A. Sugunan, J. Sommertune, M. Varón, L.K. Bogart, O. Posth, L. Zeng, D. González-Alonso, C. Balceris, J. Fock, E. Wetterskog, C. Frandsen, N. Gehrke, C. Grüttner, A. Fornara, F. Ludwig, S. Veintemillas-Verdaguer, C. Johansson, M.P. Morales. Colloidal Flower‐Shaped Iron Oxide Nanoparticles: Synthesis Strategies and Coatings. Particle & Particle Systems Characterization, 34, 1700094, 2015. doi: 10.1002/ppsc.201700094.

[9] Satoshi Ota, Tsutomu Yamada, and Yasushi Takemura, Dipole-dipole interaction and its concentration dependence of magnetic fluid evaluated by alternating current hysteresis measurement, *J. Appl. Phys.*, 117, 17D713, 2015. doi.org/10.1063/1.4914061.

[10] Satoshi Ota and Yasushi Takemura, Evaluation of easy-axis dynamics in a magnetic fluid by measurement and analysis of the magnetization curve in an alternating magnetic field, *Appl. Phys. Express*, 10, 085001 2017. doi.org/10.7567/APEX.10.085001.

[11] Suko Bagus Trisnanto, Satoshi Ota, and Yasushi Takemura, Two-step relaxation process of colloidal magnetic nanoclusters under pulsed fields, *Appl. Phys. Express*, 11, 075001, 2018. doi.org/10.7567/APEX.11.075001.

[12] Satoshi Ota, Yuki Matsugi, Takeru Nakamura, Ryoji Takeda, Yasushi Takemura, Ichiro Kato, Satoshi Nohara, Teruyoshi Sasayama, Takashi Yoshida, and Keiji Enpuku, *J. Magn. Magn. Mater.*, Effects of size and anisotropy of blood-pooling magnetic nanoparticles associated with dynamics of easy axis for magnetic particle imaging, in press, 2018. doi.org/10.1016/j.jmmm.2018.11.043.

[13] Satoshi Ota and Yasushi Takemura, Dynamics of magnetization and easy axis of individual ferromagnetic nanoparticle subject to anisotropy and thermal fluctuations, submitted, 2018.

probes to avoid any non-specific heating. Heating data was analyzed and the ILP was calculated using the Wildeboer corrected-slope method [5].

III. Results and Discussion

The measured MPS amplitudes are plotted as a function of the corresponding measured ILPs in Figure 1.

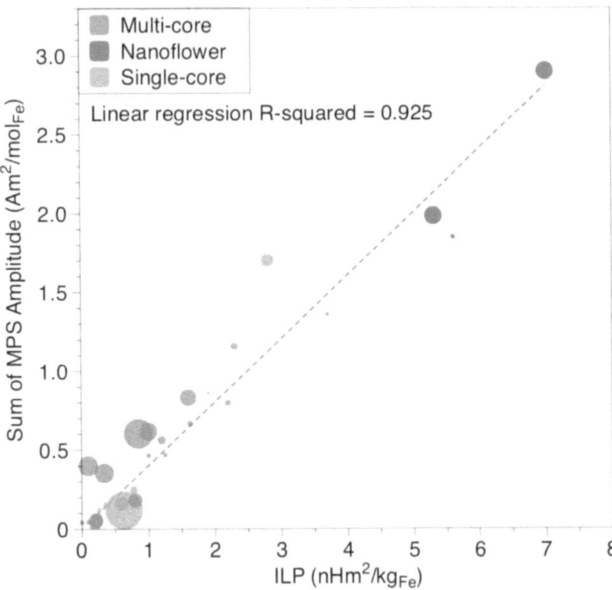

Figure 1: *Sum of MPS odd harmonics (ΣA$_i$) versus ILP values in 28 different MNP systems. The dashed line is the best-fit linear approximation to the correlation. The size of each datapoint represents the median core diameter of each sample, which ranged from 5 to 60 nm. The data are also color-coded to distinguish single-core and multicore systems, with a further distinction of the 'nanoflower' class of multicore MNPs.*

It is evident from Figure 1 that there is a clear correlation between the measured ΣA$_i$ and ILP values across all 28 samples, and across all three classes of MNP system (single-core, multicore, and multicore/nanoflower). It is also clear that there is no obvious correlation with the magnetic core size, as both small and large core-diameter MNPs appear along the entire range, that perhaps can instead be explained by the internal core-core magnetic interactions in the MNPs. The exact nature of the ΣA$_i$-to-ILP correlation cannot be determined from the available data, but to a first approximation it appears to be linear.

The observation of such a correlation between the two metrics is both striking and intriguing. At first sight, there are many reasons why one might expect there to be no such correlation. These include:

(a) that the MPS field amplitude is 2-4 times larger than the ILP field, and at a magnitude that in MFH is known to generate non-linear hysteresis loops [6];

(b) that the MPS driving frequency is ca. 40 times lower than the ILP frequency, which might be expected to elicit quite different dynamic responses; and

(c) that the MPS data were measured at 37 °C while the MFH heating curves ranged from 20 to 50 °C. (MPS spectra are known to be temperature dependent, differing by ca. 5 % from 20 to 37 °C [7].)

However, the existence of the correlation is an indication that the governing process are sufficiently similar that parallels may be drawn between these two quite difference measurement techniques, despite their inherent differences.

This provides us with the prospect of applying theoretical methods such as the kinetic Monte-Carlo simulations used previously [2], as well as analytical models, to explore the behavior of magnetic hyperthermia materials with respect to both MPS and ILP measurement conditions. This dual approach may allow us to achieve better definition and understanding of the underlying processes.

Our findings also underline the necessity for thorough thermal safety checking of promising MPI tracers.

IV. Conclusions

An experimental study of 28 different iron-oxide magnetic nanoparticle sample, covering a broad range of single-core and multicore systems (the latter including the 'nanoflower' class of multicore particles), has revealed a near-to-linear correlation between two standard performance metrics commonly used in magnetic particle imaging and in magnetic field hyperthermia. This intriguing result may allow a deeper understanding of the underlying physical process to be discerned and formulated into useful models, which may in turn lead to design rules for the future development of agents for both of these important healthcare technologies.

ACKNOWLEDGEMENTS

This work was additionally funded by the EMPIR program co-financed by the Participating States, and from the European Union's Horizon 2020 research and innovation program "MagNaStand: Towards an ISO standard for magnetic nanoparticles" (grant no. 16NRM044).

AUTHOR'S STATEMENT

Conflict of interest: none reported. Informed consent: not applicable.

REFERENCES

[1] Q.A. Pankhurst et al., Progress in applications of magnetic nanoparticles in biomedicine. *J. Phys. D* **2009**, *42*, 284001.
[2] C. Jonasson et al., Modelling the effect of different core sizes and magnetic interactions inside magnetic nanoparticles on hyperthermia performance, *JMMM* **2018**, at press.
[3] EU FP7 NMP project NanoMag, grant agreement no: 604448.
[4] J. Wells et al., Probing particle-matrix interactions during magnetic particle spectroscopy, *JMMM* **2018**, *S0304-8853*, 31898-5.
[5] R. R. Wildeboer et al., On the reliable measurement of specific absorption rates and intrinsic loss parameters in magnetic hyperthermia materials, *J. Phys. D* **2014**, *47*, 495003.
[6] R.E. Rosensweig, Heating magnetic fluid with alternating magnetic field, *JMMM* **2002**, *252*, 370–374.
[7] J. Wells et al., Temperature dependence in magnetic particle imaging, *AIP Advances* **2018**, *8*, 056703.

III. Results

The effects of nanoparticle size on MPI image quality, as approximated by MPS, were investigated. The PSF was simulated for a range of particle sizes and applied fields, and the PSF peak and FWHM were extracted.

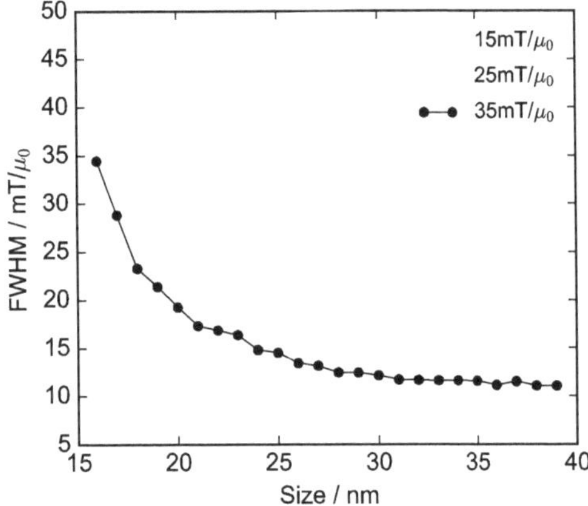

Figure 1: *Simulation results indicating initial resolution improvement with core size for three different applied field amplitudes. The FWHM asymptotes at large sizes.*

It is clear from Fig. 1 that the FWHM initially decreases significantly with increasing size, indicating that larger particles result in better image resolution. However, beyond a certain core size (e.g. ~30 nm for a 35 mT/μ_0 field amplitude) there is minimal improvement as the size continues to increase, and the FWHM value appears to asymptote. The maximum height of the PSF, indicating the signal intensity, follows a similar trend: the peak height increases significantly between core sizes ~15-25 nm, but then shows minimal improvement beyond core sizes of ~30 nm.

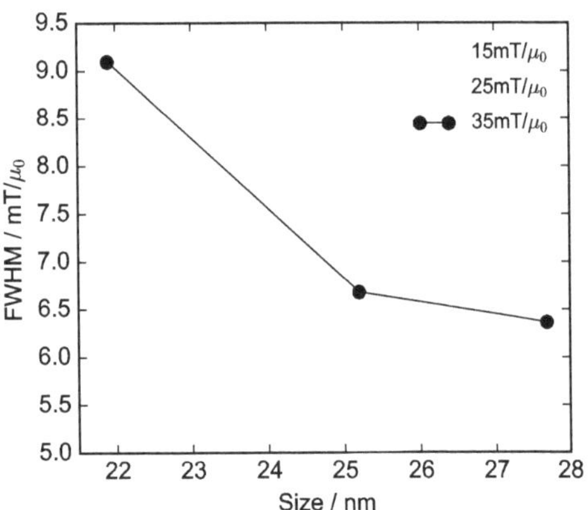

Figure 2: *MPS data indicating resolution improvement with core size for three different field amplitudes.*

Results from MPS are consistent with the simulations. Increasing particle core size from ~22 nm to ~25 nm shows a significant improvement in signal, both in resolution (see Fig. 2) and signal intensity. A much smaller improvement is seen when the size is increased from ~25 nm to ~28 nm.

IV. Discussion

The results indicate that a transition occurs at a certain core size d_c' beyond which a further size increase will not result in significant improvements to the MPI signal. Due to practical difficulties in fabricating large monodisperse particles, as well as increased likelihood for particle agglomeration (resulting in signal drop) for large particles, identifying d_c' is desirable. This transition occurs when relaxation behavior starts to dominate. At this point, the adiabatic term (Eq. 4) will be approximately equal to the relaxation term (Eq. 3). We can extract the relaxation time at which this transition occurs by setting $\Delta x_{\text{adiab}} = \Delta x_{\text{relax}}$:

$$\tau' = \frac{4.16\,k_B T}{\ln(2)v_s \mu_0 M_S V_c} \tag{5}$$

When $\tau > \tau'$, relaxation behavior will dominate. From simulations, the size at which $\tau = \tau'$, which we label d_c', can be extracted. Increasing the core size past d_c' will result in minimal improvements to the signal. d_c' for a range of applied field strengths and frequencies is shown in Table 1. For field parameters typically used for MPI, $d_c' = $ ~28 nm, and generally decreases with increasing field amplitude.

Table 1: *d_c' for different applied field conditions.*

		Applied field amplitude			
		15 mT	20 mT	25 mT	30 mT
Applied field frequency	3 kHz	28.5 nm	28.2 nm	27.9 nm	27.7 nm
	10 kHz	28.9 nm	28.6 nm	28. 5 nm	28.3 nm
	25 kHz	28.0 nm	28.0 nm	28.1 nm	27.9 nm

V. Conclusions

In this work, the effects of nanoparticle relaxation on MPI signal were studied. We found that for typical MPI field conditions, increasing core size to ~28 nm will result in significant signal improvements; however, when core size is increased beyond ~28 nm, relaxation effects dominate and improvements to the MPI signal are minimal.

ACKNOWLEDGEMENTS

C. Shasha was supported by NSF Grant No. DGE-1256082.

REFERENCES

[1] P. W. Goodwill, et al. Ferrohydrodynamic relaxometry for magnetic particle imaging. *Applied Physics Letters,* 98(26), 262502, 2011.

[2] H. Arami, R. M. Ferguson, A. P. Khandhar, and K. M. Krishnan, Size-dependent ferrohydrodynamic relaxometry of magnetic particle imaging tracers in different environments, *Medical Physics,* 40, 071904, 2013.

[3] Croft, Laura R., et al. Low drive field amplitude for improved image resolution in magnetic particle imaging. *Medical Physics* 43.1:424-435, 2016.

[4] S. J. Kemp, R. M. Ferguson, A. P. Khandhar, and K. M. Krishnan. Monodisperse magnetite nanoparticles with nearly ideal saturation magnetization. *RSC Advances,* 6(81), 77452-77464, 2016.

[5] R Matthew Ferguson, Amit P Khandhar, and Kannan M Krishnan. Tracer design for magnetic particle imaging. *Journal of Applied Physics,* 111(7):07B318, 2012.

[6] C. Shasha, E. Teeman, and K. M. Krishnan. Harmonic Simulation Study of Simultaneous Nanoparticle Size and Viscosity Differentiation. *IEEE Magnetics Letters,* 8, 1-5, 2017.

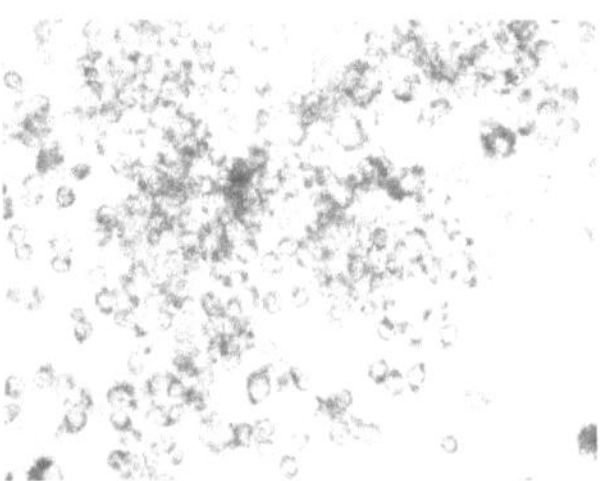

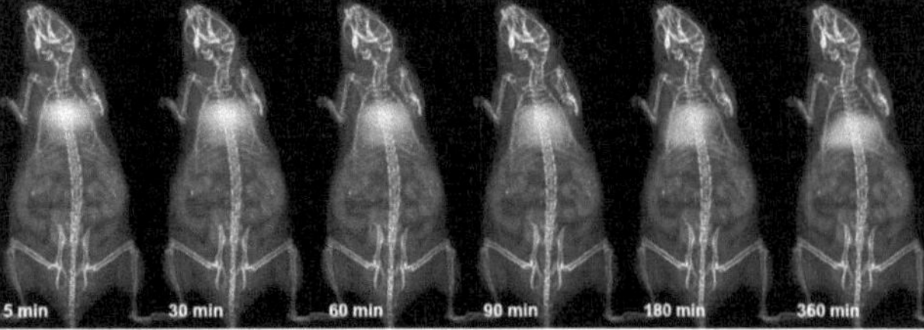

(c) Time course projection MPI images of mice post macrophage injection, overlaid onto x-rays

Figure 1: (a) 10x and (b) 20x microscopy images, respectively, of Prussian Blue stained RAW 264.7 macrophages incubated with Vivotrax SPIOs. (c) MPI leukocyte scans in vivo mice over six hours. SPIO-labeled leukocytes are initially uptaken to the lung vasculature due to their large size; over time, the cells clear to the liver and spleen. X-ray anatomical reference.

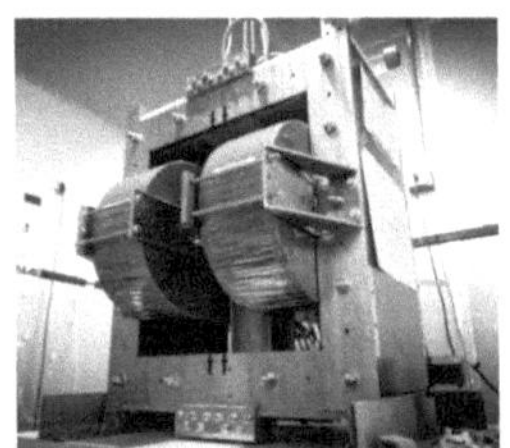
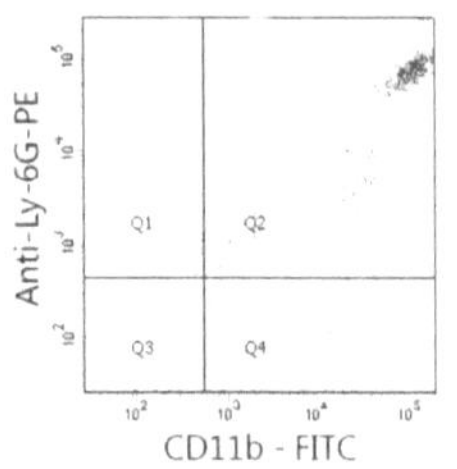

(a) 6.3 T/m FFL MPI Scanner   (b) Neutrophil FACS

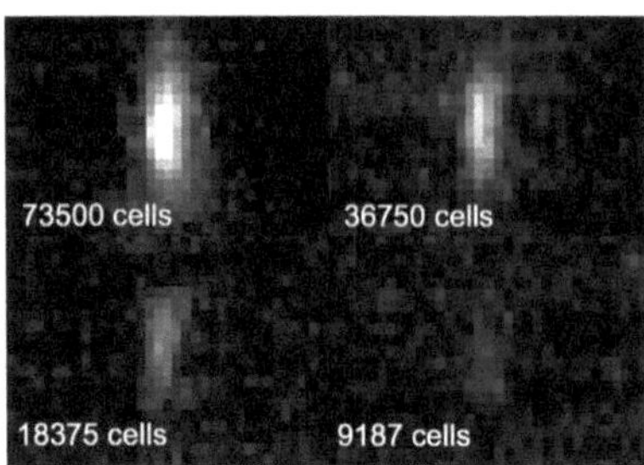

(c) MPI Neutrophil Phantom Scans

Figure 2: (a) UCB MPI 6.3 T/m FFL scanner. (b) Flow cytometry of isolated neutrophils. Neutrophils were confirmed with flow cytometry to have CD11b and Ly6G surface markers. (c) MPI neutrophil phantom scans. Test tubes of SPIO-labeled were scanned and MPI signal was correlated to cell number ($R^2 = 0.967$)

IV. Discussion

Established macrophage cell lines are simple to label and image *in vivo*, but have poor translatability to future clinical use because of they are isolated from tumorigenic origin. Isolation and labeling of autologous cells from peripheral blood for MPI is more clinically translatable, but it is difficult to isolate a high number of cells because of the differences in physiology between humans and mice. Additionally, electroporation resulted in poor viability, while incubation of nanoparticles with the peripheral blood neutrophils (data not shown) resulted in poorer uptake. Future work will require increasing viability post labeling and using optimized SPIOs for MPI in order to increase labeled cell signal.

V. Conclusions

Time course imaging of cultured macrophages and initial work on tracer labeling of neutrophils isolated from whole mouse blood demonstrates that MPI WBC imaging has potential to provide a radiation-free diagnostic complement to Indium-111 WBC and Technetium-99m WBC scans. Future work is needed to optimize cell labeling and viability of autologous cells before further evaluation of the diagnostic potential of MPI WBC scans. Because there is no decay in magnetic signal over time, there is no tradeoff between radioactive half-life, SNR and time constant for optimal pathophysiologic contrast.

AUTHOR'S STATEMENT

Research funding: Research was funded by the USA National Institutes of Health and the National Science Foundation Graduate Research Fellowship Program. Conflict of interest: Prof. Steven Conolly holds equity interest in Magnetic Insight, Inc. Elaine Y. Yu is now an employee of Magnetic Insight holding equity interest, but Dr. Yu's contributions to the abstract occurred while she was a graduate student at UC Berkeley. Ethical approval: All animal procedures were conducted according to the National Research Council's Guide for the Care and Use of Laboratory Animals and approved by UC Berkeley's Animal Care and Use Committee.

REFERENCES

[1] Lewis, S. S., Cox, G. M., & Stout, J. E. (2014). Clinical Utility of Indium 111-Labeled White Blood Cell Scintigraphy for Evaluation of Suspected Infection. *Open Forum Infectious Diseases*, 1(2), ofu089-ofu089. http://doi.org/10.1093/ofid/ofu089

[2] Censullo, A., & Vijayan, T. (2017). Using Nuclear Medicine Imaging Wisely in Diagnosing Infectious Diseases. *Open Forum Infectious Diseases*, 4(1), ofx011. http://doi.org/10.1093/ofid/ofx011

[3] Ziessman, H. A., O'Malley, J. P., Thrall, J. H., & Fahey, F. H. (2013). *Nuclear medicine: the requisites.* Elsevier Inc. Retrieved from https://jhu.pure.elsevier.com/en/publications/nuclear-medicine-fourth-edition-4

[4] B. Gleich and J. Weizenecker. Tomographic imaging using the nonlinear response of magnetic particles. *Nature*, 435(7046):1217-1217, 2005. doi: 10.1038/nature03808.

[5] Zheng, B., Vazin, T., Goodwill, P. W., Conway, A., Verma, A., Ulku Saritas, E., … Conolly, S. M. (2015). Magnetic Particle Imaging tracks the long-term fate of in vivo neural cell implants with high image contrast. *Scientific Reports*, 5(1), 14055. https://doi.org/10.1038/srep14055

[6] Maldiney, T., Bessière, A., Seguin, J., Teston, E., Sharma, S. K., Viana, B., … Richard, C. (2014). The in vivo activation of persistent nanophosphors for optical imaging of vascularization, tumours and grafted cells. *Nature Materials*, 13(4), 418–426. https://doi.org/10.1038/nmat3908

[7] Yu, E. Y., Chandrasekharan, P., Berzon, R., Tay, Z. W., Zhou, X. Y., Khandhar, A. P., … Conolly, S. M. (2017). Magnetic Particle Imaging for Highly Sensitive, Quantitative, and Safe in Vivo Gut Bleed Detection in a Murine Model. *ACS Nano*, 11(12), 12067–12076. https://doi.org/10.1021/acsnano.7b04844

II.III. Image Analysis and Histology

All analysis was performed using VivoQuant software (inviCRO, MA, USA). MRI and MPI image co-registration was performed using OsiriX (Pixmeo, Switzerland). Iron was identified in tissue through Perls Prussian Blue (PPB) staining and microscopy.

III. Results

III.I. *Ex vivo* imaging

MRI signal voids were observed throughout the 4T1 tumor (Fig. 1A), predominately in the tumor periphery. Fewer signal voids were detected in the 168FARN model tumors with MRI (Fig 1D). MPI signal was visualized in the 4T1 (Fig 1B) vs 168FARN (Fig 1E) tumors and quantification or iron indicated a higher uptake in the highly aggressive 4T1 model. Strong MPI signal was also observed within the liver, consistant with clearance through the mononuclear phagocytic system.

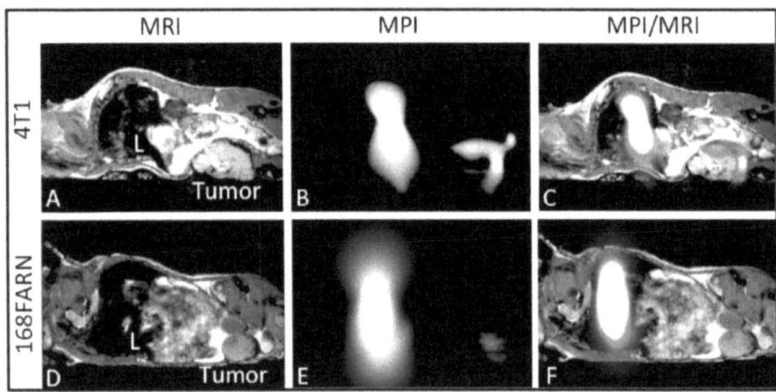

Figure 1: *Iron oxide is visible in the sagittal slices of both tumors with MRI and MPI. Both the 4T1 (A) and 168FARN (B) show signal voids in the tumor and liver. MPI of the 4T1 tumor (B) shows higher uptake of nanoparticles then the 168FARN (E). Co-registered MRI/MPI (C&F) provides the advantages of high specificity, quantification, and resolution.*

MRI of the animals that received the USPIO had a larger signal void area in the tumor compared to the SPIO cohort. Quantification with MPI showed more iron in the 4T1 tumors injected with USPIO vs SPIO, consistent with the MRI findings. Pulmonary metastases were also visualized in the 4T1 mice cohort pre-iron injection (Fig 2A), but this information was lost post-IV iron injection due to loss of contrast (Fig 2B). MPI provided information about differences in iron nanoparticle uptake within the lungs; more iron was quantified in the 168FARN model vs the 4T1.

III.II. Histology results

Visually, the histological images agree with the MRI/MPI data. More PPB+ cells were present in the USPIO 4T1 tumor and within the 168FARN SPIO lungs. F4/80 staining will be performed to verify uptake of the iron agent by macrophages.

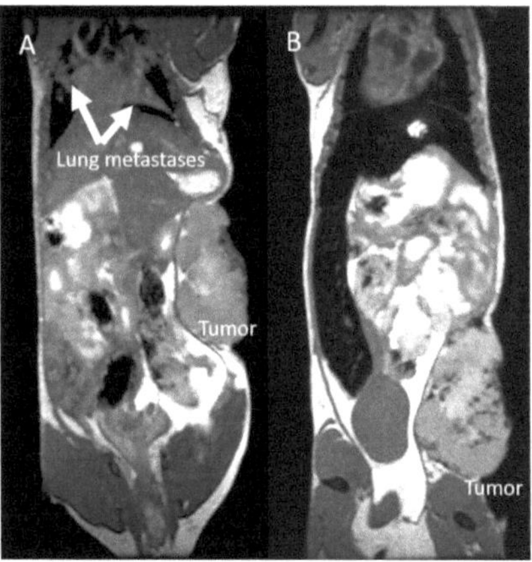

Figure 2: *Lung metastases are visible as bright masses in the MRI before administration of USPIO (A). After systemic SPION administration, the lung metastases are no longer detectable due to the loss of contrast between the lung and iron containing metastasis (B).*

IV. Discussion/Conclusions

Following systemic injection, TAMs were detectable in both the metastatically aggressive 4T1 tumor and the 168FARN tumor which only forms micrometastasis. Multi-modality imaging with MRI and MPI was found to be particularly important when looking at the metastasis to the lungs. The lung metastasis would have been missed when looking only at the post-injection MRI. MRI/MPI overcomes the necessity to obtain a pre- and post- injection scan, a current limitation of clinical SPION cellular MRI. Suprisingly, MPI quantified higher signal in the less aggressive 168FARN lungs compared to the 4T1 model. Future work aims to investigate this further.

By combining the high spatial resolution of MRI with the accurate quantification and specificity of MPI, information can be obtained on TAM presence and distribution. In addition to aiding therapeutic development, this information could be utilized as a biomarker to non-invasively predict the aggressiveness of a tumor.

Author's statement

Conflict of interest: Authors state the following conflict of interests: JMG is an employee of Magnetic Insight with equity interest. Ethical approval: The research related to animal use complies with all the relevant regulations and institutional policies and has been approved by the authors' institutional review board.

References

[1] Obeid E, Nanda R, Fu YX, Olopade OI. The role of tumor-associated macrophages in breast cancer progression. *Int J Oncol.* 2013;43(1):5-12. doi:10.3892/ijo.2013.1938

[2] Bingle L, Brown NJ, Lewis CE. The role of tumour-associated macrophages in tumour progression: Implications for new anticancer therapies. *J Pathol.* 2002;196(3):254-265. doi:10.1002/path.1027.

[3] Makela A V., Gaudet JM, Foster PJ. Quantifying tumor associated macrophages in breast cancer: a comparison of iron and fluorine-based MRI cell tracking. *Sci Rep.* 2017;7(42109)

[4] Goodwill PW, Konkle JJ, Zheng B, Saritas EU, Conolly SM. Projection X-space magnetic particle imaging. *IEEE Trans Med Imaging.* 2012;31(5):1076-1085. doi:10.1109/TMI.2012.2185247.

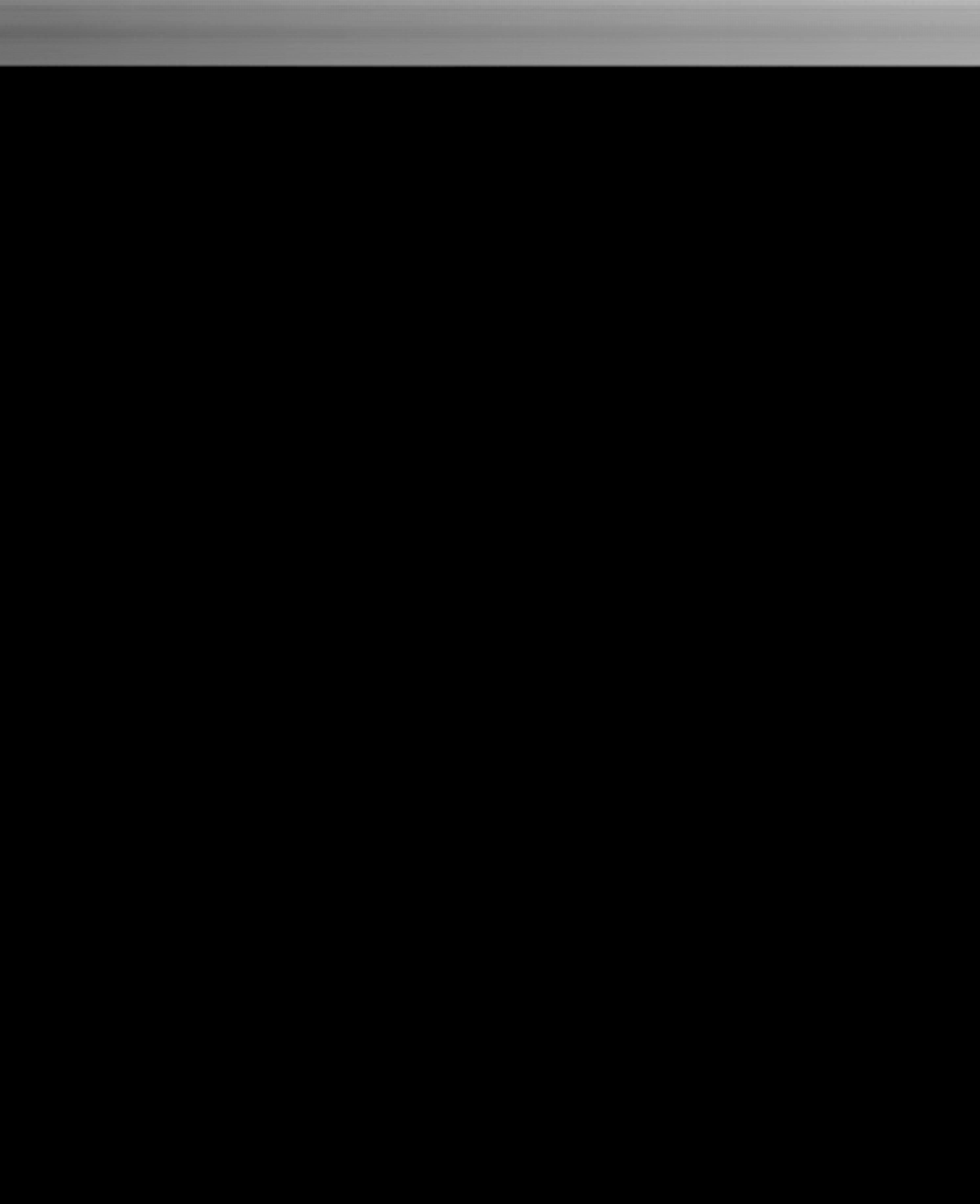

Sandvika, Norway) to a dilution of 100x. Samples were placed in the VIBE apparatus and subjected to a vertical 12 mT field for 5 min. A CaCl₂ solution was added to crosslink the alginate and preserve cell alignment, and the samples were removed from the field for bright-field microscopy.

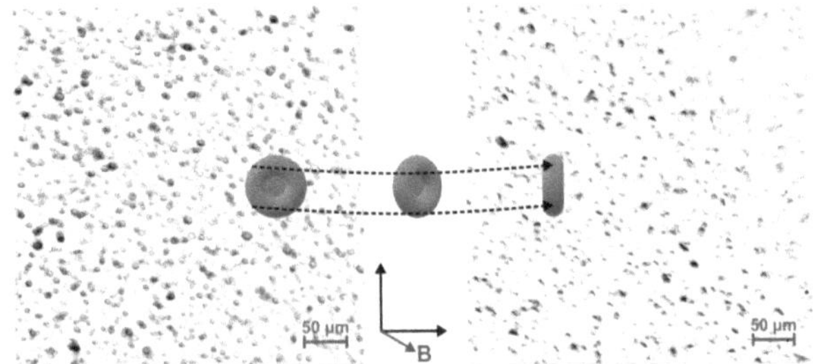

Figure 1: *RBCs in 12 mT vertical field (normal to the page).* **Left:** *Unloaded cells oriented with their disk planes parallel to the slide surface, unaffected by the field.* **Right:** *Loaded cells oriented with their disk planes normal to the slide surface, aligned with the field.*

III. Results

Analysis by a Ferene-s assay indicates that the amount of encapsulated iron increases with the volume of nanoparticles present in dialysis, with 0, 100, 200, 400, and 800 µL of ferucarbotran (per 1 mL RBCs at 70% hct) producing 0.0 ± 0.0, 1.8 ± 1.0, 4.3 ± 0.3, 6.4 ± 1.2, and 10.7 ± 2.7 mM iron in 44% hct RBC suspensions. Subsequent experiments were performed using samples loaded at the optimal ratio of 800 µL/mL. TEM shows that the encapsulated magnetite is monodisperse and well distributed throughout the cells.

Microscopy of alginate-embedded RBCs reveals that unloaded cells remain flat, with the disk plane parallel to the surface of the slide, as expected in stationary fluid. Conversely, loaded cells appear on edge, with the disk plane normal to the surface of the slide, having rotated to align with the vertically oriented magnetic field (**Fig. 1**).

The ability of this RBC alignment to manipulate the conductivity of blood was confirmed by subjecting loaded and unloaded samples to fields alternating between 0° and 90° (i.e., parallel and orthogonal to current flow). Non-flowing samples were subjected to fields of increasing strength (3, 6, 9, 12 mT). In this context, the conductivity of loaded samples increases as cells align with current, and decreases as they align against it, changing by >5% for field transitions of 6 mT or higher (**Fig. 2**). The conductivity of unloaded samples does not change significantly. When subjected to similarly alternating fields of 12 mT, loaded samples flowing at 0.78 mm/s displayed similar modulation of conductivity, though at lower magnitude (~0.5%).

IV. Discussion

The homogenous distribution of SPIO within disk-shaped RBCs creates anisotropic objects that are susceptible to alignment in relatively weak magnetic fields. This enables noninvasive manipulation of the electrical conductivity of blood. Because blood conductivity is significantly higher than that of solid tissues (particularly at the low frequencies of electrophysiological signals), its changes have relatively strong effects on overall tissue conductivity.

By inverting the wiring of the prototype apparatus, a steerable field-free point could be generated, allowing selective modulation of a voxel of tissue, effectively encoding electrophysiological signals generated therein. Demodulation would yield spatially specific EEG signals.

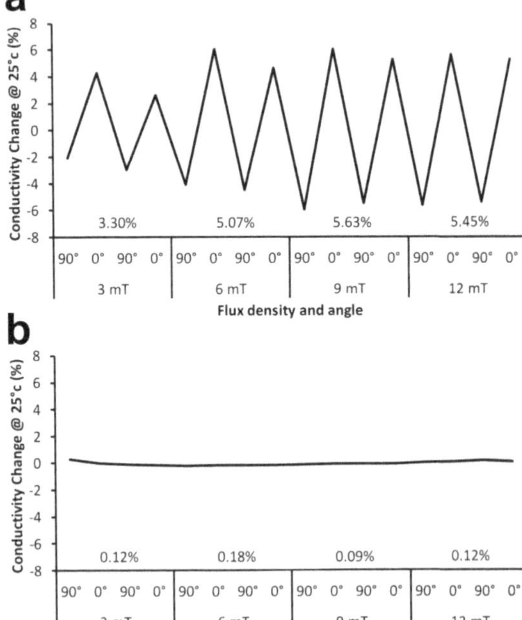

Figure 2: *Conductivity changes of stagnant SPIO loaded (**a**) and unloaded (**b**) RBCs at orthogonal field transitions.*

V. Conclusions

The proposed method expands upon the principles of MPI to reveal a promising path to noninvasive isolation, and thus localization, of EEG signal sources.

AUTHOR'S STATEMENT
Research funding: NIH R24 MH109085. Conflict of interest: Authors state no conflict of interest. Ethical approval: The research related to human use complies with all the relevant national regulations, institutional policies and was performed in accordance with the tenets of the Helsinki Declaration, and has been approved by the authors' institutional review board.

REFERENCES
[1] A. D. Seagar, D. C. Barber, and B. H. Brown. Electrical impedance imaging. *IEE Proc. A*, 134(2):201-210, 1987. doi: 10.1049/ip-a-1.1987.0028.

[2] R. Grech *et al*. Review on solving the inverse problem in EEG source analysis. *J. Neuroeng. Rehabil.*, 5(25), 2008. doi: 10.1186/1743-0003-5-25.

[3] A. Antonelli *et al*. New biomimetic constructs for improved in vivo circulation of superparamagnetic nanoparticles. *J. Nanosci. Nanotechnol.*, 8(5):2270-2278, 2008. doi: 10.1166/jnn.2008.190.

[4] M. Hedayati *et al*. An optimized spectrophotometric assay for convenient and accurate quantitation of intracellular iron from iron oxide nanoparticles. *Int. J. Hyperth.*, 2017. doi: 10.1080/02656736.2017.1354403.

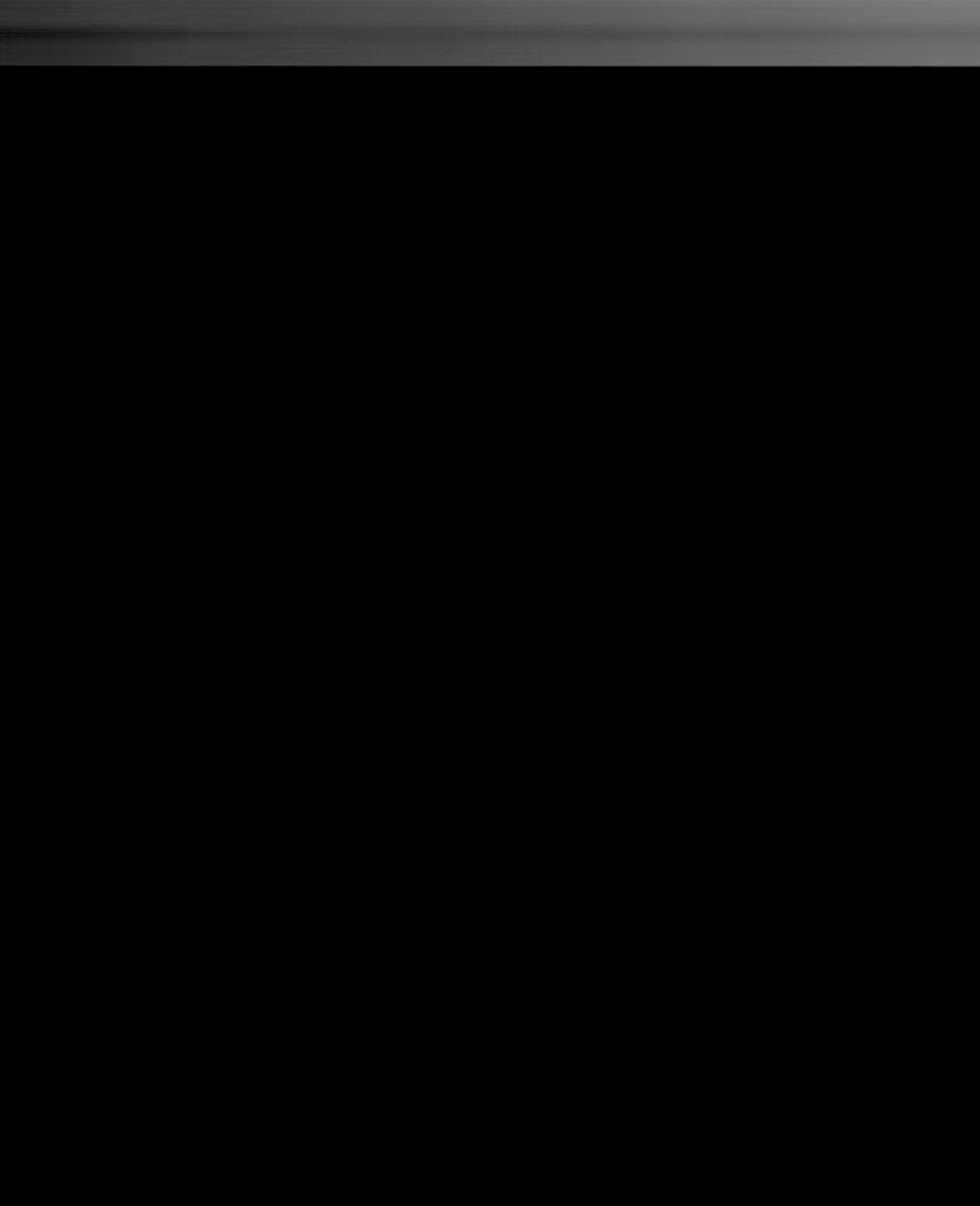

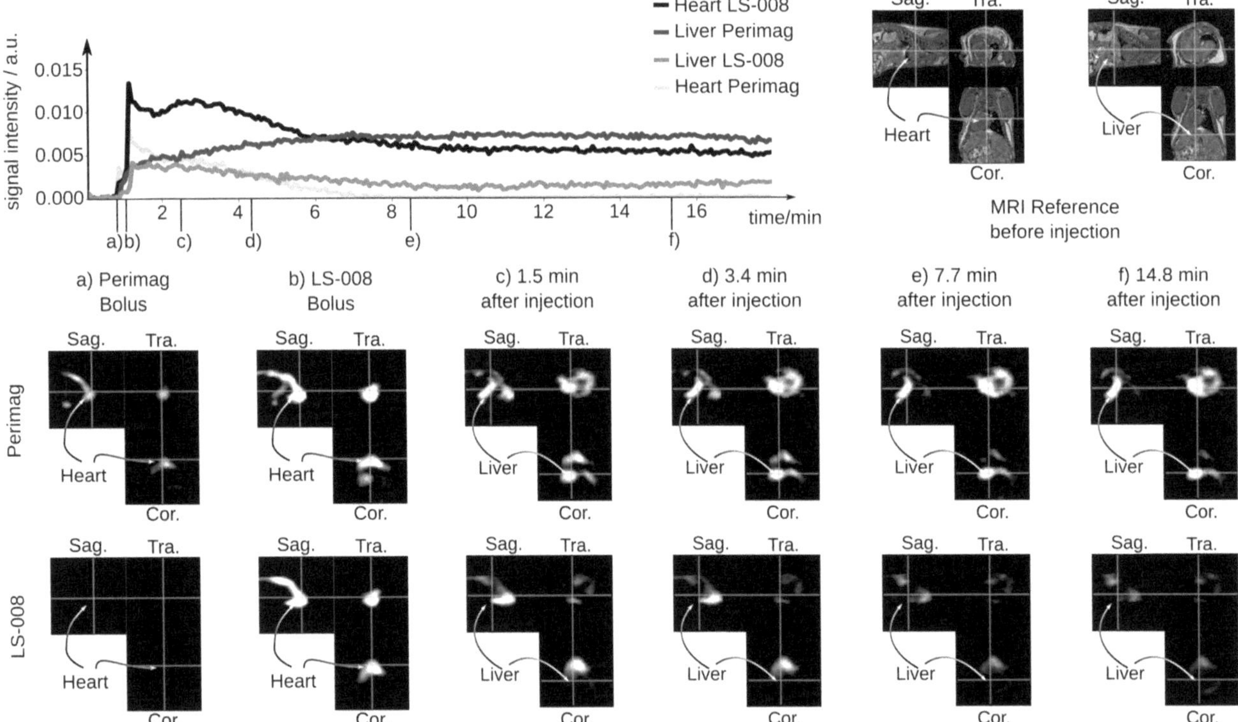

Figure 1: *Dynamic multi-contrast reconstruction results. On top left the signal intensities in the liver and the heart over the first 18 minutes of the measurement for Perimag and LS-008 are shown. In these plots the accumulation of Perimag in the liver and the nearly constant distribution of LS-008 in the blood is visible. Additionally, in a) - f) different time points from the reconstructed data are selected and visualized at the bottom. In a) and b) the focus is set to the heart to image the incoming bolus, while in c) - f) the focus is set to the liver to visualize the accumulation of Perimag over the scan time. In the first row the results from the Perimag reconstruction channel and in the second row the results from the LS-008 reconstruction channel are given. For reference, on the top right, MRI images with annotations on the liver and the heart are shown.*

in the liver over time. After 7 minutes Perimag is mostly eliminated from the vascular system and is accumulated in liver and spleen (not shown).

IV. Discussion

The results demonstrate that both tracer materials, could be visualized *in-vivo* with MPI. However, there are still some outstanding issues that require further analysis. First, the investigation of the signal leakage across the channels is necessary. One can see that e.g. the Perimag bolus is only visible in the Perimag channel, while the LS-008 bolus seems also to influence the Perimag channel in the reconstruction. This might be affected by the experiment design were the materials could not strictly be separated in the preparation of the injection, or it might be an issue of the reconstruction parameters. Second, the investigation of behavior of the MNP inside the body is needed. Dedicated system matrices with e.g. immobilized tracers might be useful to match the binding conditions in the liver and the viscosity changes in the blood. Since the particle behavior depends on the surrounding medium and the accumulation in the organs, the last part is most challenging for multi-contrast MPI. Nevertheless, with functionalized tracers MPI might be a very helpful diagnostic tool e.g. for the detection and perfusion of cancer.

V. Conclusion

With a multi-contrast reconstruction, MPI is capable of visualizing the mixing and the segregation of different tracer materials *in-vivo*. This work provides a proof of principle that MPI has a great potential as a real-time diagnosis tool in combination with functionalized tracer materials.

AUTHOR'S STATEMENT

Research funding: The authors thankfully acknowledge the financial support by the DFG (grant number KN 1108/2-1) and the BMBF (grant number 05M16GKA). Ethical approval: The animal experiment was performed using a healthy mouse approved by local animal care committees (Behörde für Lebensmittelsicherheit and Veterinärwesen Hamburg, Nr. 42/14,70/14,16/41).

REFERENCES

[1] B. Gleich and J. Weizenecker. *Nature*, 435(7046):1217-1217, 2005.
[2] J. Weizenecker et al. *Phys. Med. Biol.*, 54(5): L1–10, 2009.
[3] A. M. Rauwerdink and J. B. Weaver. *J. Magn. Magn. Mater*, 322(6): 609–613, 2010.
[4] M. Möddel et al. *New J. Phys.*, 20 (8): 083001, 2018.
[5] A. M. Rauwerdink and J. B. Weaver, *Phys. Med. Biol.*, 54(6):L51–L55, 2009.
[6] C. Stehning et al. *IJMPI*, 2(2): 16120012, 2016.
[7] J. Rahmer et al. *Phys. Med. Biol.*, 60(5):1775–1791, 2015.
[8] D. Hensley et al. *In Proceedings IWMPI 2018*, p. 185, 2018.
[9] M. Graeser et al. *Sci. Rep.*, 7:6872, 2017.
[10] M. G. Kaul et al. *Phys. Med. Biol.*, 62(9): 3454-3469, 2017.

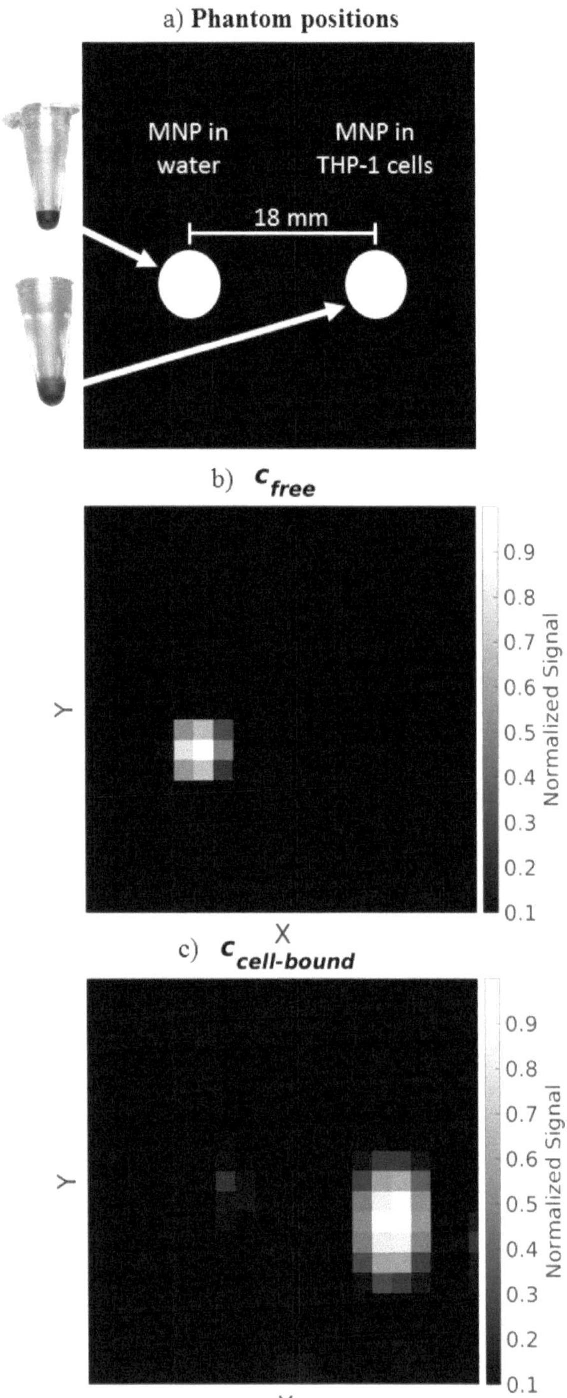

Figure 1: a) *Nominal phantom positions of the water and cell samples b,c) reconstructed particle distributions weighted for free and cell-bound MNPs respectively. Presented are normalized maximum intensity projections along the z-axis.*

III. Results and Discussion

The reconstruction results are presented as normalized, maximum intensity projections for both particle distributions in Fig. 1b and c. For both reconstructed images a clear signal spot can be identified at the correct position of the corresponding sample. A small contribution at the position of the fluid sample in the cell-bound particle distribution can be found (about 10% compared to the signal generated at the location around the cell sample). This might be corrected by optimizing the reconstruction parameters and further post processing steps. However, it is also possible that a proportion of the MNPs in the cell sample, used for the SF acquisition, were still unbound and were not removed in the washing steps during the sample preparation. For an ideal separation two samples would be optimal containing only free and cell-bound MNP respectively.

The results show the potential of fMPI for separating signals of free and cell-bound MNPs. Based on the high temporal resolution of MPI, this technique can be employed to image and quantify the uptake of MNPs into cells starting directly from MNP-cell contact, thereby providing information about the uptake dynamics. Since it is assumed that the uptake dynamics of MNP correlate with pathological changes of the pericellular matrix in diseased tissue, the further development of this technique is highly interesting for diagnostic purposes.

V. Conclusions

In this work we demonstrated, that the MPI image reconstruction can be adapted to discriminate between free and cell-bound MNPs. This enables the acquisition of additional information about the MNPs environment, which potentially can be correlated to pathological conditions. Further phantom studies as well as in-vitro cell uptake measurements will be performed and presented at the conference.

ACKNOWLEDGEMENTS

This project was supported by the DFG research grants "AMPI: Magnetic particle imaging: Development and evaluation of novel methodology for the assessment of the aorta in vivo in a small animal model of aortic aneurysms" (grant SHA 1506/2-1), "quantMPI: Establishment of quantitative Magnetic Particle Imaging (MPI) application oriented phantoms for preclinical investigations" (grant TR 408/9-1) and "Matrix in Vision" (SFB 1340/1 2018, no 372486779, projects A02 and B02).

REFERENCES

[1] N. Löwa, M. Seidel, P. Radon, F. Wiekhorst, J. Magn. Magn. Mater. 427 (2017) 133–138. doi:10.1016/j.jmmm.2016.10.096.

[2] J. Rahmer, A. Halkola, B. Gleich, I. Schmale, J. Borgert, Phys. Med. Biol. 60 (2015) 1775–1791. doi:10.1088/0031-9155/60/5/1775.

[3] C. Stehning, B. Gleich, J. Rahmer, IJMPI. 2 (2016) 1–6. doi:10.18416/ijmpi.2016.1612001.

[4] M. Möddel, C. Meins, J. Dieckhoff, T. Knopp, New J. Phys. 20 (2018) 083001. doi:10.1088/1367-2630/aad44b.

[5] H. Paysen, J. Wells, O. Kosch, U. Steinhoff, J. Franke, L. Trahms, T. Schaeffter, F. Wiekhorst, Phys. Med. Biol. (2018). doi:10.1088/1361-6560/aacb87.

[6] J. Weizenecker, J. Borgert, B. Gleich, Phys. Med. Biol. 52 (2007) 6363–6374. doi:10.1088/0031-9155/52/21/001.

Images were reconstructed by a system function approach using the in-house developed framework (MPILib) with the following parameters: regularization factor 0.5, iterations 5, averages 1, SNR threshold 1.8, bandwidth 80-125 kHz, and spectral cleaning. The system function measurement was performed with a point probe volume of 2 µl containing 100 mM of the same tracer using the same hardware settings as during the dynamic scan measurements. The robot scanned $28 \times 26 \times 16$ positions with 400 averages over 36 hours.

The reconstructed images were analyzed using an image processing software (ImageJ, NIH, USA). Regions of interest (ROI) were placed for each mouse into the right and left ventricle as well into the lung including one pulmonary artery.

III. Results

The injections were in all mice successful. As can be seen in Fig. 2, the temporal extent at half maximum was 591 ± 71 µs in the right ventricle allowing differentiating between right and left ventricle and the intermediate time points. In Fig. 3 an example of the reconstructed images is shown. The three phases show locally separated tracer distributions in the right ventricle, the lungs, and the left ventricle.

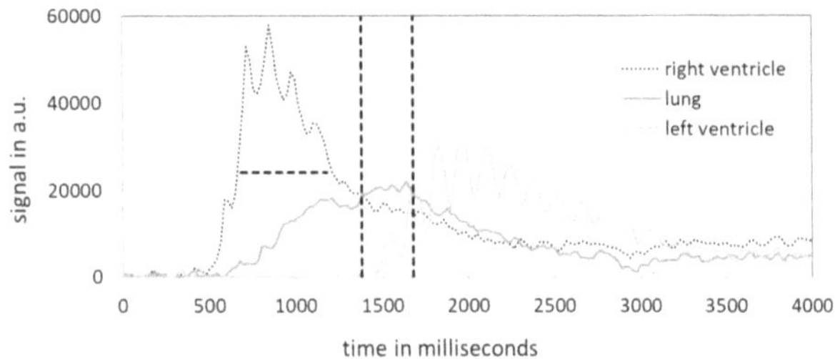

Figure 2: *Example of the inflow of tracer into the right ventricle followed by lung and left ventricle. The width at half maximum of the bolus was 600 µs, so that the signal distributions of different regions can be distinguished. In between the vertical lines, the lung shows the highest signal level. Its maximum is significantly smaller than in the right and left ventricle at other time points.*

IV. Discussion

The sub-second bolus allows to analysis each region on disjunctive time points separating the influence of signal distributions. Perimag was used in a very high concentration of one molar which was diluted during its propagation through the cardiac cycle. A volume of 1 µl is sufficient to reach the ascending aorta. The dedicated mouse coil supports the approach of a sub-second bolus. The tracer volume was decreased substantially in comparison to former examinations using the in-build receiver coils [3–5].

V. Conclusions

MPI is a fast imaging modality offering high temporal resolution. A sub-second bolus can be used to improve the spatial information as signal levels are temporal distinct. Improved reconstruction algorithms may overcome the limitation of restricted dynamic range in future. Short bolus imaging with high concentration is a practical way of improvement in mice, but may not applicable in humans because of safety reasons.

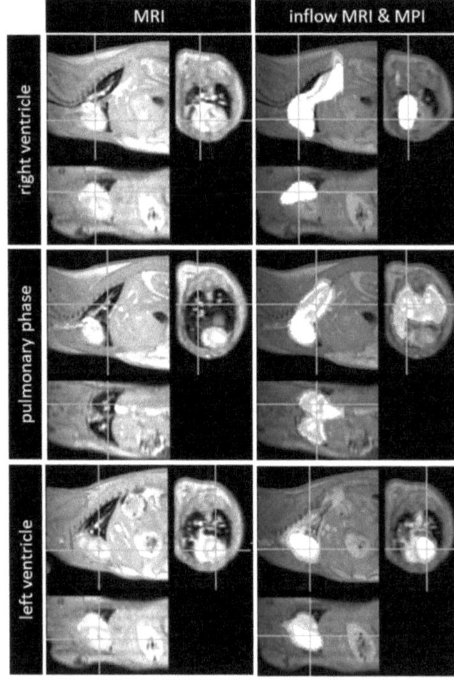

Figure 3: *Example of MRI and fused MRI-MPI-data at three distinct time points showing the inflow of tracer into the right ventricle, the passage through the lungs and the arrival at the left ventricle. The pulmonary phase is not suppressed by high tracer content present previously in the right ventricle.*

ACKNOWLEDGEMENTS
We thank the Free and Hanseatic city of Hamburg for funding.

AUTHOR'S STATEMENT
Research funding: The author state funding involved. Conflict of interest: Authors state no conflict of interest. Informed consent: Informed consent has been obtained from all individuals included in this study. Ethical approval: The research related to animal use complies with all the relevant national regulations, institutional policies as was performed in accordance to the local animal care committee.

REFERENCES
1. Graeser M, Knopp T, Szwargulski P, Friedrich T, von Gladiss A, Kaul M, Krishnan KM, Ittrich H, Adam G, Buzug TM. Towards Picogram Detection of Superparamagnetic Iron-Oxide Particles Using a Gradiometric Receive Coil. Sci Rep. 2017;7: 6872.
2. Weizenecker J, Gleich B, Rahmer J, Dahnke H, Borgert J. Three-dimensional real-time in vivo magnetic particle imaging. Phys Med Biol. 2009;54: L1–L10.
3. Kaul MG, Salamon J, Knopp T, Ittrich H, Adam G, Weller H, Jung C. Magnetic particle imaging for *in vivo* blood flow velocity measurements in mice. Phys Med Biol. 2018;63: 064001.
4. Ludewig P, Gdaniec N, Sedlacik J, Forkert ND, Szwargulski P, Graeser M, Adam G, Kaul MG, Krishnan KM, Ferguson RM, Khandhar AP, Walczak P, Fiehler J, Thomalla G, Gerloff C, Knopp T, Magnus T. Magnetic Particle Imaging for Real-Time Perfusion Imaging in Acute Stroke. ACS Nano. 2017;11: 10480–10488.
5. Kaul MG, Mummert T, Jung C, Salamon J, Khandhar AP, Ferguson RM, Kemp SJ, Ittrich H, Krishnan KM, Adam G, Knopp T. *In vitro* and *in vivo* comparison of a tailored magnetic particle imaging blood pool tracer with Resovist. Phys Med Biol. 2017;62: 3454–3469.

suppression of Brownian relaxation leads to a broadening of the point spread function, which is also more pronounced for 25 kHz.

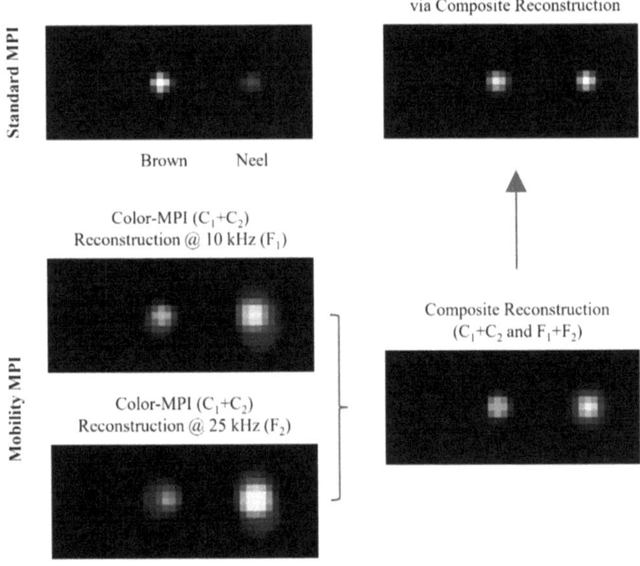

Figure 1: *Standard MPI (top left), multi-spectral MPI at individual frequencies (bottom left), composite reconstruction (bottom right) and resulting concentration estimate (top right).*

Combining the two calibration states (mobile vs. immobile) and the two drive field frequencies (10 kHz and 25 kHz) into a 2×2 composite system matrix, improves separation of different particle mobilities and restores quantitative estimation of the iron content.

IV. Conclusions

Multi-spectral (or composite) reconstruction in MPI enables the simultaneous determination of iron concentration and calibrated particle properties in a time-resolved manner.

ACKNOWLEDGEMENTS

Financial support by the German Research Foundation DFG via SPP1681 (VI892/1-1) and "Niedersächsisches Vorab" through "Quantum- and Nano-Metrology (QUANOMET)" initiative within the project NP-2 are acknowledged.

AUTHOR'S STATEMENT

Research funding: The authors state no funding involved, other than acknowledged above. Conflict of interest: Authors state no conflict of interest.

REFERENCES

[1] B. Gleich and J. Weizenecker. Tomographic imaging using the nonlinear response of magnetic particles. *Nature*, 435(7046):1217-1217, 2005. doi: 10.1038/nature03808.

[2] J. Rahmer, A. Halkola, B. Gleich, I. Schmale, and J. Borgert. First experimental evidence of the feasibility of multi-color magnetic particle imaging. *Phys. Med. Biol.*, 60(5):1775-1791, 2015. doi: 10.1088/0031-9155/60/5/1775.

[3] J. Haegele, S Vaalma, N. Panagiotopoulos, J. Barkhausen, F.M. Vogt, J. Borgert, J. Rahmer. Multi-color magnetic particle imaging for cardiovascular interventions. *Phys. Med. Biol.*, 61(16):N415-426, 2016. doi: 10.1088/0031-9155/61/16/N415.

[4] C. Stehning, B. Gleich, J. Rahmer. Simultaneous magnetic particle imaging (MPI) and temperature mapping using multi-color MPI. *Int. J. Magn. Part. Imag.*, 2(2), 2016. doi: 10.18416/ijmpi.2016.1612001.

[5] T. Viereck, C. Kuhlmann, S. Draack, M. Schilling, F. Ludwig. Dual-frequency magnetic particle imaging of the Brownian particle contribution. *J. Magn. Magn. Mater.*, 427:156-161, 2017. doi: 10.1016/j.jmmm.2016.11.003.

[6] T. Knopp, J. Rahmer, T. F. Sattel, S. Biederer, J. Weizenecker, B. Gleich, J. Borgert and T. M. Buzug. Weighted iterative reconstruction for magnetic particle imaging. *Phys. Med. Biol.*, 55(6), 2010. doi: 10.1088/0031-9155/55/6/003.

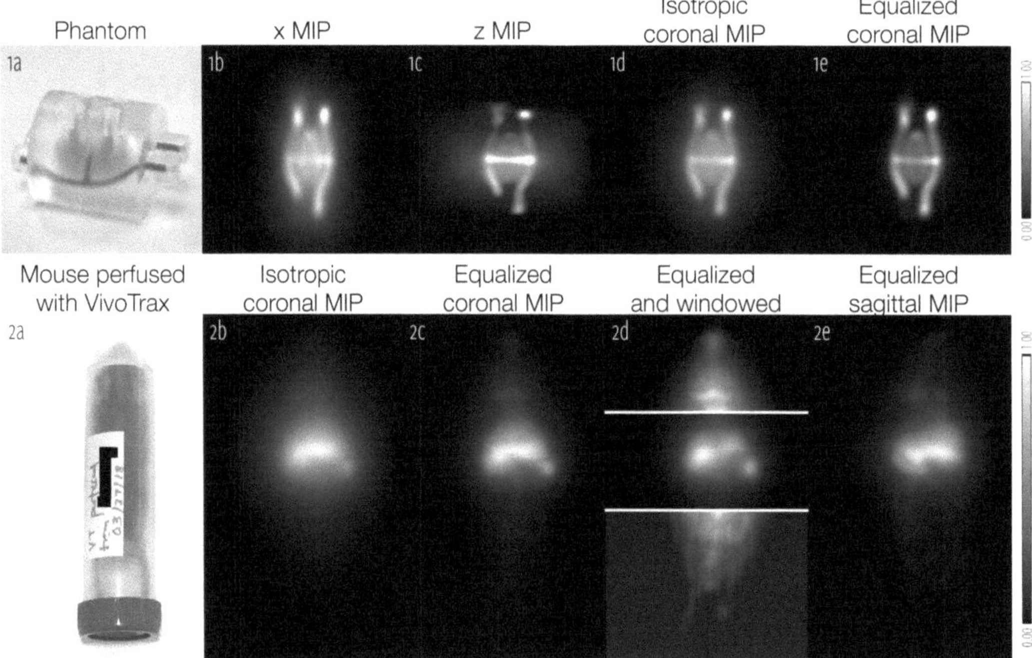

Figure 1: *Particle derived filtered and FISTA-reconstructed Magnetic Particle Imaging (MPI) images to remove $^1/_d$ component of the MPI point spread function in a 3D printed brain phantom and a perfused mouse. 1a) Phantom filled with 0.2 mg/mL VivoTrax in the hemisphere-like lobes, while the "arteries" were filled with 5 mg/mL VivoTrax. 1b) X-only excitation/receive maximum intensity projection (MIP). 1c) Z-only excitation/receive MIP. 1d) Combined x and z channel images results in an isotropic image. 1e) Particle based filter removes the bloom seen in (1d) without introducing artifacts. 2a) C57BL/6 mouse perfused with 100 mL of 5 mg/mL VivoTrax via tail vein injection and sacrificed after 20 minutes. 2b) Isotropic image. 2c) Particle derived filter removes the $^1/_d$ haze seen in (2b) without introducing artifacts. The vascular structure in the brain is more pronounced in this image due to the haze removed from the liver. 2d) Different window and leveling on the filtered data highlights the features in each region. 2e) Sagittal view of the mouse with particle derived filter.*

particles. Step size is automatically calculated from the Lipschitz constant.

III. Results and Discussion

Our phantom data demonstrates that we are able to separate the different components ($^1/_d{}^2$ and $^1/_d$) of the PSF and isolate the higher resolution $^1/_d{}^2$ component. The filtered phantom images clearly differentiate the lobes of the brain and the virtual carotid arteries. In the *in vivo* data, we see that particle derived filtering reduces the liver signal blooming, and that smaller structures are now visible in the brain and the body. The signal from the liver is also clearer, and we can discern the lobes of the liver and the spleen in a slice image. For SNR, the filter reduces the peak signal modestly (70% of prior peak signal), while the signal integrated across the entire sample is reduced. We anticipate the loss in signal may limit applying filtering to more SNR sensitive applications such as cell tracking.

IV. Conclusions

The results presented here demonstrate that FISTA and particle derived filtering of MPI images improves MPI's image quality and dynamic range by preventing larger signals, such as those in the liver, from overwhelming nearby smaller signals such as those from the brain or the rest of the body. While FISTA reconstruction can be used in all images, we anticipate applying particle derived image filtering primarily in higher SNR situations (e.g. blood pool or liver imaging) and with more nuanced application to sensitivity limited applications such as cell tracking.

AUTHOR'S STATEMENT
Research funding: Research reported in this publication was supported by NIBIB of the NIH under award number R43EB020463. The content is solely the responsibility of the authors and does not necessarily represent the official views of the NIH. Conflict of interest: Authors state the following conflict of interests: JMG, RO, PWG, RBK, PP, JJK, DWH, MW are employees of Magnetic Insight with equity interest. Informed consent has been obtained from all individuals included in this study. Ethical approval: The research related to animal use complies with all the relevant regulations and institutional policies and has been approved by the authors' institutional review board.

REFERENCES
[1] B. Gleich and J. Weizenecker. Tomographic imaging using the nonlinear response of magnetic particles. *Nature*, 435(7046):1217-1217, 2005. doi: 10.1038/nature03808.
[2] Zheng, Bo, et al. "Magnetic Particle Imaging." Design and Applications of Nanoparticles in Biomedical Imaging. Springer, Cham, 2017. 69-93.
[3] Goodwill, Patrick W., and Steven M. Conolly. "Multidimensional x-space magnetic particle imaging." IEEE transactions on medical imaging 30.9 (2011): 1581-1590.
[4] Lu, Kuan, et al. "Reshaping the 2D MPI PSF to be isotropic and sharp using vector acquisition and equalization." Magnetic Particle Imaging (IWMPI), 2015 5th International Workshop on. IEEE, 2015.
[5] Konkle et al. "A Convex Formulation for Magnetic Particle Imaging X-Space Reconstruction", PLoS ONE 10.10(2015)

II.II. System Matrix Encoding and Subsampling

We encode each complex number of the SM as RGB vector converted from the HSV color model. First, we encode the phase with hue (H), while saturation (S) and value (V) are set to one. Afterwards, we converted from HSV to RGB color; the amplitude is encoded with the intensity. For training recovery of high resolution (HR) SMs, we subsample a given HR SM equidistantly by using only every second or forth voxel in each dimension to generate a LR SM.

III. Experiments

For evaluation, we conduct two experiments. First, we train our 3d-LapSRN with a subsampled SM and test it on a new LR SM. Secondly, we employ bicubic interpolation as a baseline method and compare it to our model.

III.I. Dataset and Preprocessing

We perform our experiments with two SMs of the particle Perimag using a 4 µL delta sample with a concentration of 100 mmol/L. First, we acquired a HR 3d-SM with 37^3 voxels (scan time 32 h 40 min 54 s) for training our 3d-LapSRN. After thresholding with a signal-to-noise ratio (SNR) of 3, the SM has 3175 frequency components. We zero-pad the HR SM to 40^3 with two rows and one row at the beginning and the end, respectively. Afterwards, we apply our subsampling strategy as in II.II. Thus, our LR SMs have the spatial dimensions 10^3 and 20^3 for the input volume and the two times upscaled volume, respectively. We split the frequencies into 90% training and 10% validation data. Secondly, we acquired a LR SM with 9^3 voxels (scan time 37 min 44 s) for testing our model. To match our models input size of 10^3, we zero-pad one row at the beginning.

III.II Training details

As in [5], we employ similar training strategies. We do not use data augmentation. In total, we train for 700 epochs with 1000 iterations. Each iteration has a minibatch size of 64. For optimization, we use ADAM with $\beta_1 = 0.9$, $\beta_2 = 0.999$, and $L_2 = 10^{-4}$. We trained with a learning rate of 10^{-4} and reduced it by two every 60 epochs. Our model is implemented in PyTorch and trained on two Nvidia GTX 1080Ti GPUs.

III.III Results and Discussion

Our model archived a mean NRMSE of 5.4%, whereas bicubic archived a mean NRMSE of 8.2%. In addition, 42% and 38% of the recovered frequency components have a NRMSE below 5% for our model and bicubic interpolation, respectively. In Fig. 2, we show recovered results for selected example frequencies (i.e. $f \in \{99.5\,\text{kHz}, 400.51\,\text{kHz}, 326.98\,\text{kHz}\}$ from top to bottom) with the NRMSE in percent. The first and second column shows the input LR SM with 9^3 voxels and the corresponding HR SM with 37^3 voxels, respectively. Whereas, the third and fourth column present the model's recovered SM and the bicubic interpolated SM, respectively.

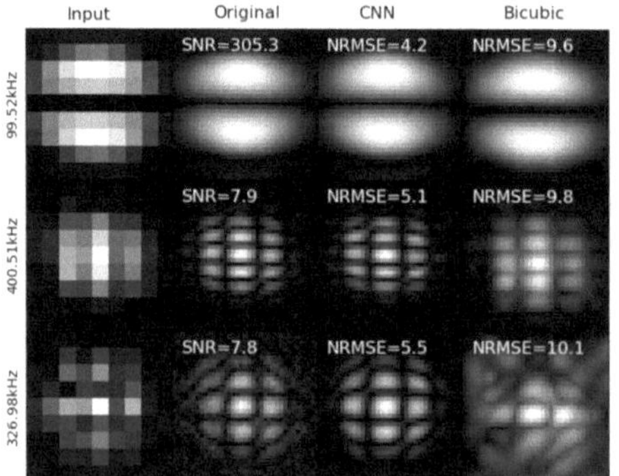

Figure 2: *Examples of some reconstructed SM for three different frequencies. The NRMSE is presented in percent.*

The results demonstrate that DL can be used to recover a SM using only 1/69 of the sampling points. Nevertheless, some frequency components seem to have a relatively high NRMSE. This can be explained by the fact, that the model was trained using only frequency components with an SNR higher than 3 such that some frequency components are misinterpreted by the model. Furthermore, for some frequency components the model corrects some measurement-based imperfections and reduces the noise in the pattern. It thus results in a higher error despite that the patterns looks visually better. In the future, it is of interest to evaluate different kinds of sampling methods, like Poisson sampling or Chebyshev grid sampling. Nevertheless, most interesting will be the application of the model on different particles types and the reconstruction of data using the model-based recovered HR SM.

IV. Conclusions

We have presented a novel method based on a 3d-Laplacian Pyramid Super-Resolution Network for system matrix recovery from a highly undersampled system matrix – i.e. 69 times less samples compared to the original. Our proposed 3d-LapSRN reduced the mean NRMSE by 34.1% compared to bicublic interpolation and sets a new state-of-the-art reduction factor.

AUTHOR'S STATEMENT
Research funding: This work was partially supported by the Forschungszentrum Medizintechnik Hamburg (02fmthh2017). Conflict of interest: Authors state no conflict of interest.

REFERENCES
[1] A. Krizhevsky, I.Sutskever, and G. E. Hinton. *Imagenet classification with deep convolutional neural networks*. Advances in neural information processing systems. 2012.
[2] O. Ronneberger, P. Fischer, and T. Brox. *U-net: Convolutional networks for biomedical image segmentation*. International Conference on Medical image computing and computer-assisted intervention. 2015.
[3] T. Knopp and A. Weber. *Spares reconstruction of the magnetic particle imaging system matrix*. IEEE Transactions on Medical Imaging. 2013.
[4] A. Weber and T. Knopp. *Reconstruction of the Magnetic Particle Imaging System Matrix Using Symmetries and Compressed Sensing*. Advances in Mathematical Physics. 2015.
[5] W. Lai, J. Huang, N. Ahuja, and M. Yang, *Deep Laplacian Pyramid Networks for Fast and Accurate Super-Resolution*. IEEE Conference on Computer Vision and Pattern Recognition. 2017.

$$c^{k+1} = \arg\min_{c \in \mathbb{R}_+^n} \left\| \begin{pmatrix} S \\ \sqrt{\frac{\rho}{2}} L \end{pmatrix} c - \begin{pmatrix} f \\ \sqrt{\frac{\rho}{2}}(u^k + z^k) \end{pmatrix} \right\|_2^2 + \| \delta\, c \|_2^2. \quad (8)$$

The entire matrix can either be split in a row-wise manner (KA I), or for the upper part with the system matrix S, a row-wise KA splitting is used, whereas for the lower part of the matrix ($\sqrt{\frac{\rho}{2}} L$) a block KA splitting is applied (KA II).

With an adaptation strategy for δ, the objective function of the problem in (3) can be minimized. The δ is increased by a factor of 2.1 if the objective function of (3) becomes higher after one ADMM iteration, otherwise it is decreased by factor 0.9. Using this, the convergence rate is better than for the standard ADMM strategy, where the subproblem (5) is solved by a gradient descent (grad. descent) method based on FISTA [7]. For comparison purposes, also an exact solver of (5) (Matlab/*lsqnonneg*), has been used. For the three inexact solvers (KA/grad. descent) for (5) an inner iteration is used, which was set in the tests to two iterations.

For evaluation, the test data have been simulated by the parameters in [8], but the FOV has been discretized to 50×50 pixels. The voltage signal has a signal-to-noise ratio of 20 dB. For the experiments, L and $\mathcal{R}(z)$ were chosen in such a way that the A-TV was optimized.

III. Results

In Fig. 1, the top row shows the phantom and reconstructions results. In the bottom left, the objective function is plotted vs. the number of ADMM iterations, where one iteration is defined by a full evaluation of the steps (5), (6), and (7). Of course, one iteration has different time consumptions for the different solvers. For comparison purposes, also a method in which (5) was solved in an exact manner is shown, which needs significantly more time than all other methods. Quite obviously, the KA solving strategies that use only two inner iterations for the approximation of problem (5) are (in terms of the objective function) nearly as good as the optimal ADMM strategy.

The gradient-based method has significant problems to follow the KAs. It should be noted that the situation becomes better if the number of inner iterations is chosen higher. However, this comes with an increase of the calculation times for one full iteration.

Interestingly, when we look at the mean squared error (MSE) in Fig. 1, bottom right, the optimal ADMM strategy starts to become a little bit worse, whereas the KA strategies always find an optimum.

IV. Discussion

The KAs clearly outperform the gradient descent method, because the system matrix rows are nearly orthogonal to each other. It should be mentioned that grad. descent can be accelerated if the system matrix rows are energy normalized. The energy normalization comes with the drawback that the noise floor is increased within the frequency components and a selection of frequency components becomes

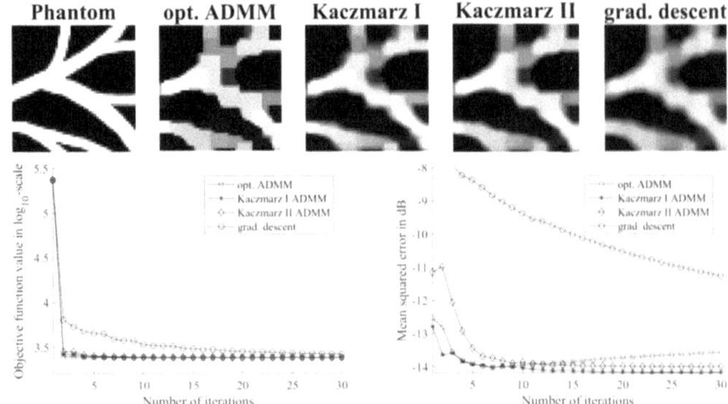

Figure 1: *Top: Reconstruction results after 100 iterations and two inner iterations for the approximation of (5). Bottom Left: The value of the objective function vs. the number of iterations for an anisotropic total variation problem solved by different solvers. Bottom Right: Mean squared error vs iterations.*

unavoidable. In contrast, KA is scale-invariant with respect to the rows of the matrix and the frequency selection is generally unnecessary, but can also help.

V. Conclusions

In this work, a strategy for the use of the Kaczmarz reconstruction in a row-wise manner with more sophisticated priors has been introduced and tested in the 2D total variation regularized setting. The method has been formulated in a generalized form and can be applied to different convex priors as well. If a closed-form solution for (6) is known or the result can be calculated, the algorithm can be efficiently implemented. The extension of the algorithm to non-convex priors is one of the next targets.

Author's statement

This work was supported by the German Research Foundation under grant number ME 1170/7-1. Authors state no conflict of interest.

References

[1] T. Knopp and T. M. Buzug. *Magnetic Particle Imaging: An Introduction to Imaging Principles and Scanner Instrumentation.* Springer, Berlin/Heidelberg, 2012. doi: 10.1007/978-3-642-04199-0.

[2] T. Knopp, J. Rahmer, T. F. Sattel, S. Biederer, J. Weizenecker, B. Gleich, J. Borgert, and T. M. Buzug. Weighted Iterative Reconstruction for Magnetic Particle Imaging. *Phys. Med. Biol.*, 55(6):1577-1589, 2010. doi: 10.1088/0031-9155/55/6/003.

[3] M. Storath, C. Brandt, M. Hofmann, T. Knopp, J. Salamon, A. Weber, and A. Weinmann. Edge Preserving and Noise Reducing Reconstruction for Magnetic Particle Imaging. *IEEE Trans. Med. Imag.*, 36(1):74–85, 2017, doi:10.1109/TMI.2016.2593954.

[4] C. Popa and R. Zdunek. Penalized Least-Squares Image Reconstruction for Borehole Tomography. *Proc. of ALGORITMY*, pp. 260-269,2005.

[5] S. Boyd, N. Parikh, E. Chu, B. Peleato, and J. Eckstein. Distributed Optimization and Statistical Learning via the Alternating Direction Method of Multipliers. *Foundations and Trends® in Machine Learning*, 3(1):1-122, 2010, doi: 10.1561/2200000016.

[6] G. T. Herman, A. Lent, and H. Hurwitz. A Storage-Efficient Algorithm for Finding the Regularized Solution of Large, Inconsistent System of Equations. *J. Inst. Maths Applics*, 25(4):361-366, 1980.

[7] A. Beck and M. Teboulle. A Fast Iterative Shrinkage-Thresholding Algorithm for Linear Inverse Problems. *SIAM J. Imaging Sci.*, 2(1):183–202, 2009, doi:10.1137/080716542.

[8] M. Maass, M. Ahlborg, A. Bakenecker, F. Katzberg, H. Phan, T. M. Buzug, and A. Mertins. A Trajectory Study for Obtaining MPI System Matrices in a Compressed-Sensing Framework. *Int. J. Magn. Part. Imaging*, 3(2), 2017, doi:10.18416/ijmpi.2017.1706005.

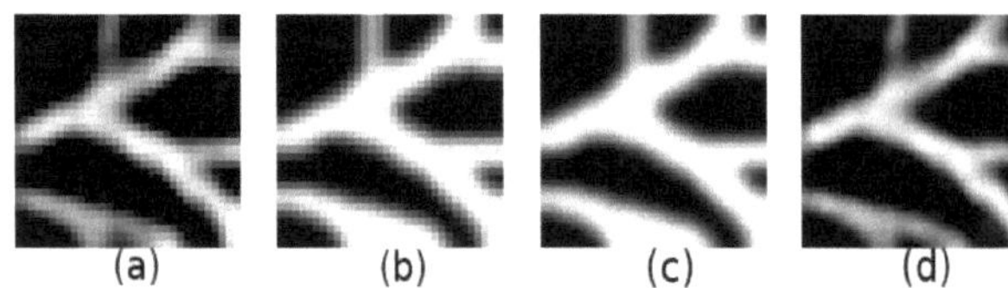

Figure 1: *Reconstruction and support detection procedure. (a) Image reconstruction at level K. (b) Estimated foreground probability at level K. (c) Upsampled foreground estimation. (d) Image reconstruction at level K-1 using (c).*

II.II Simulation

For evaluation, simulated data are used. The MPI scanner simulation uses the Langevin model of paramagnetism and a Lissajous FFP-trajectory with frequency ratio $f_x/f_y = 32/33$. The approach was tested on two vessel phantoms shown in Fig. 2 (left). The phantoms have a size of 250×250 pixels with value 0 (black) at background and 1 (white) and 0.4 (dark gray) in the structures. We used a 9/7 wavelet decomposition in four levels. The constant C was set to 15. The algorithm needs foreground and background seeds, which were chosen automatically as the smallest 40 % of values for the background seed and the highest 20 % values for the foreground seed. For each phantom, a simulated voltage signal with signal-to-noise ratios (SNRs) between 5 and 35 dB was used for reconstruction. A multilevel reconstruction without foreground detection was performed for comparison, which is referred to as baseline. The structural similarity index (SSIM) and the mean absolute error (MAE) of the reconstructions were computed. An SSIM near 1 indicates highly similar structures, while an MAE near to 0 means low errors in the concentration values.

III. Results

In Fig. 2, the reconstructed SPIO distributions for an SNR of 5 dB for the two approaches are shown. The experiments reveal that the proposed method suppresses the noise in the background effectively. For Phantom A less blurred edges are observed. In Fig. 3, the SSIM and MAE for the different SNRs are shown. The parameter λ which produced the best result for SSIM or MAE among the tested values was chosen. The SSIM value of the level-wise segmentation method outperforms the baseline on all phantoms and for all SNRs. The MAE is better for low SNRs using the support detection approach.

IV. Discussion

The proposed multiresolution segmentation method improves the SSIM of the reconstructions. For low SNRs an improvement of the MAE can be seen as well. This is due to the deletion of noise in the background and a tendency to less blurring around the edges of the structures. Although some structures in phantom B have low intensities, they are detected as foreground. It is thinkable that small, isolated structures with low intensities could be removed by the method. For low SNRs those structures are hardly reconstructed by the baseline method either.

V. Conclusions

The multilevel segmentation method provides a reconstruction with improved SSIM. Especially at signals with low SNR it can help to enhance image quality. The results are promising and let one expect that they might further improve with a more sophisticated segmentation method.

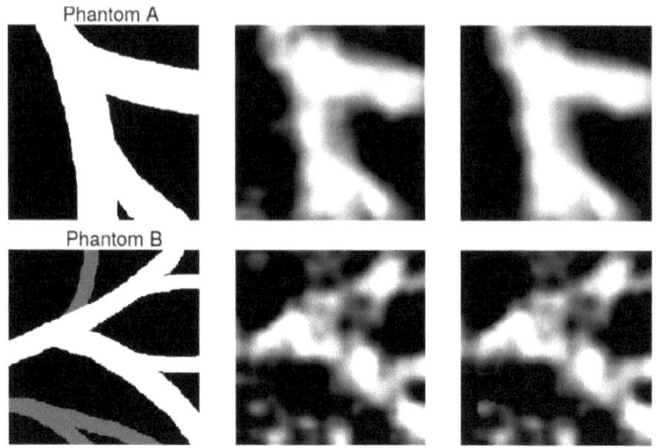

Figure 2: *Reconstructions of the phantoms (left) with best MAE value of the baseline method (middle) and the multilevel segmentation method (right) at an SNR of 5 dB.*

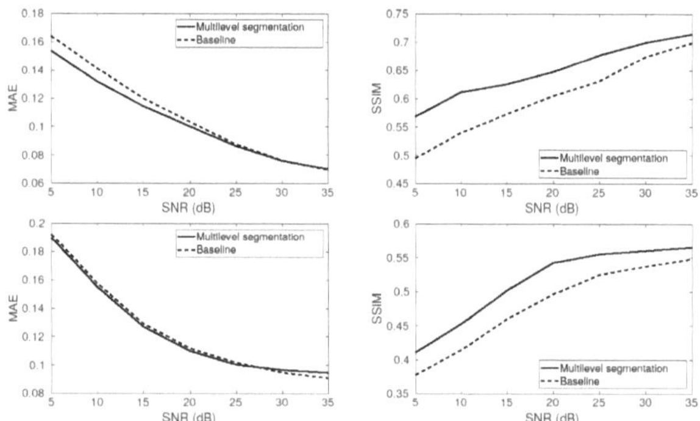

Figure 3: *MAE (left) and SSIM (right) of the phantom reconstructions A (top) and B (bottom).*

AUTHOR'S STATEMENT

This work was supported by the German Research Foundation under grant number ME 1170/7-1. Authors state no conflict of interest.

REFERENCES

[1] B. Gleich and J. Weizenecker. Tomographic imaging using the nonlinear response of magnetic particles. *Nature*, 435(7046):1217-1217, 2005. doi: 10.1038/nature03808.

[2] M. Maass, C. Mink and A. Mertins. Joint multiresolution magnetic particle imaging and system matrix compression. *Int. J. Magn. Part. Imaging*, 4(2), 2018, doi:10.18416/ijmpi.2018.1811002.

[3] H. Siebert, M. Maass, M. Ahlborg, T. M. Buzug and A. Mertins. MMSE MPI Reconstruction Using Background Identification. *Int. Workshop Magn. Part. Imaging*, 58, 2016.

[4] C. Bathke, T. Kluth, C. Brandt and P. Maass. Improved image reconstruction in magnetic particle imaging using structural a priori information. *Int. J. Magn. Part. Imaging*. 3(1), 2017.

[5] Storath, A. Weinmann, J. Frikel and M. Unser. Joint image reconstruction and segmentation using the Potts model. *Inverse Problems*, 31(2), 2015. doi: 10.1088/0266-5611/31/2/ 025003.

[6] L. Grady. Random walks for image segmentation. *IEEE Trans.Pattern Anal. Mach. Intell.*, 18(11): 1768-1783, 2006. doi: 10.1109/tpami.2006.233.

[7] A. Beck and M. Teboulle. A fast iterative shrinkage-thresholding algorithm for linear inverse problems. *SIAM J Imaging Sci.*, 2(1): 183-202, 2009. doi: 10.1137/080716542.

First, the system functions are decomposed by the SVD,

$$S_i = U_i \Sigma_i V_i^T, (i = 1,2,\cdots,N) \tag{1}$$

where S_i is a system function observed while changing the position of field free point (FFP) when the MNPs are arranged at the ith image matrix point, U_i is the left-singular vector, Σ_i is the singular value matrix, V_i is the right-singular vector, V_i^T is the transpose of the matrix V_i, i is sequential matrix number, and N is total number of pixels. The characteristic concept of our image reconstruction method is to newly expand each system function S_j with orthogonal vectors U_i and V_i obtained by expanding other system functions.

$$A_{i,j} = U_i^{-1} S_j V_i^{T-1}, (j = 1,2,\cdots,N) \tag{2}$$

$$V_i = (\boldsymbol{v}_{i;1} \quad \cdots \quad \boldsymbol{v}_{i;r}), (1 \leq r \leq M) \tag{3}$$

where $A_{i,j}$ is the singular vector matrix, j is sequential matrix number, $v_{i;r}$ is the rth right-singular vector, r is indicated which column vector was selected, M is the number of points for observing the magnetization signal generated from the MNP. When the system function S_i is expanded with the orthogonal basis U_i and V_i, the singular value matrix Σ becomes only the diagonal elements, whereas the difference between S_j and S_i is reflected in singular vector matrix $A_{i,j}$ as diagonal elements and non-diagonal elements. Therefore, if information of $A_{i,j}$ is used efficiently, image reconstruction using few orthogonal bases is considered to be possible. So, right-singular vectors were reduced from high-order singular vectors as shown in Fig.1 or equation (3), and image reconstruction was performed using minimum data.

Next, by using the same orthogonal basis U_i, V_i, the observed signals obtained from the unknown MNP's distribution are orthogonally expanded and the singular value matrix B_i is calculated.

$$B_i = U_i^{-1} O V_i^{T-1} \tag{4}$$

where B_i is the singular value matrix. When matrix $A_{i,j}$ and B_i obtained by orthogonal expansion is organized as a column vectors $\boldsymbol{A}_{i,j}$ and $\boldsymbol{B}_i$, the following equation holds,

$$\begin{pmatrix} \boldsymbol{B}_1 \\ \vdots \\ \boldsymbol{B}_N \end{pmatrix} = \begin{pmatrix} A_{1,1} & \cdots & A_{1,N} \\ \vdots & \ddots & \vdots \\ A_{N,1} & \cdots & A_{N,N} \end{pmatrix} P \tag{5}$$

where $\boldsymbol{P}$ is unknown MNP's distribution. An image is reconstructed by applying an inverse matrix solution to the equation (5).

II.II. Conditions of Numerical Analysis

In order to confirm the effectiveness of the proposed method, we performed numerical experiments. A field of view (FOV) was set to 30 mm × 30 mm with a matrix size of 9 × 9. A gradient magnetic field of 2.5 T/m was generated, and an alternating magnetic field of 20 mT was applied. The MNPs (particle diameter: 20 nm) were arranged as shown in Fig. 2.

In order to perform image reconstruction with as few orthogonal bases as possible, in this study, we reduced the number of orthogonal bases of right-singular vectors and examined whether image reconstruction is possible only with low-order orthogonal bases. Also, the number of points for observing the magnetization signal generated from the MNP was 81.

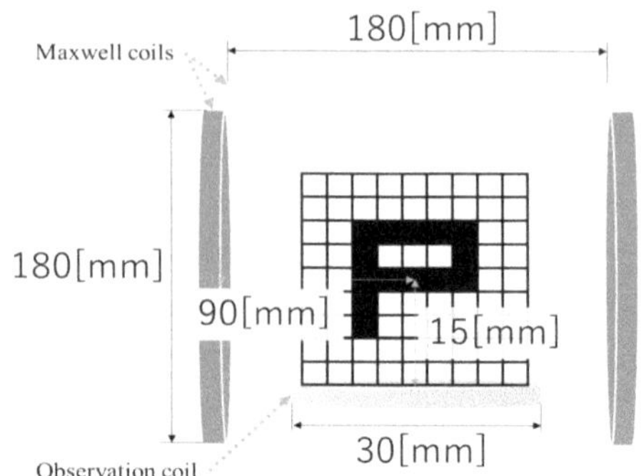

Figure 2: Analysis condition and ideal MNP position

III. Results

Table 1 shows the reconstructed images by the proposed method. In this table, it can be seen that image reconstruction is possible even if the number of orthogonal bases is reduced to 1/81. In this case, the analysis time can be reduced to 1/250.

Table 1: *Results of analysis time and reconstructed image*

Right-singular vectors	Calculation time [sec]	Reconstructed image
One column vector	1.4	
Five column vectors	21.7	
Eighty-one column vectors	358.7	

IV. Conclusions

We proposed a new image reconstruction method using the orthogonal basis obtained by SVD. It was confirmed that image reconstruction was possible with one column vector of right-singular vectors. Based on this, we will consider the use of several orthogonal bases that can reconstruct images for any particle arrangement.

REFERENCES

[1] B. Gleich and J. Weizenecker: Tomographic imaging using the nonlinear response of magnetic particles. *Nature*, vol.435, no.30, pp.1217-1217, 2005.

[2] J. Weizenecker, J. Borgert and B. Gleich: A simulation study on the resolution and sensitivity of magnetic particle imaging. Physics in medicine and biology, vol.52, no.21, pp.6363-6374, 2007.

[3] T. Takagi, H. Tsuchiya, T. Hatsuda, Y. Ishihara, Inverse problem image reconstruction method for magnetic nanoparticle imaging using orthogonal basis by singular value decomposition, Japanese Society for Medical and Biological Engineering, vol.53, no.5, pp.276-282, 2015.

A simulation approach is not recommended for a final implementation, since the simulation has to include every detail of the receive coil and the field generating coil setup. It is however a good start to get an idea of the problem at hand.

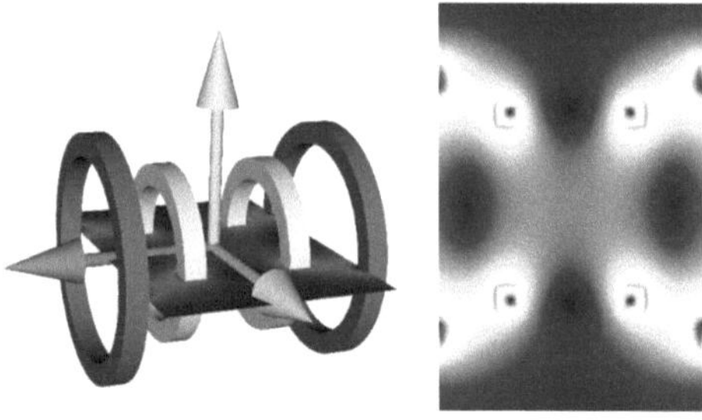

Figure 1: Left: *The coil setup consists of a center coil pair (bright) and a competing coil pair (dark).* **Right:** *A magnetic flux is produced in the center of the setup. Huge magnetic flux is produced between center coil pair and competing coil pair (higher values are brighter).*

We propose a solution, implementing a measurement-based method similar to the one used to design a gradiometric receive coil published in [3]. In figure 1 (right) one realizes the increased magnetic flux between center coil pair and compensation coil pair, leading to increased power demand. To reduce this effect the center coil pair is put as close as possible to the region-of-interest and the compensation coil pair as far away as possible from it.

Following the method in [3], for each of the coil pairs a single loop, with radius of the respective coil pair, is moved along the central axis. Simultaneously, a current is applied to the coils in which the destructive voltage is assumed to be induced in later applications. The induced voltage in the single loop is measured for every position along the central axis with a distance of 1 mm, resulting in an induced-voltage profile for each of the coil pairs.

An algorithm determines position and winding direction of the windings of the self-compensating coil setup, such that it minimizes the induced voltage of the setup. Due to reciprocity, minimizing the voltage induced in the self-compensating coil setup also minimizes the voltage in the receive coils during hyperthermia. The asymmetry of the induced-voltage profiles (see fig. 2) results in an asymmetric coil (see fig. 3)

A prototype has been built and the transmission coefficient from the compensating coil setup to the LNA outputs of the imaging system has been measured.

III. Results & Discussion

Table 1: *Transmission coefficients of the self-compensating coil prototype for different frequencies and imaging coils.*

	Gain/Loss in x-channel coil	Gain/Loss in y-channel coil	Gain/Loss in z-channel coil
300 kHz	−56.05 dBm	−72.62 dBm	−62.55 dBm
500 kHz	−61.19 dBm	−74.44 dBm	−60.44 dBm
700 kHz	−70.25 dBm	−85.02 dBm	−70.25 dBm

The results given in table 1 have been corrected for the gain of the LNA and indicate good performance for all channels of the imaging system, proofing the presented approach is suitable for a self-compensating coil design. The best damping is achieved for a frequency of 700 kHz.

V. Conclusions

In conclusion, for effective protection of the receive chain electronics the self-compensating coil has to be driven at a frequency of 700 kHz. The question remains, whether the specific absorption rate of tissue is too high to conduct in vivo experiments. Although the compensation values are satisfactory, a filter should be integrated in the receive chain for further protection.

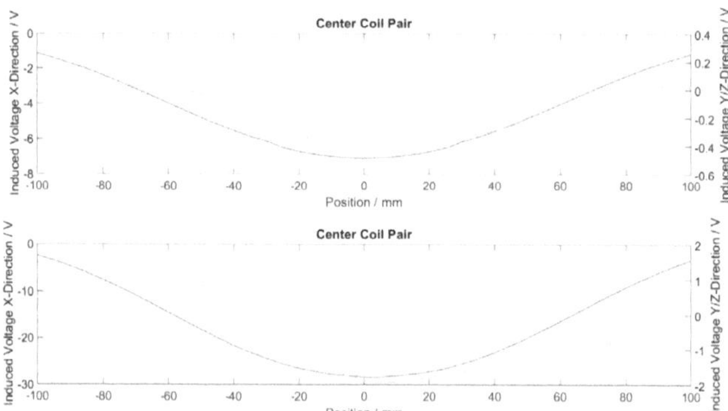

Figure 2: *Profile of the voltage induced in a single loop of the center pair coils (top) and the compensation pair coils (bottom) for different positions in x-direction (dark), y-direction (bright), z-direction (bright dashed) to the loop. The asymmetry of the y- and z-profiles is apparent.*

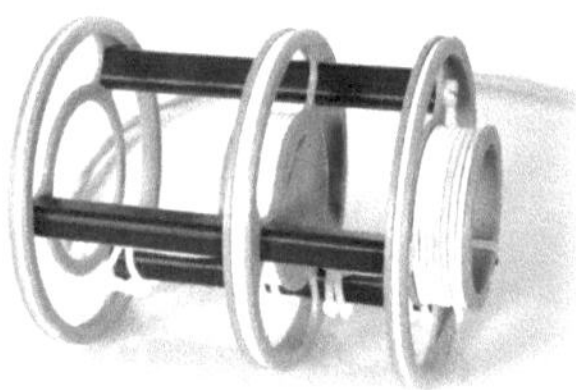

Figure 3: *Photo of the derived self-compensating coil prototype. The center of the coil is between the middle and right windings.*

ACKNOWLEDGEMENTS

We acknowledge the support of the Federal Ministry of Education and Research, Germany (BMBF) under the grant numbers 13GW0230B, 13GW0071D and 13GW0069A.

REFERENCES

[1] C. Stehning, B. Gleich and J. Rahmer. *Simultaneous magnetic particle imaging (MPI) and temperature mapping using multi-color MPI.* International Journal on Magnetic Particle Imaging, 2(2), doi:10.18416/ijmpi.2016.1612001.

[2] D. Hensley, Z. W. Tay, et al. *Combining magnetic particle imaging and magnetic fluid hyperthermia in a theranostic platform*, Physics in Medicine and Biology, 62(9), 3483. doi:10.1088/1361-6560/aa5601.

[3] M. Graeser, T. Knopp, et al. *Towards Picogram Detection of Superparamagnetic Iron-Oxide Particles Using a Gradiometric Receive Coil.* Scientific Reports, 7, 6872, doi: 10.1038/s41598-017-06992-5

To excite magnetic nanoparticles, a low field 1D excitation of a few mT would be sufficient. To complete the MPI scanner setup a receive unit needs to be integrated. Both can be realized either with solenoidal coils or D-shaped coils in single-sided geometry [11].

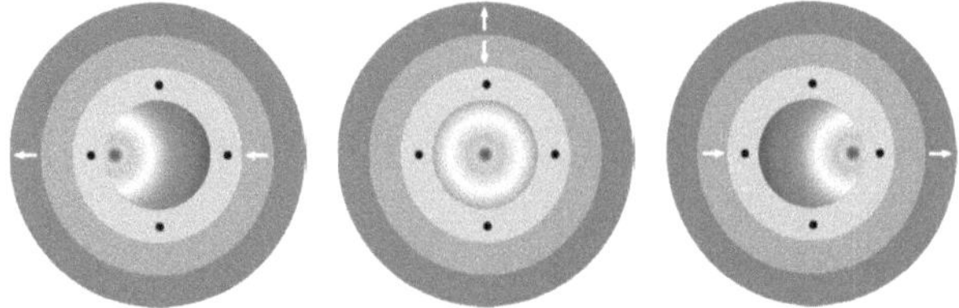

Figure 1: *A schematic drawing of the basic principle of the suggested MPI system. A Halbach quadrupole (innermost cylinder, the four poles are indicated by the four dots) produces the selection field forming an FFP in the illustrated plane. Two counter rotating dipoles (their field directions are indicated by the arrows) move the FFP, here, from left to right. By applying different rotation frequencies, a flower shaped trajectory is obtained, which can be adjusted by choosing the velocity difference.*

II.I. Simulations

Simulations are performed with Comsol Multiphysics (Comsol AB, Stockholm, Sweden) to calculate the needed remanences of the permanent magnets and to validate the magnetic field configurations achieved.

III. Results

The described MPI scanner concept generates the selection field, the drive field and the focus field solely with permanent magnets. It features the adjustability of the gradient strength and enables to switch between a real time imaging mode, an imaging mode for detailed visualization with high resolution and overview scanning with a large FOV.

IV. Discussion

One of the major drawbacks of MPI systems with permanent magnets, so far, is their lack of adjustability. Conceptually the system we propose is almost as flexible as an electromagnetically operated system. However, since the mechanical rotation frequencies are limited the image acquisition rate will be lower. Probably real-time imaging with an acquisition rate of a few Hz will be possible by choosing a coarse trajectory. Since permanent magnets provide high field strengths and steep gradients without excessive power loss, the strength of this MPI system will lie in its resolution rather its acquisition speed.

This concept can be further extended towards 3D imaging. The first approach would be the continuous movement of the object through the 2D imaging system. A second possibility is to utilize the sensitivity profile of an excitation or receive coil. Alternatively, multiple 2D systems in a row could also be combined.

A combination of this MPI system with magnetic manipulation is also investigated. Since Halbach quadrupoles

in combination with dipoles can generate strong uniform gradients as shown in [12]. Magnetic nanoparticles with a magnetic moment $\vec{m}$ experience a force $\vec{F} = \nabla(\vec{m} \cdot \vec{B})$ along the field gradient, which can be used to guide them to predetermined positions, which could be controlled with MPI.

V. Conclusions

A concept for MPI with permanent magnets is presented which will reduce the power requirements dramatically, because only mechanical rotations as well as the generation of a low amplitude excitation field are necessary. Despite using permanent magnets, this system provides high flexibility in adjusting all encoding fields, making it a valid alternative to electromagnetically driven MPI systems with the potential of upscaling. Furthermore, such a system can be used to guide magnetic particles for theranostic treatments.

ACKNOWLEDGEMENTS

The authors gratefully acknowledge the Federal Ministry of Education and Research, Germany (BMBF) for funding this project under Grant Nos., 13GW0071D (SKAMPI) and 13GW0230B (FMT).

AUTHOR'S STATEMENT

Authors state no conflict of interest.

REFERENCES

[1] J. Borgert, J. D. Schmidt, I. Schmale, C. Bontus, B. Gleich, B. David, J. Weizenecker, J. Jockram, C. Lauruschkat, O. Mende, M. Heinrich, A. Halkola, J. Bergmann, O. Woywode and J. Rahmer. Perspectives on clinical magnetic particle imaging, Biomed Tech, 58(6): 551–556, 2013. doi: 10.1515/bmt-2012-0064.

[2] M. Graeser, F. Thieben, P. Szwargulski, F. Werner, N. Gdaniec, M. Boberg, F. Griese, M. Möddel, P. Ludewig, D. van de Ven, O. M. Weber, O. Woywode, B. Gleich, T. Knopp. Human-sized Magnetic Particle Imaging for Brain Applications. ArXiv: 1810.07987, 2018

[3] https://www.bruker.com/products/preclinical-imaging/mpi-welcome.html (visited 15-11-2018)

[4] https://www.magneticinsight.com/ (visited 15-11-2018)

[5] M. Weber, K. Bente, A. von Gladiß and T. M. Buzug. MPI with a mechanically rotated FFL. In International Workshop on Magnetic Particle Imaging 2015.

[6] M. Weber, T. M. Buzug, *Magnetic Field-Generating Device for Magnetic Particle Imaging*, 2017, PCT, WO 2017/050789 A1

[7] M. Weber, J. Beuke, A. von Gladiss, V. Behr, P. Vogel, K. Gräfe, T. M. Buzug, Novel Field Geometry featuring a Field Free Line for Magnetic Particle Imaging, *International Journal on Magnetic Particle Imaging*, vol 4(2), 2018 (in press).

[8] A. Tonyushkin. Single-sided hybrid selection coils for field-free line magnetic particle imaging. International Journal on Magnetic Particle Imaging, 3(1), 2017, doi:10.18416/ijmpi.2017.1703009

[9] H. Bagheri, C. A. Kierans, K. J. Nelson, B. A. Andrade, C. L. Wong, A. L. Frederick, and M. E. Hayden. A mechanically driven magnetic particle imaging scanner. Appl. Phys. Lett. 113, 183703 (2018); doi: 10.1063/1.5052646

[10] P. Blümler. Proposal for a permanent magnet system with a constant gradient mechanically adjustable in direction and strength. Concepts in Magnetic Resonance Part B, 46(1) 41-48, 2016, doi: 10.1002/cmr.b.21320

[11] K. Gräfe, A. von Gladiß, G. Bringout, M. Ahlborg, and T. M. Buzug. 2D Images Recorded with a Single-Sided Magnetic Particle Imaging Scanner, IEEE Transactions on Medical Imaging, 35(4), 1056-1065, 2016, doi: 10.1109/TMI.2015.2507187.

[12] O. Baun, P. Blümler. Permanent magnet system to guide superparamagnetic particles. Journal of Magnetism and Magnetic Materials, 439 (2017) 294–304, doi: 10.1016/j.jmmm.2017.05.001

III. Results

Three consecutive 3D blocks of image data were obtained and merged. As the tracer volume in each test tube was rather small, the tracer was detected in the center slice only (Fig. 2a). The selected slice was merged with a photograph (Fig. 2b).

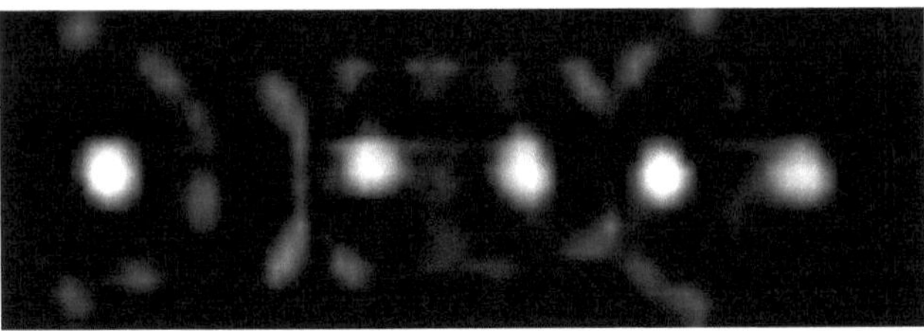

a

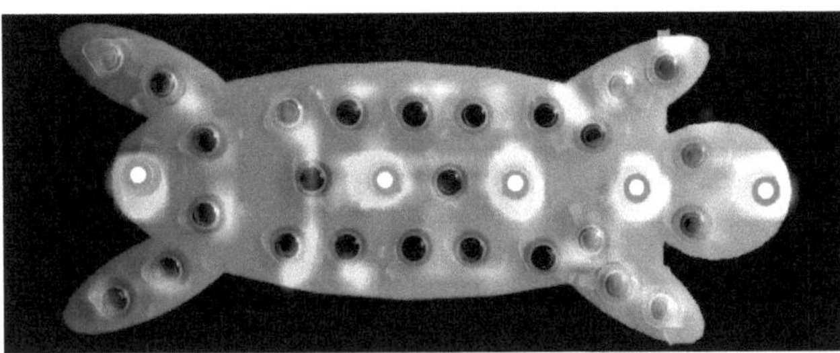

b

Figure 2: a) Three merged MPI scans. b) An overlay of the MPI scan with a photograph of the phantom.

This simple experiment proved that sequential scanning of larger objects with a small FOV is possible and feasible with minimal hardware modifications.

IV. Discussion

Field of view limitations (mainly low drive field and missing focus field) caused by hardware settings may be easily overcome by sequential scanning. Essentially no special hardware is required for the precise movement of the scanned object, provided the scanner is equipped with a robot (an inseparable part of FFP machines requiring calibrations).

The method demonstrated in this study enables work with smaller FOVs, therefore allowing higher selection field gradients to be used, which increases spatial resolution.

Another approach for scanning of larger FOVs is the utilization of focus fields [1]. This option may suffer from image distortions caused by possible field imperfections far away from the center of the scanner. Sequential scanning overcomes these problems by scanning of small FOVs always placed in the scanner center.

Usage of smaller FOVs also eliminates time-consuming calibration of large matrices.

However, the proposed method decreases temporal resolution. As the movement itself requires just a fraction of a second, the most time-consuming part of the measurement is repetitive preparation and setting of the scanner. Nevertheless, if the sequential scanning is implemented directly into the scanner software (thus avoiding manual control of the robot and unnecessary repetitive settings), each single step of the sequential scan (including a move of the scanned object) should last less than 1 s (unless more acquisitions are required).

The presented study is a proof-of-principle, confirming that this straightforward approach can be implemented on any MPI scanner with minimal effort. However, its utilization in routine practice will require further optimization of gradient strength and FOV settings, considering also the overlap of partial FOVs and more sophisticated post-processing.

V. Conclusions

Hardware limitations of our MPI scanner do not enable scanning of large FOVs. This was overcome by the simple movement of a scanned object and repeated scanning. A robot, originally dedicated for calibration measurements, was used for precise repositioning of the object in the scanner. Sequential measurements represent a convenient and accessible method of scanning without usage of the focus field.

ACKNOWLEDGEMENTS

Research funding:

Project GAČR No. 19-02584S funded by Czech Science Foundation

Projects Czech-BioImaging LM2015062 and SVV 260371/2017 funded by Ministry of Education Youth and Sports, Czech Republic

REFERENCES

[1] B. Gleich, et al., Fast MPI Demonstrator with Enlarged Field of View. *Proc. Intl. Soc. Mag. Reson. Med.* 18:218, 2010.

[2] P. Bornert, and B. Aldefeld, Principles of whole-body continuously-moving-table MRI. *Journal of Magnetic Resonance Imaging*, 28(1):1, 2008.

[3] P. Szwargulski, et al., Enlarging the Field of View in Magnetic Particle Imaging using a Moving Table Approach. *Medical Imaging 2018: Biomedical Applications in Molecular, Structural, and Functional Imaging*, 10578, 2018.

[4] P. Szwargulski, et al., Moving table magnetic particle imaging: a stepwise approach preserving high spatio-temporal resolution. *Journal of Medical Imaging*, 5(4): 046002, 2018.

[5] C. T. Rueden, J. Schindelin, M. C. Hiner, et al. ImageJ2: ImageJ for the next generation of scientific image data. *BMC Bioinformatics* 18:529, 2017.

Similar values were calculated by determining the minimum instead of the maximum values for each individual measurement.

III. Results

The averaged minima and maxima values of each system function are presented over time in Fig. 1 for all three implemented receive channels.

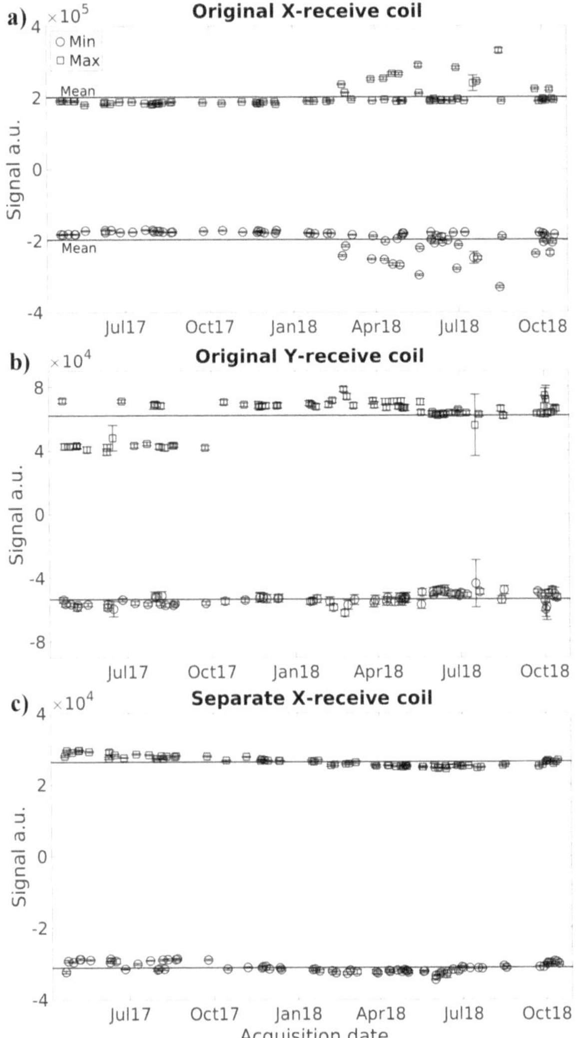

Figure 1: *Averaged maximum or minimum values of the signal for each SF over the last 1.5 years (see (1)). The uncertainty bars present the standard deviation during the acquisition. The horizontal lines depict the mean value over all SFs.*

Ideally, an empty scanner measurement would yield the same result every time. However, due to changing environmental conditions (temperature, humidity, …) and possible wear of hardware components over time, signal fluctuations and signal drifts can be observed. Such effects can be seen e.g. in Fig 1c) for the minimum and maximum values acquired with the gradiometric separate receive coil. During the last 1.5 years, a slow signal drift towards lower signal amplitudes could be observed. However, the maximum deviation from the mean value is below 12%. Additional causes for non-

stable empty scanner signals could be permanent hardware changes or external distortions. These might be the reasons for the rather high deviations of the original x- and y-receive coils of our scanner in the last 1.5 years, for which a maximum deviation of 67% and 27% compared from their mean values were determined (Fig. 1 a, b). Especially around July 2017 and starting from March 2018 strong deviations can be observed for the y- and x-receive coils respectively. The exact causes for these effects have not been clearly identified so far.

IV. Discussion

The results presented here represent only the first step towards a full characterization of the long-term system performance. Next, additional investigations will be performed in the frequency domain by analyzing the signal stability of all frequency components over time. The results will be correlated with appropriate phantom measurement data, to review the influence of the observed signal drifts and fluctuations on the qualitative and quantitative information of MPI images.

Additional information can be extracted from these datasets to investigate a number of other issues: Does the total acquisition time effect the system stability? What is the influence of the measurement parameters? Are diurnal changes observable in the data? All these questions will be addressed, and the results will be presented at the conference.

V. Conclusions

A method for analyzing the system stability of a MPI scanner over time is presented. For this purpose, empty scanner measurement data, acquired over the last 1.5 years, were collected and analyzed in the time domain. Analysis of the data revealed signal drifts and fluctuations up to 67% of the acquired raw signals. In the near future, additional investigations will be performed and the influence of these signal drifts on reconstructed MPI images will be evaluated.

ACKNOWLEDGEMENTS

This project was supported by the DFG research grants "AMPI: Magnetic particle imaging: Development and evaluation of novel methodology for the assessment of the aorta in vivo in a small animal model of aortic aneurysms" (grant SHA 1506/2-1), "quantMPI: Establishment of quantitative Magnetic Particle Imaging (MPI) application oriented phantoms for preclinical investigations" (grant TR 408/9-1) and "Matrix in Vision" (SFB 1340/1 2018, no 372486779, projects A02 and B02). This project has received funding from the EMPIR programme co-financed by the Participating States and from the European Union's Horizon 2020 research and innovation programme under grant number 16NRM04 MagNaStand.

REFERENCES

[1] N. Löwa, J.-M. Fabert, D. Gutkelch, H. Paysen, O. Kosch, F. Wiekhorst, J. Magn. Magn. Mater. 469 (2019) 456–460. doi:10.1016/J.JMMM.2018.08.073.

[2] L. Wöckel, J. Wells, O. Kosch, S. Lyer, C. Alexiou, C. Grüttner, F. Wiekhorst, S. Dutz, J. Magn. Magn. Mater. 471 (2019) 1–7. doi:10.1016/J.JMMM.2018.09.012.

[3] H. Paysen, J. Wells, O. Kosch, U. Steinhoff, J. Franke, L. Trahms, T. Schaeffter, F. Wiekhorst, Phys. Med. Biol. (2018). doi:10.1088/1361-6560/aacb87.

time method" and second the "phase method", and compared the results.

In the arrival time method, we determine the displacement of the cube by using the difference of the time the ultrasonic waves took to reflect back. On the other hand, in the phase method, we calculated the displacement using the phase change amount from the reference when the irradiated ultrasonic wave returns.

First, we tried five experiments to measure the displacement by raising the piezo stage by 6 μm from the initial state. We then analyzed the waveform data obtained by each method and calculated the displacement.

Next, we performed the experiment with the stage raised by 0.6 μm from the initial state to 6 μm, and measured the change. The data obtained was analyzed with the same procedure, and the displacement was calculated.

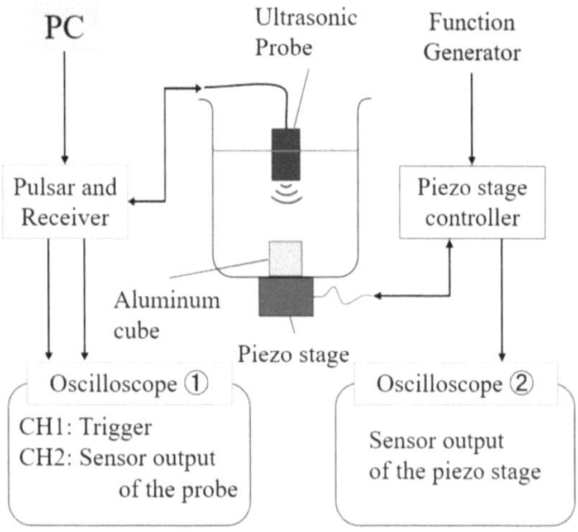

Figure 2: Experimental measurement system

***Table 1:** Experimental conditions*

Frequency of ultrasound	5	[MHz]
PRF of ultrasound	5	[kHz]
Record length	20	[K]
Sampling rate	500	[MS/s]
Water temperature	20.9	[°C]

IV. Results

Fig. 3 shows the measurement results when raising the piezo stage by the setting value of 6 μm. Fig. 4 shows the average of the two results obtained when raised in increments of 0.6 μm and the resulting error rate. Table 2 shows the standard error calculated from the results. From these results, it was confirmed that using both the arrival time method and the phase method, the displacement could be measured with sub-micron order accuracy. The phase method measurement was smaller than the arrival time method in both error and dispersion. This is because the arrival time method is largely

influenced by the sampling rate of the oscilloscope and it is considered that the resolution is large.

These measurement precisions are considered sufficient to measure the MNP oscillation of several tens to several hundreds of microns, and we think that both these methods are effective in the proposed MPI system.

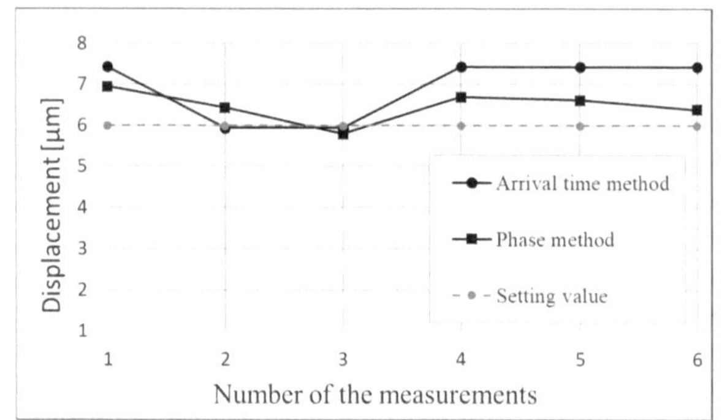

***Figure 3:** Result of the measurements of 6 μm displacement*

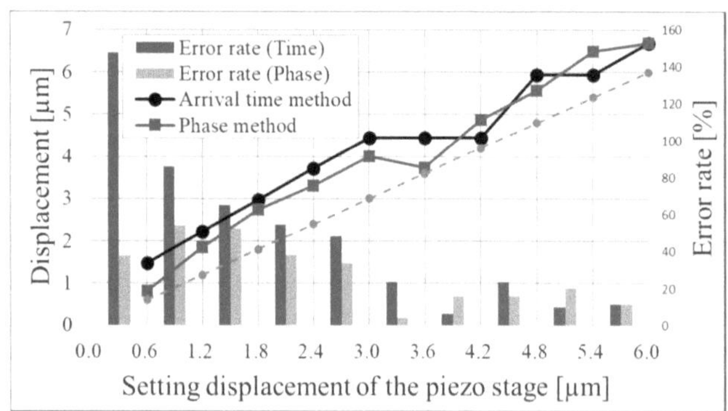

***Figure 4:** Result of the measurements of 0.6-6 μm displacement*

***Table 2:** Standard error*

	Standard error
Arrival time method [μm]	0.93 ± 0.29
Phase method [μm]	0.47 ± 0.14

V. Conclusion and Future work

We indicated the promising prospect of observing vibration of an MNP in accordance with these proposed measurement concepts (methods of arrival time and phase). We aim to make these possible by constructing a system and data flow program that controls measuring equipment using a PC. In addition, we will evaluate the influence of the vibration of the object on the observation accuracy of the phase method in the near future.

REFERENCES

[1] B. Gleich and J. Weizenecker. Tomographic imaging using the nonlinear response of magnetic particles. *Nature*, 435 (7046):1214-1217, 2005.

[2] S. Urushibata, T. Takagi, T. Hatsuda, A. Matsuhisa, M. Arayama, and Y. Ishihara. Improvement of detection sensitivity for MPI system based on vibrating particles. 7th International Workshop on Magnetic Particle Imaging IWMPI 2017, 2017, Prague.

transducer used in the experiment. In this simulation, the perfectly matched layer (PML) boundary was considered to preclude the reflection of ultrasound waves outside this boundary. The performance parameters of the ultrasound transducer are listed in Table 1, and the performance parameters of the hydrophone are shown in Table 2. The parameters of water are listed in Table 3. Furthermore, Table 4 shows the experimental ultrasound conditions.

Fig. 4 shows the experimental and simulation sound pressure variations around the focus point, as summarized in Table 5.

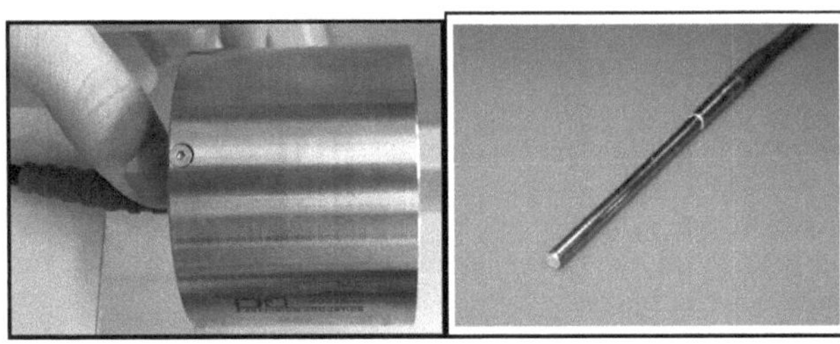

(a)   (b)

Figure 2: *Experimental device.*
(a) Ultrasound transducer, (b) Hydrophone

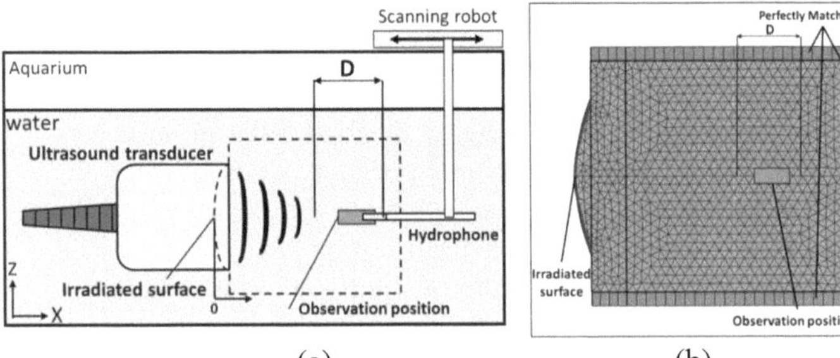

(a)   (b)

Figure 3: *Measurement setup.*
(a) Experiment, (b) Simulation

Table 1: *Performance of ultrasound.*

Radius of transducer [mm]	30
Nominal center frequency [MHz]	1
Acoustic path length [mm]	75
Signal amplitude [V]	30
Electrical impedance [Ω]	50

Table 2: *Performance of hydrophone.*

Element diameter [mm]	0.5
Sensitivity [nV/Pa]	250
Directionality [°]	30

Table 3: *Water characteristics.*

Density [kg/m³]	998
Sound velocity [m/s]	1483
Damping coefficient [1/m]	0.025

Acoustic impedance	1.48×10^6

Table 4: *Operating conditions of ultrasound.*

Voltage [Vpp]	30
Frequency [MHz]	1
Sampling frequency [MHz]	20
Observation position D [mm]	31.6*
Drive waveform	Sine wave burst
Interval [μs]	500

31.6* : The point of 61.8 mm from the irradiation surface is the starting point of the measurement range.

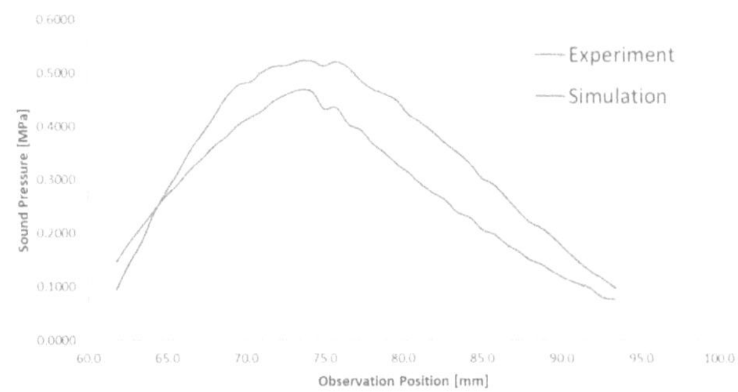

Figure 4: *Sound pressure variations for experiments and simulations around the focus point.*

Table 5: *Estimates of sound pressure at the focus point.*

	Experiment	Simulation
Sound Pressure [MPa]	0.469	0.522

IV. Conclusion and Future works

We confirmed the results shown in Fig. 4 with FEM simulations and experiments. Considering the elastic modulus of the living body, MNP vibrations of the order of tens of micrometers are expected from the obtained sound pressure in this study. In the future, we will establish a system that can verify the displacement induced owing to the vibrations of the MNPs.

REFERENCES
[1] B. Gleich and J Weizenecker: Tomographic imaging using the nonlinear response of magnetic particles. *Nature*, 435(30), 1214–1217, 2005.
[2] A. Matsuhisa, T. Hatsuda, T. Takagi, M. Arayama and Y. Ishihara. Magnetic signal detection method based on active vibration of magnetic nanoparticles. In 6th International Workshop on Magnetic Particle Imaging, Lübeck, 2016.
[3] S. Urushibata, T. Takagi, T. Hatsuda, A. Matsuhisa, M. Arayama, and Y. Ishihara. Improvement of detection sensitivity for MPI system based on vibrating particles. In 7th International Workshop on Magnetic Particle Imaging Prague, 2017.

III. Materials

Iron oxide Fe_3O_4 silicon-coated nanoparticles, 20-30 nm, were purchased from US Research Nanomaterials Inc. The particles were embedded in to epoxy resin to create various 3D objects. Solution of trityl (GE, 1mM) radical was used for EPR imaging.

IV. Experiment and Results

In our experiment, nanoparticles (24 % by mass) were mixed with an epoxy resin and injected into a 3D- printed plastic sphere with an inner diameter of 1 mm. Then, the spherical sample was inserted into 12 mm tube containing a 1mM aqueous solution of trityl radical. The trityl radical is an EPR spin probe to measure oxygen concentration. The linewidth of the RS EPR spectrum of trityl increases with increasing oxygen concentration, but the position of the line depends on the value of the local magnetic field created by the nanoparticles (Fig.2).

Functional EPR images are four-dimensional, containing three spatial components and one spectral. The images were reconstructed from sets of projections using the standard filtered back-projection method. The gradients were varied in amplitude and direction to acquire several thousand projections of data. The spectra in the images were post-processed to extract EPR line intensity, width and position. An example of the magnetic field image is shown in Fig. 3.

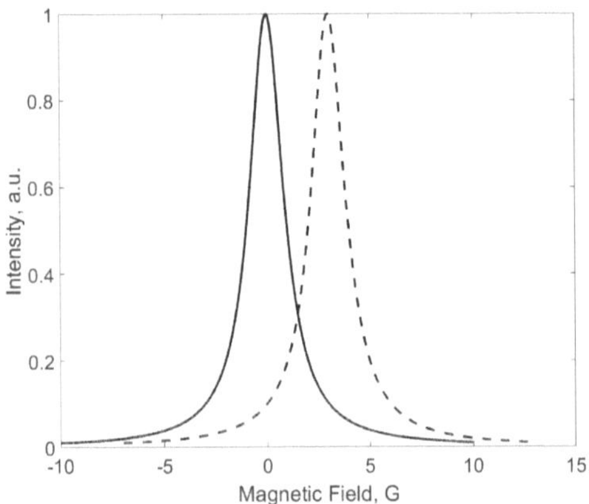

Figure 2: *Absorption EPR spectrum (solid line) shifts to a new position (dashed line) along the magnetic field axis. The new line position reports the value of the magnetic field offset.*

V. Discussion

MPI and EPR co-imaging has a potential to become a valuable tool for pre-clinical and clinical studies. Co-registration will enrich both modalities. For practical implementation of co-imaging, the external magnetic field used in EPR will have to be attenuated. A set of receiving coils and all supporting electronics need to be developed. The available digital feed-back system can be used to control amplitude and phase in the excitation coil.

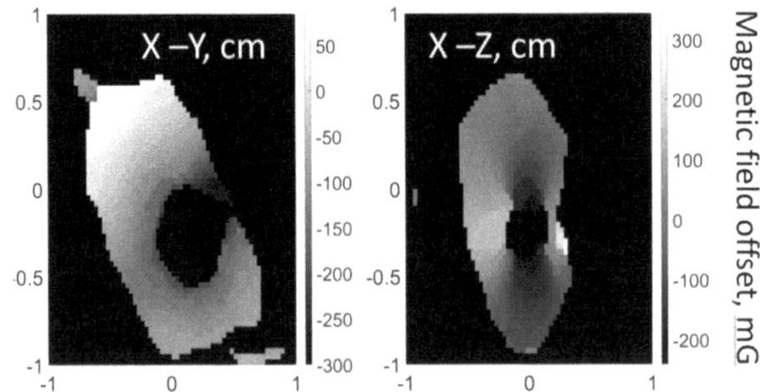

Figure 3: *Magnetic field distribution (two cross-sections) around a spherical sample (OD=2 mm). The external magnetic field is in the z-direction.*

The proposed method of mapping of the magnetic field created by iron nanoparticles can be a valuable tool in pre-clinical imaging. An inverse problem can be solved to find the location of the magnetic nanoparticles based on the measured magnetic field distribution. In this case, EPR will permit indirect imaging of the particles.

ACKNOWLEDGEMENTS

The support of this work by NIH/NIBIB R21 EB022775, NIH/NIBIB R01 EB023888, NIH/NIGMS U54GM104942 and NIH/NIGMS, P20GM121322 are gratefully acknowledged.

AUTHOR'S STATEMENT

Authors state no conflict of interest.

REFERENCES

[1] U. Sanzhaeva, X. Xu, P. Guggilapu, M. Tseytlin, V.V. Khramtsov, B. Driesschaert, Imaging of Enzyme Activity by Electron Paramagnetic Resonance: Concept and Experiment Using a Paramagnetic Substrate of Alkaline Phosphatase, *Angew Chem Int Ed Engl*, 57 (2018) 11701-11705.

[2] M. Tseytlin, Full cycle rapid scan EPR deconvolution algorithm, *J Magn Reson*, 281 (2017) 272-278.

[3] M. Tseytlin, A.V. Stolin, P. Guggilapu, A.A. Bobko, V.V. Khramtsov, O. Tseytlin, R.R. Raylman, A combined positron emission tomography (PET)- electron paramagnetic resonance imaging (EPRI) system: initial evaluation of a prototype scanner, *Phys Med Biol*, (2018)

experiments, the AC excitation field amplitude was changed from 2 mT to 20 mT in steps of 1 mT, while the frequency was fixed at 20 kHz.

III. Results and Discussion

The estimated magnetic moment distributions for the two samples are shown in Fig. 1. As indicated by the dashed line, there are two large peaks in the magnetic moment distribution for Resovist®. In contrast, the peak with the small magnetic moment disappears for MS1. This means that MNPs with small magnetic moments could be eliminated by magnetic fractionation and the MS1 sample mainly consists of MNPs with large magnetic moments.

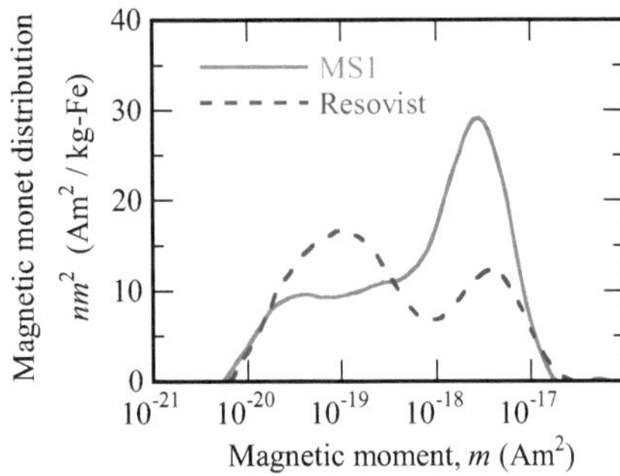

Figure 1: *Estimated magnetic moment distribution. The vertical axis represents the square of the magnetic moment weighted number distribution.*

Figure 2 shows the dependence of the maximum dM/dt value on the AC excitation field amplitude. As the figure shows, the maximum values for both samples are almost proportional to H_{ac}. This indicates that the signal intensities from both samples are almost proportional to the slew rate, i.e., to $2\pi f H_{ac}$. The MS1 sample showed more than a twofold increase in signal intensity when compared with that of the Resovist® sample. This can be attributed to the large proportion of MNPs with large magnetic moments in the MS1 sample when compared with the Resovist® sample.

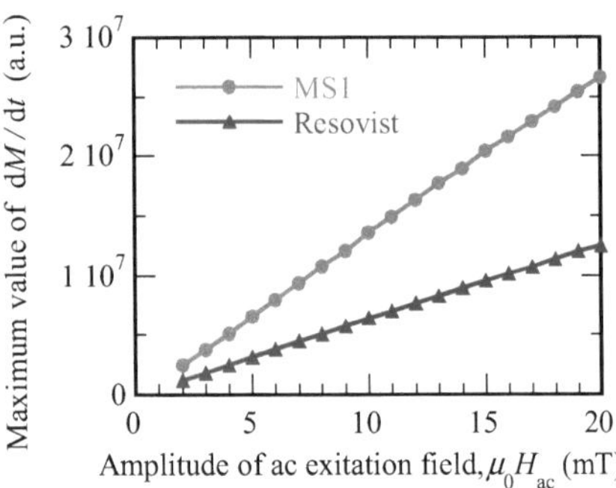

Figure 2: *Dependence of maximum value of dM/dt on AC excitation field amplitude.*

Figure 3 shows the $dM/dH - H$ curves for two samples. These curves were plotted for $H_{ac} = 20$ mT/μ_0. Following convention, only half of the full period, i.e., a forward scan with respect to H, is shown. As shown, the $dM/dH - H$ curves for both samples are not symmetrical about $H = 0$. This is caused by the finite relaxation times of the two samples. The full width at half maximum (FWHM) values of the $dM/dH - H$ curves were 9.4 and 12.1 mT/μ_0 for the MS1 and Resovist® samples, respectively. The wider FWHM of the Resovist® sample will be caused by the MNPs with smaller magnetic moments. These results indicate that the spatial resolution can be improved by a factor of 1.3 when using the MS1 sample rather than Resovist® sample.

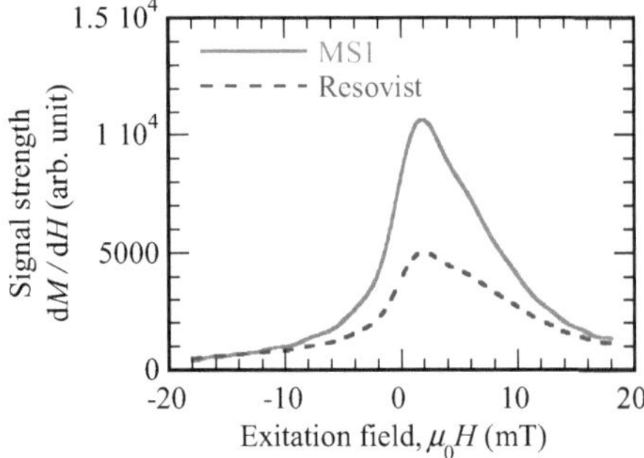

Figure 3: *dM/dt – H curves.*

V. Conclusions

In this study, we investigated the sensitivity and spatial resolution in MPI for original Resovist® and magnetically fractionated samples called MS1. We showed that the Resovist® sample consists of MNPs with small and large magnetic moments, while the MS1 sample mainly consists of MNPs with large magnetic moments. Because of the large proportion of MNPs with large magnetic moments, MS1 provides better performance in MPI with respect to both sensitivity and spatial resolution.

ACKNOWLEDGEMENTS

This work was supported by JSPS KAKENHI JP15H05764 and JP18K04170.

REFERENCES

[1] B. Gleich and J. Weizenecker. Tomographic imaging using the nonlinear response of magnetic particles. *Nature*, 435(7046):1214-1217, 2005. doi: 10.1038/nature03808.

[2] T. Yoshida, K. Enpuku, F. Ludwig, J. Dieckhoff, T. Wawrzik, A. Lak, and M. Schilling. Characterization of Resovist® Nanoparticles for Magnetic Particle Imaging. *Springer Proc. Phys.*, 140:3-7, 2012. doi: 10.1007/978-3-642-24133-8_1.

[3] T. Yoshida, N. B. Othman, and K. Enpuku. Characterization of magnetically fractionated magnetic nanoparticles for magnetic particle imaging. *J. Appl. Phys.*, 114: 173908, 2013. doi: 10.1063/1.4829484.

[4] N. Löwa, P. Knappe, F. Wiekhorst, D. Eberbeck, A. F. Thünemann, and L. Trahms. Hydrodynamic and magnetic fractionation of superparamagnetic nanoparticles for magnetic particle imaging. *J. Magn. Magn. Mater.*, 380:266–270, 2015. doi: 10.1016/j.jmmm.2014.08.057.

[5] J. van Rijssel, B. W.M. Kuipers, B. H. Erné. Non-regularized inversion method from light scattering applied to ferrofluid magnetization curves for magnetic size distribution analysis. *J. Magn. Magn. Mater.*, 353:110–115, 2014. doi: 10.1016/j.jmmm.2013.10.025.

the equation system by the Kaczmarz-algorithm using 20 iterations and a regularization factor $\lambda_r=10^{-9}$.

III. Results

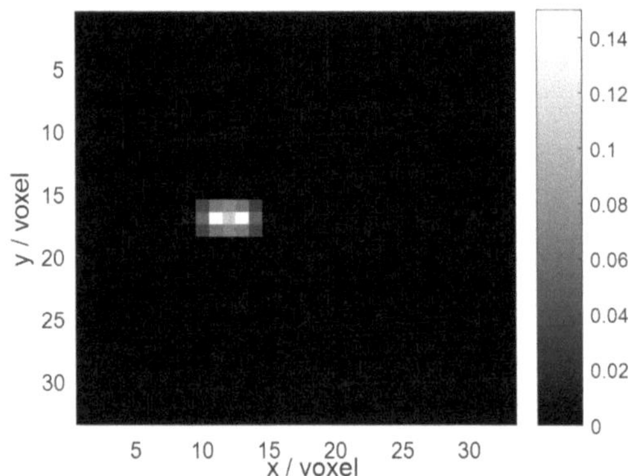

Figure 1: *Reconstructed MPI image of Resovist at voxel layer z=17 using a synthetic measurement vector $\bar{u}$ combining the two voxels (x=11 and 13, y= 17, z=17) of the measured SF.*

Fig.1 depicts the reconstruction result of Resovist in the xy-plane and Fig. 2 for all tracer systems in x-direction, respectively.

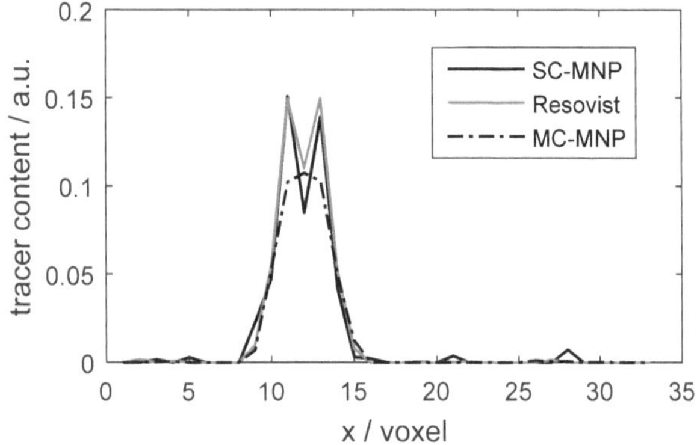

Figure 2: *Reconstructed voxel content of the three tracer systems along the line (x, y=17, z=17)$|_{x=1...33}$.*

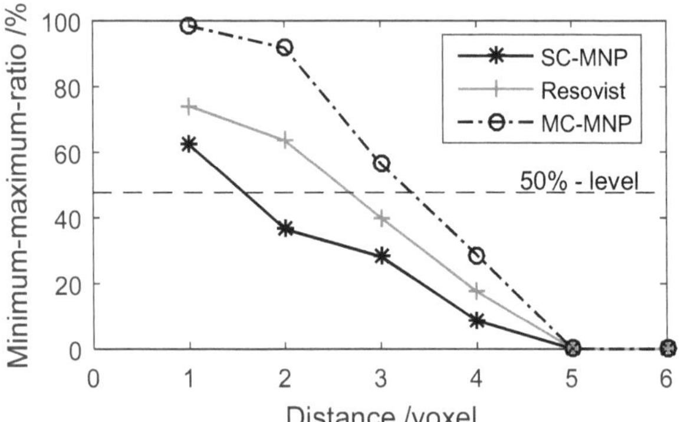

Figure 3: *Minimum-maximum-ratio as a function of the voxel distance.*

The distance between the two "MNP containing" voxels of $\bar{u}$ was then increased up to six "empty voxels". The relative difference between minimum and mean of the maxima as a function of this distance is shown in Fig. 3. Using the full width at half maximum criterion (FWHM), we achieve the following resolutions for each tracer:

Table 1: *Tracer resolution.*

Resovist	MC-MNP	SC-MNP
2.6 voxel	3.24 voxel	1.5 voxel
2.1 mm	2.6 mm	1.2 mm

IV. Discussion

In our method we generate the measurement vector u by using the SF and avoid the noise influence of an additional phantom measurement. Further to minimize the influence of the SF noise on the resolution results, we used in our method an SNR at least better than 4. In [2] we have determined by MPS-measurements at 10 mT an increase of the amplitude of the third harmonics in comparison to Resovist by a factor 2.3 for the MC-MNPs and a factor 5.8 for the SC-MNPs. Furthermore, we observed an improved imaging performance for the SC-MNPs using a pipe phantom. However, the imaging performance of the MC-MNPs was only like Resovist and at a higher concentration (5 mmol/L) even worse. Now by the proposed method in combination with MPS measurements we can predict the imaging performance, correctly.

V. Conclusions

The presented method enables MPI-tracer characterization based on the best achievable image resolution without scanner noise. By applying this method, we are able to resolve the discrepancy in tracer characterization by MPS measurements as reported in [2]. The MPS measurement leads to a characterization of the tracer more focusing on the detection limit, the here presented method provides complementary information on the image resolution quality of the tracer independent of the instrumentation.

ACKNOWLEDGEMENTS

This work was supported by the Deutsche Forschungsgemeinschaft research program "quantMPI" (DFG grant TR408/9-1) and "Matrix in Vision", (DFG SFB 1340/1 2018, projects A02 and B02).

REFERENCES

[1] S. Biederer, T. Knopp, T.F. Sattel, K. Lüdtke-Buzug, B. Gleich, J. Weizenecker, J. Borgert, T.M. Buzug, Magnetization response spectroscopy of superparamagnetic nanoparticles for magnetic particle imaging, *J. Phys. D. Appl. Phys.* 42 (2009) 205007. doi:10.1088/0022-3727/42/20/205007.

[2] S. Ziemian, N. Löwa, O. Kosch, D. Bajj, F. Wiekhorst, G. Schütz, Optimization of Iron Oxide Tracer Synthesis for Magnetic Particle Imaging, *Nanomaterials.* 8 (2018) 180. doi:10.3390/nano8040180.

[3] J. Rahmer, J. Weizenecker, B. Gleich, J. Borgert, Signal encoding in magnetic particle imaging: properties of the system function, *BMC Med. Imaging.* 9 (2009) 4. doi:10.1186/1471-2342-9-4.

[4] J. Rahmer, J. Weizenecker, B. Gleich, J. Borgert, Analysis of a {3-D} system function measured for magnetic particle imaging, *IEEE Trans. Med. Imaging.* 31 (2012) 1289–1299. doi:10.1109/TMI.2012.2188639.

[5] N. Löwa, P. Radon, O. Kosch, F. Wiekhorst, Concentration Dependent MPI Tracer Performance, *IJMPI*, 2 (2016) 1–5. https://journal.iwmpi.org/index.php/iwmpi/article/view/26/6.

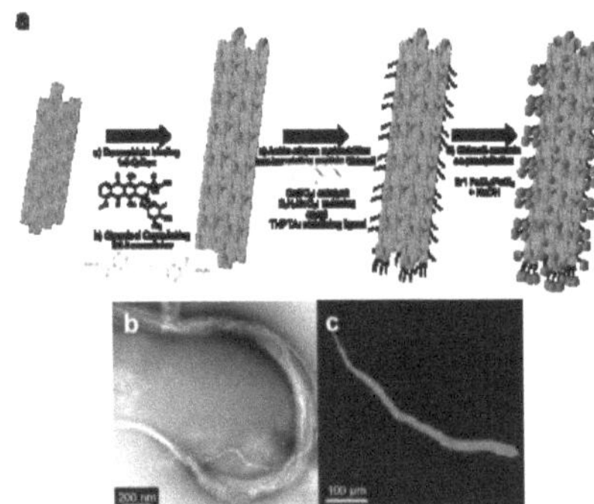

Figure 1: (a) Schematic depiction of iron oxide-bound drug-carrying protein Q biomaterial from nanofiber assembly, to doxorubicin (Dox) binding and crosslinking, to cycloaddition with iron-templating peptide CMms6 and CMms6-mediated iron oxide templation. (b) TEM confirms the nanofiber protein assembly achieved after buffer exchange into acid buffer conditions and fluorescence microscopy reveals micron-scale protein constructs following Dox binding and BS^3-crosslinking (c).

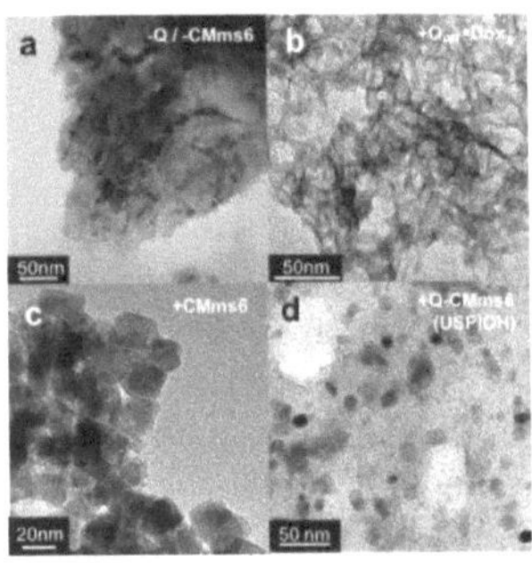

Figure 2: TEM of iron synthesized (a) in the absence of Q protein and CMms6 peptide, (b) in the presence of Q_{WT} protein, (c) in the presence of CMms6, and (d) in the presence of Q-CMms6, demonstrating CMms6-organized USPIOs in panels (c) and (d).

Diffraction rings of USPIOs templated by CMms6 demonstrated distinct concentric rings typically seen in polycrystalline samples composed of randomly oriented crystallites[49] , while Q-CMms6 revealed templated USPIOs with spot-like patterns typical of single crystals[49] with well-defined spots arranged in rings. Both diffraction patterns revealed *d*-spacing measurements in agreement with well-described magnetite composition [6]. Feraheme and USPIOH showed minimal T_1 brightening (**Fig. 3**), with a longitudinal relativity (r_1) for USPIOH of 0.17 ± 0.01 mM^{-1}s^{-1} that is significantly lower than 1.63 ± 0.15 mM^{-1}s^{-1} for Feraheme (**Fig. 5**).

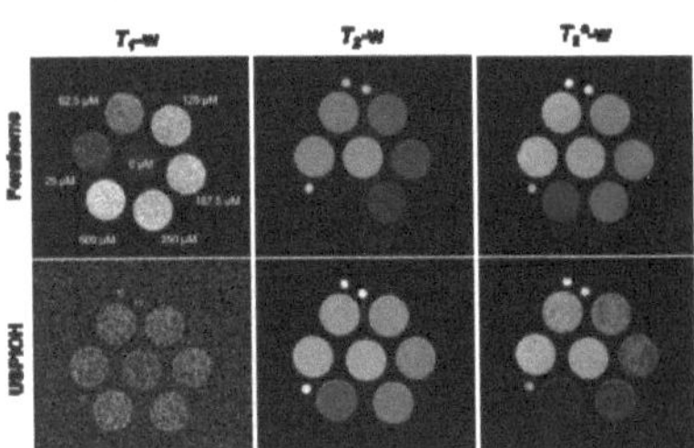

Figure 3 2D MRI Feraheme and USPIO templated by Q-CMms6. Representative inversion time for the Look-Locker sequence (for T_1 relaxation) and echo times for MSME (for T_2 relaxation) and MGE (for T_2^* relaxation). The presence of the CMms6 construct and its ability to biosynthesize USPIOs results in effective T_2^* signal dampening compared to the clinical agent Feraheme.

T_2-we MRI (**Fig. 3&4**) showed a stronger darkening effect for Feraheme (r_2=87.03 ± 4.74 mM^{-1}s^{-1}) than USPIOH (r_2=17.69 ± 1.00 mM^{-1}s^{-1}). However, the hybrid biomaterial demonstrated a 1.91-fold higher apparent transverse relaxivity (r_2^*=177.25 ± 10.17 mM^{-1}s^{-1}) over Feraheme (r_2^*=93.04 ± 6.76 mM^{-1}s^{-1}) resulting in superior T_2^* darkening.

Sample	r_1 (mM^{-1} s^{-1})	r_2 (mM^{-1} s^{-1})	r_2^* (mM^{-1} s^{-1})	r_2/r_1	r_2^*/r_2
Feraheme	1.63 ± 0.15	87.03 ± 4.74	93.04 ± 6.76	53.66 ± 4.87	1.07 ± 0.04
USPIOH	0.17 ± 0.01	17.69 ± 1.00	177.25 ± 10.17	104.06 ± 9.15	10.03 ± 0.53

Figure 5 Table summarizing the quantified relaxivity values of Feraheme and USPIOH, all described in Figure 4. The commonly used r2/r1 relaxivity ratio to characterize the effectiveness of MRI agents confirms the notable T_2/T_2^*-weighting illustrated in Fig.4 with a greater T_2^* effect for USPIOH compared to Feraheme.

IV. Discussion & Conclusions

By biosynthesizing a coiled-coil protein and utilizing bio-inspired iron oxide templation, we engineered a trackable USPIO-functionalized drug carrying hybrid scaffold, USPIOH. TEM studies confirmed that its ability to organize USPIOs is due to conjugation to iron-templating CMms6 and imaging studies revealed that organized USPIOs resulted in an appreciable T_2^* relaxation effect. Our USPIOH was validated by its 1.91-fold higher r_2^* relaxivity than Feraheme, resulting in an r_2/r_1 value of USPIOH that was 1.94-fold higher than that of Feraheme and r_2^*/r_2 ratio 9.37-fold higher, suggesting its use as a theranostic agent enabling chemotherapeutic delivery to be visualized via T_2^*-weighted MRI. We are currently analyzing the response of the amplitudes of the MPI's harmonics of the iron crystals emanating from this construct and how they compare with Feraheme as well as previously published magnetosomes [7]. Importantly, the latter magnetosomes have shown to exceed the performance of Resovist®; which is the other clinical agent and current "gold standard" in MPI. Moreover, the amplitude of the third harmonic of the magnetosomes was higher by a factor of 7; the highest value reported so far for iron oxide nanoparticles. We are currently characterizing both bio-mineralized iron bound to our construct and Feraheme.

Acknowledgements

This work was supported, in part, by ARO (W911NF-11-1-0449), NSF DMR-0820341 NSF DMR-1728858. It was also performed at the NYU Langone Health Preclinical Imaging Laboratory, a shared resource partially supported by the NIH/SIG 1S10OD018337-01, NIH/NCI 5P30CA016087 and the NIBIB NIH P41 EB017183.

AUTHOR'S STATEMENT

Research funding: The author state no further funding involved. Conflict of interest: Authors state no conflict of interest. Informed consent: Informed consent has been obtained from all individuals included in this study. Ethical approval: No research related to human has been performed in this study.

REFERENCES

[1] Hume J, Sun J, Jacquet R, Renfrew PD, Martin JA, Bonneau R, Gilchrist ML, Montclare JK. 2014 Oct 13;15(10):3503-10.
[2] Arakaki A, Webb J, Matsunaga T. J Biol Chem 2003; 278:8745–8750.
[3] Link AJ, Tirrell DA. J Am Chem Soc. 2003;125(37):11164-5.
[4] Hong V, Presolski SI, Ma C, Finn MG. Angew Chem Int Ed Engl. 2009;48(52):9879-83.
[5] Mérida F, Chiu-Lam A, Bohórquez AC, Maldonado-Camargo L, *et al.* J Magn Magn Mater. 2015; 394:361-371.
[6] JCPDS- International Centre for Diffraction Data. 1986. Power Diffraction. Swathmore, PA:
[7] Kraupner A, Eberbeck D, Heinke D, Uebe R, Schüler D, Briel A. Nanoscale. 2017;9(18):5788-5793.

III. Results and Discussion

MPS harmonic spectra of each sample of the viscosity series were acquired for $f_0 = 1$ kHz and $H = 25$ mT/μ_0. The complex-valued harmonic spectra were assembled into a system matrix for a given number of reference samples. Subsequently, all contributions were reconstructed via Truncated Singular Value Decomposition (TSVD) of the system matrix for the whole sample series.

In [2], each particle mixture was directly represented as an additive superposition of the pure particle references. For continuous viscosity dependences, a complex-valued reconstruction must be consulted, i.e. intermediate values are not composed of the exact references.

Fig. 2 shows reconstructed contributions for two references. Real and imaginary parts of the reconstruction results are in the same range of values indicating that a functional relationship could be derived.

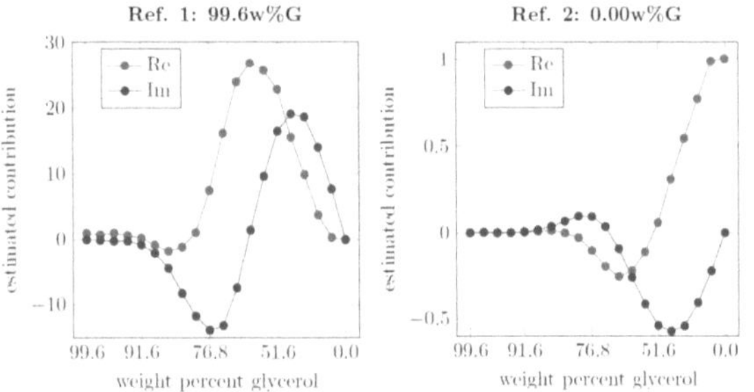

Figure 2: *Reconstructed contributions of reference 1 (left) with 99.6 w% glycerol and reference 2 (right) with 0.0 w% glycerol content for the viscosity sample series.*

Similar dependences are observed for reconstructions using more than two references as exemplarily shown in Fig. 3 for three references.

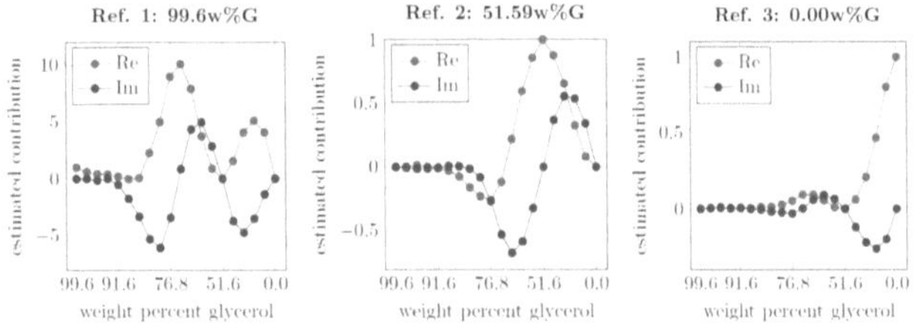

Figure 3: *Reconstructed contributions of three references with 99.6 w% (left), 51.6 w% (center) and 0.0 w% (right) glycerol content for the viscosity sample series.*

As can be seen, reconstructed contributions reveal real positive values for samples at reference points. All other samples exhibit complex-valued contributions with in part large values (Fig. 2 and Fig. 3, left) for the first reference.

V. Conclusions

MPI requires calibrations to represent a quantitative imaging modality with respect to particle concentration and particle mobility or further influencing factors like temperature. MPS

provides a powerful tool to study such relationships detached from time-consuming acquisitions of dedicated system functions and even more complex spatial dependences. The multispectral decomposition approach enables the investigation of mapping functions, which are of high importance for multispectral reconstruction in MPI. Experimental data show that complex-valued reconstruction is required to determine arbitrary viscosity values between reference points. Our investigations cover the number of required references as a function of reconstruction quality and quantitativity for influences of the particle mobility using tailored magnetic nanoparticles as model systems. Furthermore, results are applied to commercially available particle systems.

ACKNOWLEDGEMENTS

Financial support by the German Research Foundation DFG via Priority Program 1681 under grant no. VI 892/1-1 and "Niedersächsisches Vorab" through "Quantum- and Nano-Metrology (QUANOMET)" initiative within the project NP-2 are acknowledged.

AUTHOR'S STATEMENT

Research funding: The author state no funding involved, which was not already referred to in acknowledgements. Conflict of interest: Authors state no conflict of interest. Informed consent: Informed consent has been obtained from all individuals included in this study. Ethical approval: The research related to human use complies with all the relevant national regulations, institutional policies and was performed in accordance with the tenets of the Helsinki Declaration, and has been approved by the authors' institutional review board or equivalent committee.

REFERENCES

[1] S. Biederer, T. Knopp, T. F. Sattel, K. Lüdtke-Buzug, B. Gleich, J. Weizenecker, J. Borgert, and T. M. Buzug. Magnetization response spectroscopy of superparamagnetic nanoparticles for magnetic particle imaging. *J. Phys. D: Appl. Phys.*, 42, 2009. doi: 10.1088/0022-3727/42/20/205007.

[2] T. Viereck, S. Draack, M. Schilling, and F. Ludwig, Multi-spectral Magnetic Particle Spectroscopy for the investigation of particle mixtures, *J. Magn. Magn. Mater.*, 2018, doi: 10.1016/j.jmmm.2018.11.021.

[3] B. Gleich and J. Weizenecker. Tomographic imaging using the nonlinear response of magnetic particles. *Nature*, 435(7046):1217-1217, 2005. doi: 10.1038/nature03808.

[4] S. Draack, N. Lucht, H. Remmer, M. Martens, B. Fischer, M. Schilling, F. Ludwig, and T. Viereck. Multiparametric Magnetic Particle Spectroscopy of CoFe$_2$O$_4$ nanoparticles in viscous media. J. Phys. Chem., submitted 2018.

[5] S. Draack, T. Viereck, C. Kuhlmann, M. Schilling, and F. Ludwig. Temperature-dependent MPS measurements. Int. J. Magn. Part. Imag., 3(1), 2017, doi: 10.18416/ijmpi.2017.1703018.

[6] S. Draack, T. Viereck, F. Nording, K.-J. Janssen, M. Schiling, and F. Ludwig. Determination of dominating relaxation mechanisms from temperature-dependent Magnetic Particle Spectroscopy measurements. J. Magn. Magn. Mater., 2018, doi: 10.1016/j.jmmm.2018.11.023.

SPIONs but also to the diamagnetic human tissue which limits the sensitivity and requires time-consuming balancing [5]. Differential Magnetometry (DiffMag), a new magnetic measurement technique was developed by our group to overcome these drawbacks, by detecting at the specific magnetic signature of SPIONs.

I.II. Technical background

This DiffMag technique utilizes nonlinear properties of SPIONs, similar to Magnetic Particle Imaging (MPI) and Magnetic Particle Spectroscopy (MPS). The main differences are that we use a smaller AC amplitude ($\pm$ 1 mT) and measure in the time domain instead of harmonic spectra. Our technique negates the magnetic field of the human body and stationary metal (surgical) instruments, making it a selective measurement for SPIONs. In contradiction to the SentiMAG® detector, stationary surgical steel can be used in close proximity to the detection probe, making DiffMag easier to use in clinical practice. A handheld probe based on our DiffMag principle was developed that contains both excitation and detection coils for use in open surgery [6].

In the Netherlands, most prostate/bladder surgeries are performed laparoscopically. However, in laparoscopic surgery, the diameter of the probe is restricted by the use of standard trocars. The depth sensitivity of a coil is determined by the diameter of the coil, according to Biot-Savart law. As a result, making the handheld probe smaller would result in inadequate depth sensitivity, making it impossible to find sentinel nodes in laparoscopic surgery. This problem is solved by separating the excitation and detection part of the DiffMag handheld system. The excitation coils will be large and placed underneath the patient, as shown in Fig. 1. The detection coils can be small enough to fit through standard laparoscopic trocars (12 mm). A first laparoscopic prototype has been developed on this principle. However, it is still too early to use in a first clinical trial. For this reason, a first clinical test will be executed with the Diffmag handheld probe for open surgery. Both probes are based on the same physical principle, ensuring the usability of the results for this trial for the further development of the laparoscopic probe.

I.III. Objectives

The primary goal of this trial is to map normally missed high risk lymph nodes during standard laparoscopic pelvic lymph node dissection. The draining lymph nodes will be visualized through the use of Magtrace® and a preoperative MRI-scan. In the ideal situation the physician would have the means to detect the Magtrace® absorbed lymph nodes during the operation. However, as explained no laparoscopic magnetic detector is yet available. For this reason the secondary goal of this study is to compare *ex vivo* our DiffMag detector with the SentiMAG®. It is our hypothesis that the new DiffMag detector is at least as accurate as the SentiMAG® when identifying lymph nodes.

II. Material and Methods

II.I. Study design

This is a prospective, interventional, single center pilot trial. Twenty patients with a primary prostate or bladder tumor will be included. One day before surgery, Magtrace® will be injected around the tumor under ultrasound guidance, followed by an MRI-scan to pre-operatively localize the draining SNs. After resection of the tumor and lymph nodes, first the DiffMag probe will be used for *ex vivo* detection of the SN, followed by the SentiMAG®. The results of both devices will be compared, in order to validate the new DiffMag technique. This research aims to increase the detection rate of tumor draining lymph nodes and prove the efficacy of the DiffMag technique.

III. Results

Before the proposed study can start, permission of the Dutch Medical Ethical Committee is obligatory. All the necessary documents are finished and submitted, approval is expected soon. This study is planned to start in April 2019.

IV. Conclusions

This clinical patient trial will give the physician a more complete map of the draining lymph nodes. It would be ideal for the physician to measure SPIONs in the lymph nodes real-time, not just beforehand based on a MRI-scan. To further our laparoscopic DiffMag prototype, we use the secondary goal of this research as input for the further development. Since most prostate/bladder operations are performed laparoscopically, a magnetic detector fit for a trocar is mandatory. The DiffMag technique will enable us to decrease the diameter of the probe while maintaining an acceptable detection depth.

ACKNOWLEDGEMENTS

Financial support from the Netherlands Organization for Scientific Research (NWO), under the research program Magnetic Sensing for Laparoscopy (MagLap) with project number 14322 is gratefully acknowledged.

REFERENCES

1. Briganti, A., et al., Updated nomogram predicting lymph node invasion in patients with prostate cancer undergoing extended pelvic lymph node dissection: the essential importance of percentage of positive cores. Eur Urol, 2012. **61**(3): p. 480-7.
2. Cagiannos, I., et al., A preoperative nomogram identifying decreased risk of positive pelvic lymph nodes in patients with prostate cancer. J Urol, 2003. **170**(5): p. 1798-803.
3. Brouwer, O., et al., De schildwachtklierprocedure bij prostaatkanker. Tijdschrift voor Urologie, 2012. **2**(4): p. 84-91.
4. Winter, A., J. Woenkhaus, and F. Wawroschek, A Novel Method for Intraoperative Sentinel Lymph Node Detection in Prostate Cancer Patients Using Superparamagnetic Iron Oxide Nanoparticles and a Handheld Magnetometer: The Initial Clinical Experience. Annals of Surgical Oncology, 2014. **21**(13): p. 4390-4396.
5. Pouw, J.J., et al., Phantom study quantifying the depth performance of a handheld magnetometer for sentinel lymph node biopsy. Physica medica, 2016. **32**(7): p. 926-931.
6. Waanders, S., et al., A handheld SPIO-based sentinel lymph node mapping device using differential magnetometry. Physics in Medicine and Biology, 2016. **61**(22): p. 8120.

in the xy plane. At each position a full 2D imaging sequence was applied. We used the joint reconstruction approach [3], where individual 1D measurements were combined prior to reconstruction. The linear imaging equation was solved iteratively using the regularized Kaczmarz algorithm.

II.I. Static Brain Experiment

In order to prove that the new imager is capable of detecting perfusion deficiencies, a human-sized brain model was designed consisting of two hemispheres. One hemisphere was the healthy control with a volume of 490 ml. The second hemisphere had a smaller volume of 440 ml due to a cut out region. A fitting insert of 42 ml was constructed, which represents a typical stroke in the middle cerebral artery territory (MCA) [5]. The used tracer within this study was perimag. The stroke part was manufactured four times to be filled with varying concentrations of 0 µg/ml, 6.37 µg/ml, 3.185 µg/ml and 9.65 µg/ml representing different degrees of stenosis. The two hemispheres were filled with 965 ng/ml iron and placed in the scanner to be measured successively with the different stroke parts. The selection field gradient was chosen to be 0.2 T/m/µ0 and the drive field amplitude was set to 6 mT/µ0.

III. Results

The results of the static brain experiment are shown in Fig. 1. As can be seen, an 100 % underperfusion related to the MCA-territory of our model is clearly identifiable. The stroke region appears as a triangular dark shape when considering the transversal cross-section through the phantom, which coincides with the CAD model of the stroke. With decreasing severity of stroke, respectively increasing tracer concentration c in the stroke part, the stroke area is worse to distinguish from the hemisphere. For the 66 % case the stroke is still clearly to identify, whereas for the 33 % case the result is less obvious. However, in direct comparison with the control image there still is a difference in concentration. To highlight the lower concentrations in the stroke parts, the middle column shows difference images Idiff resulting from subtracting the control image from the respective stroke images. As the phantom was taken out of the scanner between consecutive measurements, the exact position of the phantom differed slightly, which leads to the artifacts in the difference images.

IV. Discussion

Within this study we developed a human brain phantom that allows to simulate different degrees of stenosis. The experiment showed that the human-sized brain imager is capable of detecting a 42 ml stroke even for a perfusion reduction of only 33 %. We further showed that the calculation of difference images provides meaningful information on the degree of stenosis and helps to identify restenosis in a surveillance scenario. The artifacts that become apparent in the difference images due to rough positioning would be the same in a real scenario and could be avoided by using rigid image registration algorithms.

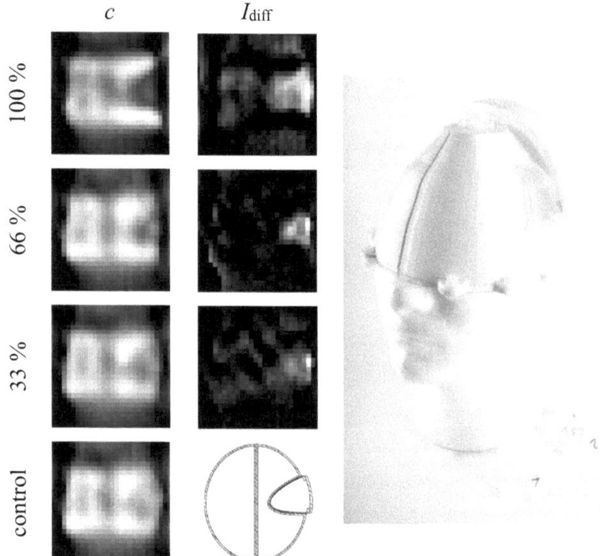

Figure 1: *Brain phantom (right) and reconstruction results (left). The control image shows both hemispheres and the stroke part filled with 965 ng/ml. From bottom to top, the concentration c in the stroke part decreases representing increasing degrees of stenosis. The upper left image displays an underperfusion of 100 %. The middle column shows the difference images I_{diff}, which result from subtracting the control image from the respective stroke image. A horizontal cut of the CAD model is shown next to the control image.*

V. Conclusions

This work shows that the new developed brain imager allows for the detection of perfusion deficits and thus for the detection of stroke. The combination of low technical requirements of the device and the imaging modality that does not require ionizing radiation makes the first MPI human-sized brain imager optimally suited for longtime monitoring on an ICU.

AUTHOR'S STATEMENT

Research funding: German Research Foundation (DFG, grant 388 number KN 1108/2-1) and the Federal Ministry of Education and Research (BMBF, grant numbers 05M16GKA, 13XP5060B). Conflict of interest: Authors state no conflict of interest. Informed consent: Informed consent has been obtained from all individuals included in this study. Ethical approval: The research related to human use complies with all the relevant national regulations, institutional policies and was performed in accordance with the tenets of the Helsinki Declaration, and has been approved by the authors' institutional review board or equivalent committee.

REFERENCES

[1] V. e. a. Feigin, "Global and regional burden of stroke during 1990-2010.", The Lancet, pp. 245-255, 2014.

[2] B. Gleich and J. Weizenecker, "Tomographic imaging using the nonlinear response of magnetic particles.", Nature, pp. 1217-1217, 2005.

[3] M. Graeser et al., "Human-sized Magnetic Particle Imaging for Brain Applications.", arXiv:1810.07987 [physics.med-ph], 2018.

[4] T. Knopp et al., "Joint reconstruction of non-overlapping magnetic particle imaging focus-field data.", Physics in medicine and biology, 2015.

[5] C. &. K. H.-O. Sperber, "Topography of acute stroke in a sample of 439 right brain damaged patients.", NeuroImage: Clinical, 2016.

with tunable flow velocity. An injector needle was mounted to the tube and connected to a second pump which injects the tracer and depending on tube diameter and injected tracer volume, tracer bolus segments of variable length are formed, see figure 1. For different tube diameters, segments of different length were adjusted in the tube and imaged by means of MPI for flow velocities up to 40 cm/s.

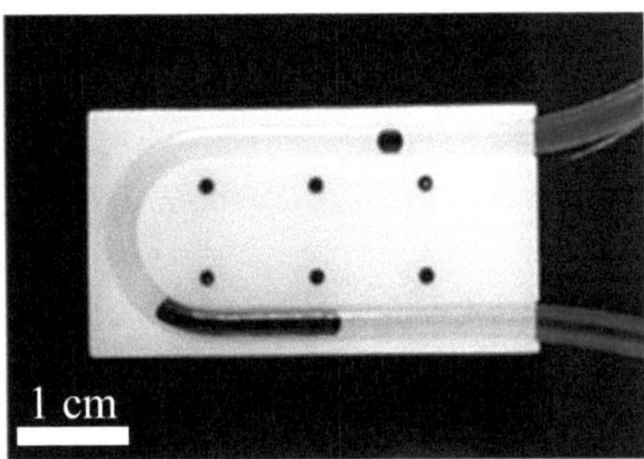

Figure 1: *Photograph of the tube phantom (D_i = 1.6 mm) with an almost spherical bolus as well as an elongated bolus.*

III. Results

MP imaging of 15 different static segments (5 different diameters x 3 different bolus lengths) revealed that all tested bolus dimensions can be visualized by of both MPI systems. Figure 2 shows the reconstruction of bolus length of 1.6 mm (a), 3.2 mm (b), and 4.8 mm (c) within a tube of D_i = 1.6 mm imaged by the MPI 25/20FF scanner.

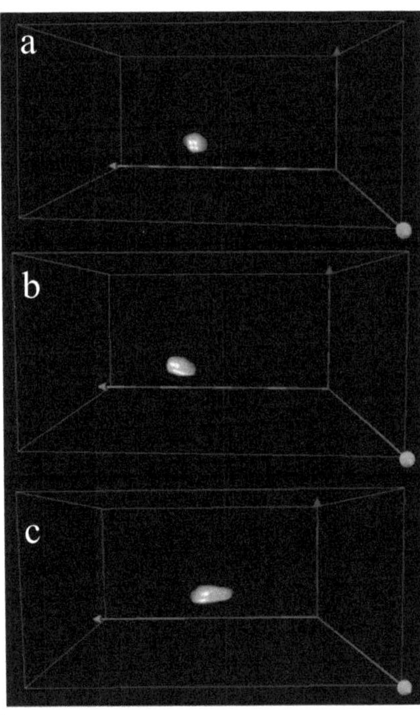

Figure 2: *3D MPI iso reconstruction of a bolus of 1.6 mm (a), 3.2 mm (b), and 4.8 mm (c) length within a tube of 1.6 mm inner diameter.*

The MPI reconstruction shows, that the entire geometry of the static bolus phantoms can be imaged. By comparing the three different bolus images, the different segment lengths in the phantom can be clearly differentiated, see Figure 2.

Moving boluses were imaged by means of both scanners successfully. The obtained temporal imaging resolution is defined by the used spatial resolution. For all tube diameters it was possible to reconstruct the moving bolus up to flow velocities of 40 cm/s. Higher flow velocities can't be realized with the present dynamic bolus phantom.

IV. Conclusions

We developed a dynamic bolus phantom system for evaluation of the temporal resolution of an MPI scanner. A tracer bolus of adjustable size, volume, concentration, and flow velocity can be realized with the presented bolus phantom system. The boluses show very good stability against leaching into the carrier liquid. This enables a reliable distinction between tracer front and carrier liquid, which is an important prerequisite for measurements of temporal resolution with high accuracy. Moving boluses were imaged by both used scanner systems.

ACKNOWLEDGEMENTS

This work was supported by Deutsche Forschungsgemeinschaft (DFG) in the frame of the project quantMPI (DU 1293/6-1 and TR 408/9-1).

AUTHOR'S STATEMENT

Research funding: The author state no funding involved. Conflict of interest: Authors state no conflict of interest. Informed consent: Informed consent has been obtained from all individuals included in this study. Ethical approval: The research related to human use complies with all the relevant national regulations, institutional policies and was performed in accordance with the tenets of the Helsinki Declaration, and has been approved by the authors' institutional review board or equivalent committee.

REFERENCES

[1] B. Gleich and J. Weizenecker. Tomographic imaging using the nonlinear response of magnetic particles. *Nature* 435/7046: 1214-1217 (**2005**).
[2] N. Gdaniec, M. Schlüter, M. Möddel, M.G. Kaul, K.M. Krishnan, A. Schlaefer, and T. Knopp. Detection and Compensation of Periodic Motion in Magnetic Particle Imaging. *IEEE TRANSACTIONS ON MEDICAL IMAGING* 36/7: 1511–1521 (**2017**).
[3] L. Wöckel, J. Wells, O. Kosch, S. Lyer, C. Alexiou, C. Grüttner, F. Wiekhorst, S. Dutz. Long-term stable measurement phantoms for magnetic particle imaging. *J. Magn. Magn. Mater.* 471: 1–7 (**2019**).
[4] P. Vogel, M.A. Rückert, P. Klauer, W.H. Kullmann, P.M. Jakob, V.C. Behr, Traveling Wave Magnetic Particle Imaging, *IEEE TMI* 33/2: 400-407 (**2014**).
[5] P. Vogel, M.A. Rückert, P. Klauer, W.H. Kullmann, P.M. Jakob, V.C. Behr, Superpseed Traveling Wave Magnetic Particle Imaging, *IEEE Trans Magn* 52/2 :6501603 (**2015**).

times, nearly 50% of samples were positive, i.e. that no favorable timespan was fixable by MPS. In contrast, the results of AAS measurement showed an increasing median iron gradient over time in the first axillary LN (Fig. 3). At the same time, iron concentration decreased in the surrounding tissue of axillary lymph nodes.

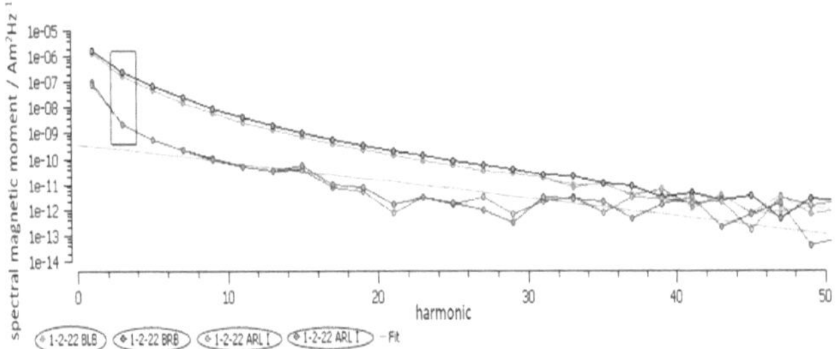

Figure 2: *Example of MPS measurement results: harmonics of four samples and median (straight line), 3 hours after intramammary SPION injection.*
ARL I = region A (axilla), Left, Lymph node level I,
BLB/BRB = region B (anterior chest), Left/Right, Breast tissue

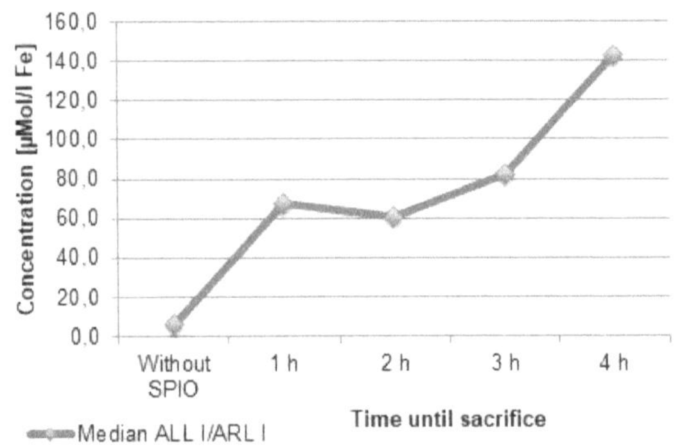

Figure 3: *AAS: Gradient (median) of the iron concentration over time in the first axillary lymph node (SNL) after mammary SPION injection.*
ALL I/ARL I = region A (axilla), Left/Right, Lymph node level I

IV. Discussion

We could detect SPIONs within the SNL by MPS measurements. However, no optimal running time for SPION enrichment within the SNL could be defined. This might be explained by the fact, that only 3-30% of the molecules contained in Resovist are suitable for the use in MPS or MPI [8,9]. Therefore, a SPION with better properties might improve the detection rate by MPS. The positive AAS gradient of the iron concentration in the first axillary lymph node over time correlates to the culmination of optimal SPION running time. A running time of 4 hours after SPION injection in the mammary gland of the healthy mouse seems to be optimal. Further investigation must show, if the same running time is feasible within a tumor bearing mouse model. This must be shown within an MPI setting.

V. Conclusions

It can be concluded that the best running time for SPIONs from breast to SNL is 4 hours within this study. There is an urgent need for better SPIONs with higher signal yield. It must be proven, if same results can be reproduced within a tumor bearing mouse model and under the use of MPI.

ACKNOWLEDGEMENTS

This work was supported in by the German Federal Ministry of Education and Research (BMBF) under Grant 01EZ0912 and by the University Research Program "Imaging of Disease Processes", University of Lübeck, Germany.

AUTHOR'S STATEMENT

Research funding: The author state no further funding involved. Conflict of interest: Authors state no conflict of interest. Informed consent: Informed consent has been obtained from all individuals included in this study. Ethical approval: The research related to human use complies with all the relevant national regulations, institutional policies and was performed in accordance with the tenets of the Helsinki Declaration, and has been approved by the authors' institutional review board or equivalent committee.

REFERENCES

[1] Ruhland, B., Baumann, K., Knopp, T., Sattel, T., Biederer, S., Lüdtke-Buzug, K., Buzug, T., Diedrich, K. and Finas, D.: Magnetic Particle Imaging durch Superparamagnetische Nanopartikel zur Sentinellymphknotendetektion beim Mammakarzinom, In: *Geburtshilfe und Frauenheilkunde*, A096, 2009, DOI: 10.1055/s-0029-1239012.

[2] Finas, D., Ruhland, B., Baumann, K., Knopp, T., Sattel, T., Biederer, S., Lüdtke-Buzug, K., Diedrich, K. and Buzug, T.: Sentinel lymphnode detection in breast cancer by magnetic particle imaging using superparamagnetic nanoparticles. In: Buzug, T., Borgert, J., Knopp, T., Biederer, S., Sattel, T., Erbe, M., Lüdtke-Buzug, K. eds. *Magnetic Nanoparticles Particle science, imaging technology, and clinical applications*. New Jersey: World Scientific Publishing 2010:205-10.

[3] Gräfe, K., von Gladiß, A., Bringout, G., Ahlborg, M. and Buzug, T. M.: 2D images recorded with a single-sided Magnetic Particle Imaging Scanner, *IEEE Transactions on Medical Imaging*, 35(4), 1056-1065, 2016, DOI: 10.1109/TMI.2015.2507187.

[4] Gräfe, K., v. Gladiss, A., Buzug. T. M.: First phantom measurements with a 3D single-sided MPI scanner. (Abstract). *International Workshop on Magnetic Particle Imaging*. Hamburg, 2018.

[5] Sattel, T. F., Erbe, M., Biederer, S., Knopp, T., Finas, D., Diedrich, K., Lüdtke-Buzug, K., Borgert, J. and Buzug, T. M.: Single-sided magnetic particle imaging device for the sentinel lymph node biopsy scenario. Medical Imaging 2011: Biomedical applications in molecular, structural, and functional imaging. San Diego, California, USA: *SPIE - The International Society of Optics and Photonics*, 2012.

[6] Finas, D., Baumann, K., Sydow, L., Heinrich, K., Rody, A., Gräfe, K., Buzug, T. M. and Lüdtke-Buzug, K.: SPIO Detection and Distribution in Biological Tissue - A Murine MPI-SLNB Breast Cancer Model, *IEEE Transactions on Magnetics*, 51(2), 5400104, 2015, DOI: 10.1109/TMAG.2014.2358272.

[7] Biederer, S., Knopp, T., Sattel, T. F., Lüdtke-Buzug, K., Gleich, B., Weizenecker, J., Borgert, J. and Buzug, T. M.: Magnetization response spectroscopy of superparamagnetic nanoparticles for magnetic particle imaging, *Journal of Physics D: Applied Physics*, 42(20), 205007, 2009, DOI: 10.1088/0022-3727/42/20/205007.

[8] Lüdtke-Buzug, K.: Magnetische Nanopartikel - Von der Synthese zur klinischen Anwendung, *Chemie in unserer Zeit*, 46(1), 32-39, 2012, DOI: 10.1002/ciuz.201200558.

[9] Lüdtke-Buzug, K., Haegele, J., Biederer, S., Sattel, T. F., Erbe, M., Duschka, R. L., Barkhausen, J. and Vogt, F. M.: Comparison of commercial iron oxide-based MRI contrast agents with synthesized high-performance MPI tracers, *Biomedizinische Technik / Biomedical Engineering*, 58(6), 527-533, 2013, DOI: 10.1515/bmt-2012-0059.

was measured at increasing field amplitudes. The heating curves for both the water and FCT samples are presented in Fig 1. The resolution of the fibre-optic thermometer was 0.1K. As a result of the slow heating rate, some digitization of the signal is observed. Artefacts and noise distortions in the heating curves result from range-switching events in the thermometer read-out electronics.

The initial slope of curve at the onset of heating was extracted and plotted against the excitation field amplitude in Fig 2.

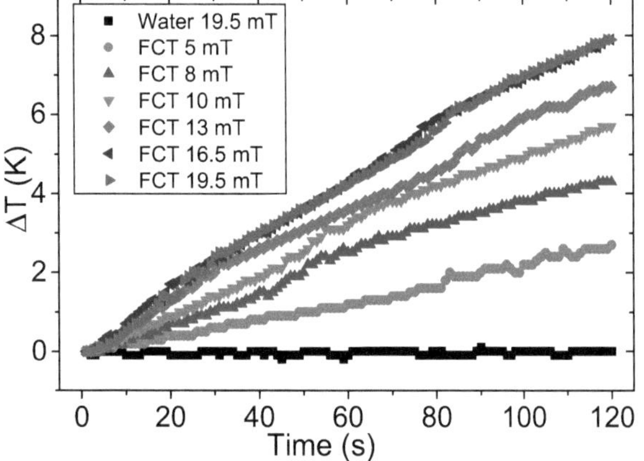

Figure 1: Heating curves measured FCT samples and pure water (control) at different excitation amplitudes.

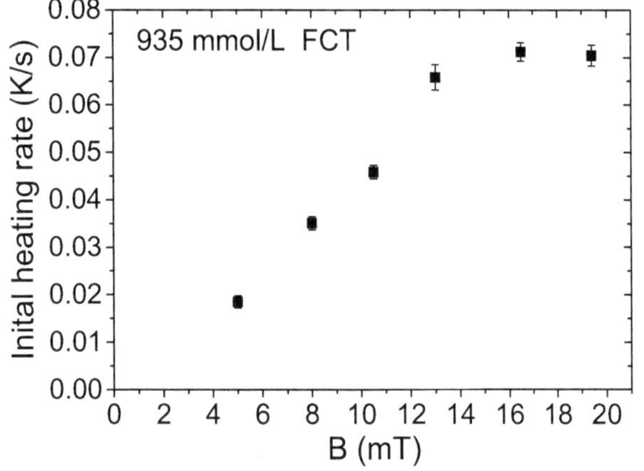

Figure 2: Initial slope of FCT heating curves plotted against field amplitude.

IV.   Discussion

The maximum change in temperature recorded after continuous field excitation for 2 minutes was ~8 K above the ambient room temperature. The measurement of pure water demonstrated no temperature increase over the same period, indicating that the whole 8 K temperature rise in FCT was caused by heat dissipated by the MNP.

The typical apoptosis region for therapeutic hyperthermia therapy is around 5 – 8 K above the body temperature of a human, while higher temperatures will induce thermoablation [7]. Thus, if the temperature rises recorded here translate into real heating in in-vivo applications, then care must be taken

when designing MPI imaging protocols to avoid unwanted damage to the subject's physiology. This will be particularly important in the case of long imaging sequences, for example for monitoring tracer transport, or for averaging low-intensity signals.

The initial gradients extracted from each heat curve suggest a linear dependence of the heating efficiency on field amplitude in the lower field range (0-14mT), with evidence for saturation at higher fields.

Further measurements will be conducted to investigate the concentration and sample-volume dependence of the observed heating. This will be used to obtain guidelines for appropriate bolus concentrations and volume for safe in-vivo MPI measurements using this tracer. The completed study will present these findings for FCT, as well as the heating behaviour of other common MPI tracer materials.

The authors acknowledge that the real field distribution during MPI image acquisition is significantly more complex than the 1D homogeneous excitation considered here. The impact of multiple excitation axes and field gradients for spatial resolution will be studied for a Bruker preclinical scanner in the near future.

V.   Conclusions

Using low-frequency calorimetry measurements, we have demonstrated significant heat dissipation in concentrated FCT nanoparticles undergoing typical MPI field excitation. The results show that heat dissipation by tracers during MPI is a topic deserving of further study.

ACKNOWLEDGEMENTS

The financial support of the DFG research grants "quantMPI: Establishment of quantitative Magnetic Particle Imaging (MPI) application oriented phantoms for preclinical investigations" (TR 408/9-1), "AMPI: "Magnetic particle imaging: Development and evaluation of novel methodology for the assessment of the aorta in vivo in a small animal model of aortic aneurysms" (SHA 1505-2/1) and "Matrix in Vision" (DFG CRC SFB 1340/1 2018, project A02) are gratefully acknowledged.

REFERENCES

[1] B. Gleich and J. Weizenecker, Tomographic imaging using the nonlinear response of magnetic particles, Nature, 435, 2005

[2] J. Weizenecker, B. Gleich and J. Borgert, Journal of Physics D: Applied Physics, Magnetic particle imaging using a field free line J. Phys D 41 10 2008

[3] Vogel P, Ruckert MA, Klauer P, Kullmann WH, Jakob PM, Behr VC. Traveling wave magnetic particle imaging IEEE Trans Med Imaging. 2014 Feb;33(2):400-7

[4] Panagiotopoulos N, Duschka RL, Ahlborg M, Bringout G, Debbeler C, Graeser M, Kaethner C, Lüdtke-Buzug K, Medimagh H, Stelzner J, Buzug TM, Barkhausen J, Vogt F, Haegele J, Magnetic particle imaging: current developments and future directions Int. J. Nanomed. 2015:10(1) Pages 3097—3114

[5] J. Wells, H. Paysen, O. Kosch, L. Trahms and F. Wiekhorst Temperature dependence in magnetic particle imaging

[6] J. Wells, N. Löwa, H. Paysen, U. Steinhoff and F. Wiekhorst, Probing Particle-Matrix Interactions during Magnetic Particle Spectroscopy, JMMM, Manuscript submitted

[7] A. Hervault and N K Tanh, Magnetic nanoparticle-based therapeutic agents for thermo-chemotherapy treatment of cancer, Nanoscale 2014; &; 11553-11573

II.III. Perfusion parameter maps

Reconstruction was performed using the system-matrix approach with a system matrix acquired with a cubic delta-sample filled with $250\,\mu l$ Perimag with an iron concentration of 17 mg/ml. The system matrix was acquired on a 2D grid of size 28×28 covering a field-of-view (FoV) of 140×140 mm^2 while applying a full 2D imaging sequence at each position. The drive-field FoV was 100×140 mm^2. The 1D measurements were combined prior to reconstruction [4] to obtain a single image for each selection-field cycle. A regularized Kaczmarz algorithm was used to iteratively solve the imaging equation. The number of iterations was eight while the relative regularization parameter was 1.5 and 1.1 for the higher concentration and 30.1 for the lower concentration. The perfusion parameter maps were calculated based on the low-pass filtered pixel-wise concentration-time series. The TTP values were extracted from the series as the time of maximum concentration values. The MTT is the first moment of the time-concentration series during bolus transition divided by the integral of the time series, while the CBV is the integral over time and the CBF is the maximum derivative of the concentration-time series. The CBV and the CBF were normalized to the maximum value in the imaging volume, thus representing relative values rCBV and rCBF.

III. Results

Perfusion parameter maps are shown in the lower part of Fig. 1. In the experiments corresponding to the first and third row, both hemispheres experience signal up-take, while it is prevented in the second and forth row in one hemisphere due to the occluded hose. The images in the first two rows were reconstructed from the data with a bolus of higher concentration, while the last two rows from lower concentrations. The distinction of the hemispheres, and the general distinction between stroke or no stroke is possible for both concentrations. The shape of the phantom is better reproduced at higher concentrations. The TTP maps accurately show bolus arrival times corresponding to the time series of specific voxels shown in the upper part of Fig.1. The bolus enters the phantom through the feeding hose and proceeds from the inner part to the outer part of the phantom and leaves through the discharge hose. The MTT describing the bolus duration is higher in the phantom than in feeding hose and increases towards the outer part of the phantom. The flow described by the rCBF is the highest near and inside the feeding hollow rod and decreases towards the periphery. The overall volume of tracer described by the rCBV has its maxima in the central part of the tube and decreases towards the outer parts of the respective tube.

IV. Discussion

The designed phantom enabled the simulation of brain perfusion and we were able to visualize it with the MPI scanner. The determined perfusion maps were plausible for the phantom, but the flow was slightly lower than expected for the human brain. These times are specific for the used experimental setup of the phantom, especially the flow rate, but not for the imaging system, which has a higher temporal resolution. In the experiments with occlusion, the hemisphere without perfusion could be determined for both concentrations of tracer material. We occluded one hemisphere completely in our experiments. In a realistic setting, vessels are also partially occluded. The influence of partial occlusion on the time series of the MPI reconstructed images needs to be explored in the future.

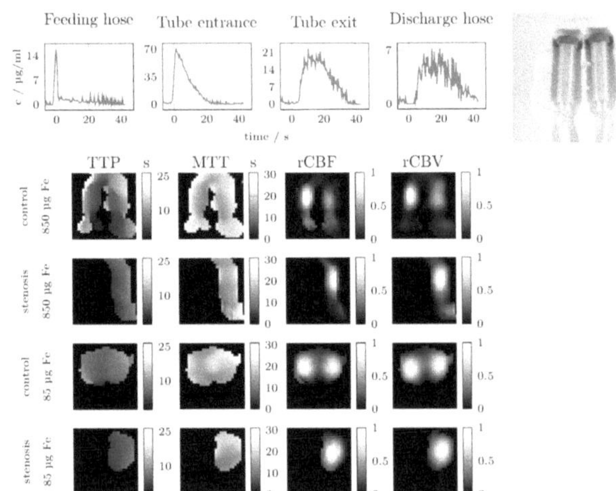

Figure 1: *Exemplary time series and perfusion parameter maps. The upper part shows the time series for voxels representing specific regions and the phantom. The parameter maps are shown in the lower part.*

V. Conclusions

We were able to detect a simulated stroke in a human-sized flow phantom with the human-sized MPI head scanner. The perfusion could be described with the help of calculated perfusion parameter maps.

AUTHOR'S STATEMENT
Research funding: German Research Foundation (DFG, grant 388 number KN 1108/2-1) and the Federal Ministry of Education and Research (BMBF, grant numbers 389 05M16GKA, 13XP5060B). Conflict of interest: Authors state no conflict of interest. Informed consent: Informed consent has been obtained from all individuals included in this study.

REFERENCES
[1] M. Gräser, F. Thieben, P. Szwargulski, F. Werner, N. Gdaniec, M. Boberg, F. Griese, M. Möddel, P. Ludewig, D. van de Ven, O. M. Weber, O. Woywode, B. Gleich, T.Knopp. Human-sized Magnetic Particle Imaging for Brain Applications. arXiv:1810.07987
[2] B. Gleich and J. Weizenecker. Tomographic imaging using the nonlinear response of magnetic particles. *Nature*, 435(7046):1217-1217, 2005. doi: 10.1038/nature03808.
[3] P. Ludewig, N. Gdaniec, J. Sedlacik, N. D. Forkert, P. Szwargulski, M. Graeser, G. Adam, M.G. Kaul, K.M. Krishnan, R.M. Ferguson, A.P. Khandhar, P. Walczak, J. Fichler, G. Thomalla, C. Gerloff, T. Knopp, T. Magnus. Magnetic Particle Imaging for real-time perfusion imaging in acute stroke. 2017 Oct 24;11(10):10480-10488. doi: 10.1021/acsnano.7b05784.
[4] T. Knopp, K. Them, M. Kaul, and N. Gdaniec. Joint reconstruction of non-overlapping magnetic particle imaging focus-field data. Physics in medicine and biology 60, L15 (2015).

III. Results

To evaluate the measured SNR values concerning their suitability for image reconstruction we applied the rose criterion (SNR > 5) [14]. The SNR values of the stents were below the threshold of 5. In comparison, 431 frequency components have been above the same threshold for the tracer solution. It was possible to visualize all of the stented vessel phantoms. There was no difference between the stented vessel phantoms and the reference phantom (Figure 1). The reconstructed images did not show any stent related artifacts.

Reference 3 mm

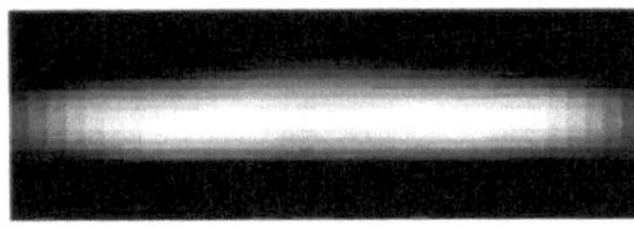

Biomatrix Neoflex 3/28

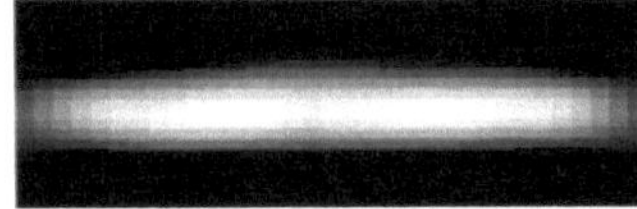

Promus Element 3/32

Figure 1: MPI images of the reference phantom and the coronary stents.

IV. Discussion

In this proof of concept study we demonstrated the potential of MPI for artifact-free visualization of the in-stent lumen of coronary stents.

MRI and CT can visualize coronary stents, but due to severe artifacts and artificial luminal narrowing the evaluation of the stent lumen and the detection of in-stent stenosis is difficult or even impossible. In contrast to these modalities stents are invisible using MPI. Therefore MPI allows for an artifact-free visualization of the in-stent lumen and the assessment of in-stent stenosis. However, the visualization of stents in MPI can be achieved using SPIO-based stent markers [12]. Furthermore multicolor MPI would be able to distinguish between the vessel lumen and the stent by encoding different particles with different colors [15], [16].

A limitation of our study is the amount of stents we investigated. To proof the concept we only tested two coronary stents made from two different materials. Further studies should prove our results with stents of different materials and dimensions. Another interesting point to address in the future is the possibility to quantify in-stent restenosis using MPI and if multicolor MPI will have an impact on the accuracy of the quantification.

V. Conclusions

MPI is able to image the in-stent lumen of coronary stents without artifacts and artificial lumen narrowing. Thus, MPI may overcome the disadvantages of MRI and CT concerning the visualization of the in-stent lumen.

ACKNOWLEDGEMENTS

The authors thank Ankit Malhotra and Kerstin Luedtke-Buzug for their help with filling the phantoms.

AUTHOR'S STATEMENT

Research funding: This work partially was funded by Federal Ministry of Education and Research BMBF grant numbers 13GW0071D, 13GW0069A and 01DL17010. Conflict of interest: Authors state no conflict of interest. Informed consent: Informed consent is not applicable. Ethical approval: The conducted research is not related to either human or animal use.

REFERENCES

[1] J. W. Moses *et al.*, "Sirolimus-eluting stents versus standard stents in patients with stenosis in a native coronary artery," *N. Engl. J. Med.*, vol. 349, no. 14, pp. 1315–1323, 2003.

[2] D. Maintz *et al.* "Imaging of coronary artery stents using multislice computed tomography: in vitro evaluation," *Eur Radiol*, vol. 13, no. 4, pp. 830–835, 2003.

[3] T. Klemm *et al.*, "MR imaging in the presence of vascular stents: A systematic assessment of artifacts for various stent orientations, sequence types, and field strengths," *J Magn Reson Imaging*, vol. 12, no. 4, pp. 606–615, 2000.

[4] J. Weizenecker *et al.*, "Three-dimensional real-time in vivo magnetic particle imaging," *Phys Med Biol*, vol. 54, no. 5, pp. L1–L10, 2009.

[5] J. Salamon *et al.*, "Magnetic Particle / Magnetic Resonance Imaging: In-Vitro MPI-Guided Real Time Catheter Tracking and 4D Angioplasty Using a Road Map and Blood Pool Tracer Approach," *PLoS ONE*, vol. 11, no. 6, p. e0156899, 2016.

[6] S. Herz *et al.*, "Magnetic Particle Imaging Guided Real-Time Percutaneous Transluminal Angioplasty in a Phantom Model," *Cardiovasc Intervent Radiol*, 2018.

[7] S. Vaalma *et al.*, "Magnetic Particle Imaging (MPI): Experimental Quantification of Vascular Stenosis Using Stationary Stenosis Phantoms," *PLoS ONE*, vol. 12, no. 1, p. e0168902, 2017.

[8] S. Herz *et al.*, "Magnetic Particle Imaging for Quantification of Vascular Stenoses: A Phantom Study," *IEEE Transactions on Medical Imaging*, pp. 1–1, 2017.

[9] M. G. Kaul *et al.*, "Magnetic particle imaging for *in vivo* blood flow velocity measurements in mice," *Phys Med Biol*, 2018.

[10] J. Haegele *et al.*, "Magnetic particle imaging: visualization of instruments for cardiovascular intervention," *Radiology*, vol. 265, no. 3, pp. 933–938, 2012.

[11] J. Haegele *et al.*, "Toward cardiovascular interventions guided by magnetic particle imaging: first instrument characterization," *Magn Reson Med*, vol. 69, no. 6, pp. 1761–1767, 2013.

[12] J. Haegele *et al.*, "Magnetic Particle Imaging: A Resovist based Marking Technology for Guide Wires and Catheters for Vascular Interventions," *IEEE Trans Med Imaging*, 2016.

[13] F. Wegner *et al.*, "First heating measurements of endovascular stents in magnetic particle imaging," *Phys Med Biol*, vol. 63, no. 4, p. 045005, 2018.

[14] A. E. Burgess, "The Rose model, revisited," *Journal of the Optical Society of America A*, vol. 16, no. 3, p. 633, 1999.

[15] J. Rahmer *et al.*, "First experimental evidence of the feasibility of multi-color magnetic particle imaging," *Physics in Medicine and Biology*, vol. 60, no. 5, pp. 1775–1791, 2015.

[16] J. Haegele *et al.*, "Multi-color magnetic particle imaging for cardiovascular interventions," *Phys Med Biol*, vol. 61, no. 16, pp. N415-426, 2016.

Fig. 2 shows the industrial polymer extruder we used to form the tube depicted in Fig. 3, a piece of catheter tube extruded from our custom MPI compound. It is 17 mm long, has an outer diameter of 3.5 mm and a wall thickness of 0.3 mm. It is made of three layers, where the middle one is MPI visible.

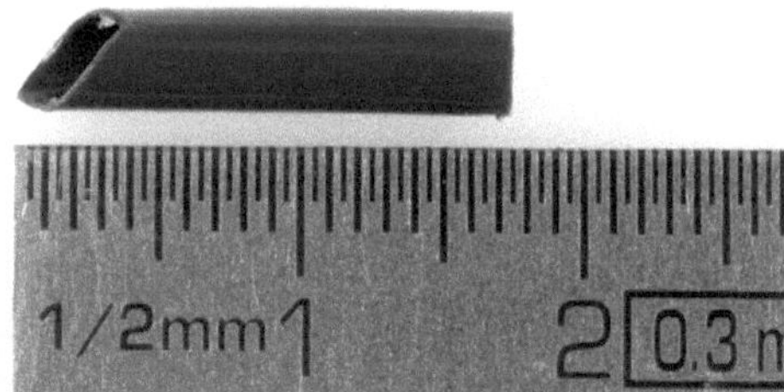

Figure 3: *Multi-material catheter tube prototype made of MPI visible polymer compound.*

In analogy to the x-ray visible markers on common interventional devices, our MPI visible compound also makes specific MPI markers for intrinsically MPI invisible devices possible.

II.III. Imaging

In order to demonstrate the MPI visibility of the compound, we use the preclinical MPI system MPI25/20FF with a gradiometric receive coil insert [4].

The exemplary part shown in Fig. 3 has been scanned using the aforementioned MPI system at a gradient strength of 1.5 T/m in z-direction and 0.75 T/m in x- and y-direction. With an isotropic drive field amplitude of 12 mT, this leads to a field of view of $(32 \times 32 \times 16)$ mm^3. For the image reconstruction, we use a $17 \times 17 \times 7$ hybrid system matrix [5, 6].

III. Results

Fig. 4 shows an MPI image of the scanned part (see Fig. 3). The reconstructed image has the same orientation as in Fig. 3. We observe that the spatial resolution of the reconstructed image is higher along the tube and significantly lower perpendicular to the tube. This leads to a visible vertical blurring.

IV. Discussion

The signal strength of the demonstrated MPI visible compound is sufficient for imaging a tubular structure as thin as 0.3 mm that incorporates nonmagnetic surface layers of biocompatible technical polymers. The compound is mechanically and chemically well suitable for the industrial manufacturing of catheters. Further the MPI signal from the compound is assumed to be easily distinguishable from the MPI signal of a bolus of liquid tracer material, due to its solid-state nature, that does not allow the particles to rotate, i.e. there is no Brownian relaxation.

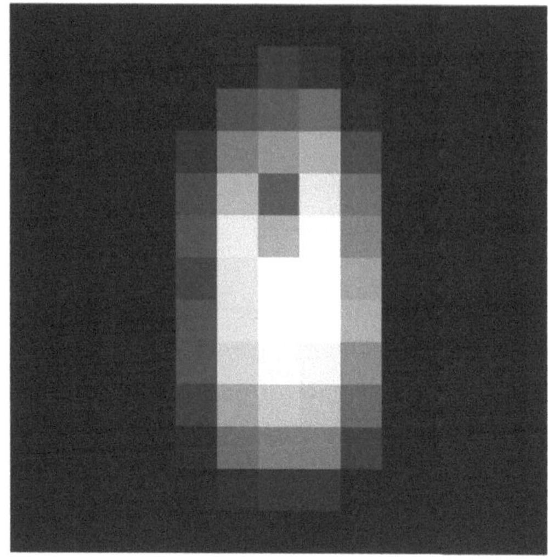

Figure 4: *MPI Image (single slice) of the tube depicted in Fig. 3.*

V. Conclusions

We developed a thermoplastic polymer compound that can be used to produce MPI visible interventional surgical devices in an industrial scale. In this contribution we show, that imaging of thin structures made of our compound is possible. In the progress of our collaboration, this will be further optimized, so that surgical devices for MPI guided interventions can be produced.

AUTHOR'S STATEMENT
The authors gratefully acknowledge the Federal Ministry of Education and Research, Germany (BMBF) for funding this project under Grant Nos. 13GW0069A (SAMBA PATI), 13GW0071D (SKAMPI) and 13GW0230B (FMT). Authors state no conflict of interest.

REFERENCES
[1] B. Gleich and J. Weizenecker. Tomographic imaging using the nonlinear response of magnetic particles. *Nature*, 435(7046):1217-1217, 2005. doi: 10.1038/nature03808.
[2] T. Knopp and T. M. Buzug. *Magnetic Particle Imaging: An Introduction to Imaging Principles and Scanner Instrumentation.* Springer, Berlin/Heidelberg, 2012. doi: 10.1007/978-3-642-04199-0.
[3] J. Haegele, et al. Multi-color magnetic particle imaging for cardiovascular interventions. *Physics in Medicine and Biology*, 61:N415, 2016. doi: 10.1088/0031-9155/61/16/N415.
[4] M. Graeser, et al. Towards Picogram Detection of Superparamagnetic Iron-Oxid Particles Using a Gradiometric Receive Coil. *Scientific Reports*, 7(6872), 2017. doi: 10.1038/s41598-017-06992-5.
[5] A. von Gladiss, et al. Hybrid system calibration for multidimensional magnetic particle imaging. *Physics in Medicine and Biology*, 62:3392, 2017. doi: 10.1088/1361-6560/aa5340.
[6] X. Chen, et al. First Measurement and SNR Results of a 3D Magnetic Particle Spectrometer. *International Journal on Magnetic Particle Imaging*, 4(1), 2018. doi: 10.18416/ijmpi.2018.1810001.

value for the compounds with 8 wt% MNP is 70 % higher than for the compounds with only 4 wt% MNP.

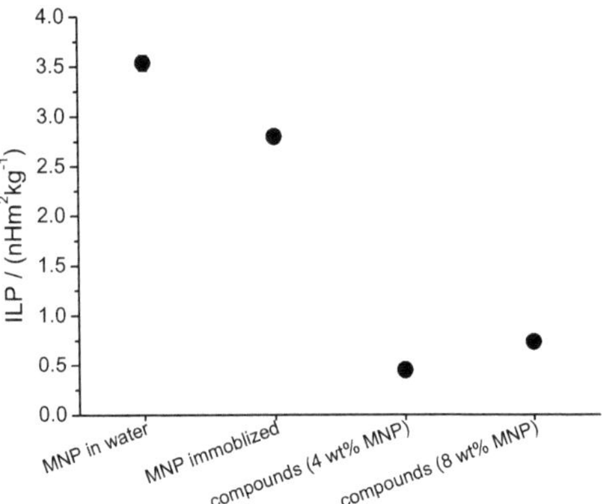

Figure 1: *Intrinsic loss power (ILP) values of (from left to right): MNP dispersed in water, MNP immobilized in polyacrylamide hydrogel, 4 wt% and 8 wt% MNP incorporated in compounds.*

Figure 2 displays the amplitude decay ratio A_5/A_3 for the same MNP states as for the ILP measurement showing the same trend as in figure 1. A_5/A_3 decreases by approximately 40 % for the compounds with 4 wt% MNP compared to one of MNP in water. Yet, the value for the compounds with 8 wt% MNP is 20 % higher than for the compounds with only 4 wt% MNP.

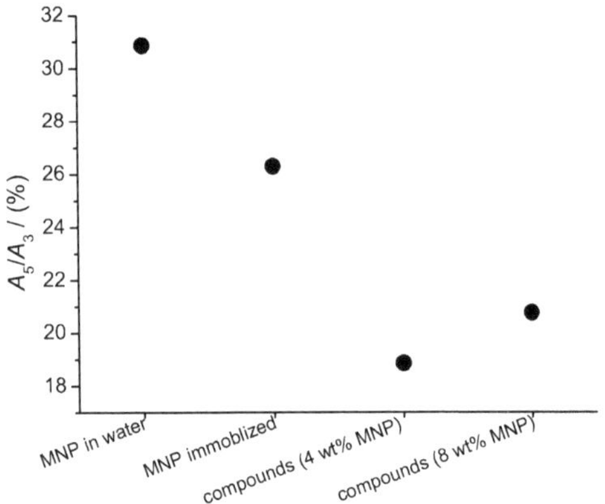

Figure 2: *A_5/A_3 amplitude decay ratio of (from left to right): MNP dispersed in water, MNP immobilized in plaster, 4 wt% and 8 wt% MNP incorporated in compounds.*

IV. Discussion

The results from hyperthermia and MPS measurements show a significant decrease in magnetic heating (ILP) and relaxation amplitude (A_5/A_3) for immobilized MNP compared to MNP dispersed in water. For MNP immobilized in compounds, Brownian relaxation is fully blocked causing a loss in heating efficiency and imaging performance. Such a decrease in ILP and A_5/A_3 was recently demonstrated for immobilized MNP inside hydrogels [5] and living cells [6], respectively.

The slight increase in ILP and A_5/A_3 for a higher MNP concentration inside the compounds (8 wt% MNP) can be attributed to particle-particle interactions which are more pronounced when agglomerates are formed. The formation of agglomerates in the compounds is expected at such high MNP concentrations [7]. For MNP agglomerates, the dipolar particle-particle interaction and the effective anisotropy energy increase, directly influencing the non-linear dynamic magnetic susceptibility of the MNP. Since hyperthermia and MPI rely on the non-linear dynamic magnetic susceptibility the same behavior is observed in both techniques [4].

V. Conclusions

For the evaluation of hyperthermia and imaging performance of hybrid stents, the effect of MNP immobilization inside the hybrid base material (compounds) on their heating and relaxation behavior were investigated. The results show that the ILP values and amplitude decay ratios A_5/A_3 decrease by up to 88 % and 40 %, respectively, for MNP immobilized inside compounds. Compared to compounds with 4 wt% MNP, an increased relaxation performance (i. e. increased ILP and A_5/A_3) is observed for compounds with higher MNP concentration (8 wt% MNP), which is attributed to the formation of bigger agglomerates.

ACKNOWLEDGEMENTS

The research project is funded as part of the program "Joint Industrial Research (IGF)" of the German Federal Ministry of Economic Affairs and Energy (contract number: 19735 N) and partly by the PTB core facility for the Measurement of Ultra-Low Magnetic Fields funded by the German Research Foundation.

AUTHOR'S STATEMENT

The authors state no conflict of interest. Informed consent was obtained from all individuals included in this study.

REFERENCES

[1] K. F. Chu and D. E. Dupuy, Thermal ablation of tumours: biological mechanisms and advances in therapy, *Nature Reviews Cancer,* 14:199-208, 2014. doi: 10.1038/nrc3672.

[2] B. Mues, E. M. Buhl, T. Schmitz-Rode and I. Slabu, Towards optimized MRI contrast agents for implant engineering: Clustering and immobilization effects of magnetic nanoparticles, *Journal of Magnetism and Magnetic Materials,* 471:432-438, 2019. doi: 10.1016/j.jmmm.2018.09.119.

[3] U. M. Engelmann, C. Shasha, E. Teeman, I. Slabu and K. M. Krishnan, Predicting size-dependent heating efficiency of magnetic nanoparticles from experiment and stochastic Néel-Brown Langevin simulation, *Journal of Magnetism and Magnetic Materials,* 471:450-456, 2019. doi: 10.1016/j.jmmm.2018.09.041.

[4] K. M. Krishnan, Biomedical Nanomagnetics: A Spin Through Possibilities in Imaging, Diagnostics, and Therapy, *IEEE Transactions on Magnetics,* 46:2523-2558, 2010. doi: 10.1109/Tmag.2010.2046907.

[5] M. Engelmann, J. Seifert, B. Mues, S. Roitsch, C. Ménager, A. M. Schmidt and I. Slabu, Heating efficiency of magnetic nanoparticles decreases with gradual immobilization in hydrogels, *Journal of Magnetism and Magnetic Materials,* 471:486-494, 2019. doi: 10.1016/j.jmmm.2018.09.113.

[6] B. W. Ficko, C. Ndong, P. Giacometti, K. E. Griswold and S. G. Diamond, A Feasibility Study of Nonlinear Spectroscopic Measurement of Magnetic Nanoparticles Targeted to Cancer Cells, *IEEE transactions on bio-medical engineering,* 64:972-979, 2017. doi: 10.1109/tbme.2016.2584241.

[7] I. Slabu, N. Wirch, T. Caumanns, R. Theissmann, M. Kruger, T. Schmitz-Rode and T. E. Weirich, Electron tomography and nano-diffraction enabling the investigation of individual magnetic nanoparticles inside fibers of MR visible implants, *Journal of Physics D-Applied Physics,* 50:315303, 2017. doi: 10.1088/1361-6463/aa77e8.

II.II. The Actuation Sequence

A rotating focus field in the y-/z-plane, which leads to a forward movement of the swimmer in x-direction, is generated by a list of discretized focus field steps. A ramping of the focus field in the direction of movement is required. The number of steps per turn, the number of turns and the amplitudes of the focus fields can be varied. An example is shown in Fig. 1. 10 turns and 50 steps per turn were applied, with the parameters shown in Fig. 1. The retention time at each field step was chosen to match one 2D drive field cycle, which is 0.65 ms. The ramping time between the focus field steps was 150 ms, resulting in a rotation frequency of 0.13 Hz.

II.III. Image Acquisition and Reconstruction

The swimmer was positioned and fixed in the center of the MPI scanner (Bruker 20/25 FF). 2D images of the x-/y-plane with 2.5 T/m z-gradient and 12 mT drive field strength were acquired. A schematic drawing of the sequence can be found in Fig. 2. The receive channel x of the scanner was replaced by a gradiometric receive coil [9]. A system matrix on a 20 x 10 x 1 grid with a 1 mm step size was acquired. One image was acquired at each focus field step position.

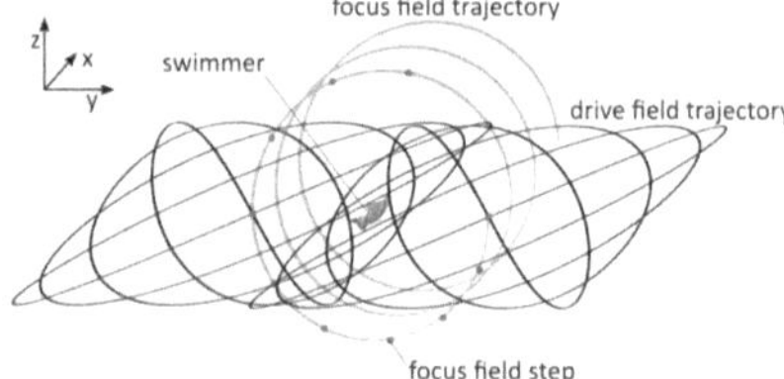

Figure 2: The simultaneous actuation and visualization sequence. The focus field steps are forming a helical focus field trajectory. The drive field Lissajous trajectory acquires 2D MPI images at every focus field step simultaneously (only two drive field trajectories are shown).

III. Results

The reconstructed images are treated as patches. The centers of the small FOVs were placed into a larger and finer matrix with a resolution of 0.5 mm/voxel according to the applied focus field steps. This results into a static image with an enlarged FOV of the swimmer (see Fig. 3).

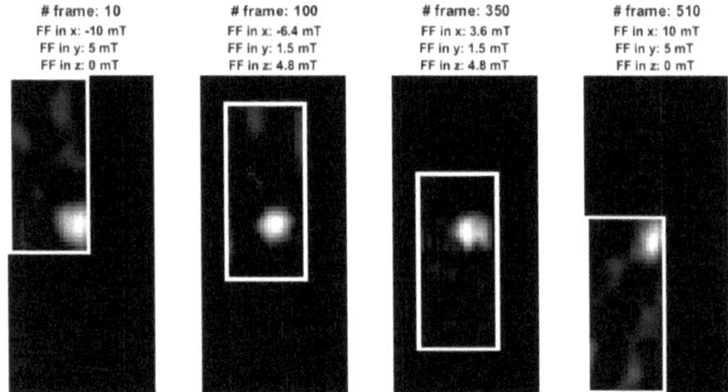

Figure 3: Reconstructed images of the x-/y-plane (4 out of 520 frames are exemplarily shown), while driving the actuation sequence. The single images with a small FOV of 20x10 mm² (white boxes) were placed into an enlarged FOV of 36x18 mm² according to the applied focus field (FF) steps.

IV. Discussion

With smaller ramping times between the focus field steps, higher rotation frequencies, leading to a forward movement of the swimmer, are achievable. It needs to be considered, that the rotation field amplitude of the y-direction needs to be smaller than the drive field amplitude in the same direction to ensure that the drive field FOV covers the object. A selective actuation also becomes possible, since both the focus fields and the selection field are used. Images of low resolution can be also reconstructed when the 2D drive field FOV is above or below the swimmer. This may be avoided by increasing the overscan of the system matrix in z-direction. Furthermore, this would enable a 3D imaging by stacking the 2D images according to the focus field strength in z-direction.

V. Conclusions

The simultaneous combination of actuation and imaging enables the real-time imaging of a moving swimmer. It has been demonstrated that the reconstruction of 2D MPI images of a static swimmer is possible while driving the drive field FOV on a helical trajectory.

ACKNOWLEDGEMENTS

The authors gratefully acknowledge the Federal Ministry of Education and Research, Germany (BMBF) for funding this project under Grant Nos. 13GW0069A (SAMBA PATI), 13GW0071D (SKAMPI), 13GW0230B (FMT) and 01DL17010A (IMAGINE), as well as the German Research Foundation (DFG) under Grant No. BU 1436/7-1.

AUTHOR'S STATEMENT

The authors state no conflict of interest.

REFERENCES

[1] F. Carpi, N. Kastelein, M. Talcott, C. Pappone, Magnetically controllable gastrointestinal steering of video capsules, IEEE Trans. Bio-med. Eng. 58 (2011) 231-4, doi: 10.1109/TBME.2010.2087332B.

[2] J. Rey, H. Ogata, N. Hosoe, K. Ohtsuka, N. Ogata, K. Ikeda, H. Aihara, I. Pangtay, T. Hibi, S. Kudo, and H. Tajiri. Feasibility of stomach exploration with a guided capsule endoscope. Endoscopy, 42(07): 541–545, 2010. doi: 10.1055/s-0030-1255521.

[3] M. Sitti, H. Ceylan, W. Hu, J. Giltinan, M. Turan, S. Yim, and E. Diller. Biomedical applications of untethered mobile milli/microrobots. Proceedings of the IEEE, 103(2): 205-224, 2015. doi: 10.1109/jproc.2014.2385105.

[4] S. Yim and M. Sitti. Shape-programmable soft capsule robots for semi-implantable drug delivery. IEEE Transaction on Robotics, 28(5):1198-1202, 2012. doi: 10.1109/TRO.2012.2197309.

[5] A. Ghosh and P. Fischer. Controlled propulsion of artificial magnetic nanostructured propellers. Nano Letters, 9(6):2243-2245, 2009. doi: 10.1021/nl900186w.

[6] B. J. Nelson, I. K. Kaliakatsos, J. J. Abbott, Microrobots for minimally invasive medicine, Annu. Rev. Biomed. Eng. 12 (1) (2010) 55-85, doi: 10.1146/annurev-bioeng-010510-103409.

[7] A. C. Bakenecker, A. von Gladiss, T. Friedrich, U. Heinen, H. Lehr, K. Lüdtke-Buzug, and T. M. Buzug, Actuation and visualization of a magnetically coated swimmer with magnetic particle imaging, Journal of Magnetism and Magnetic Materials, vol 473, 2019, 495-500, doi: 10.1016/j.jmmm.2018.10.056.

[8] J. Rahmer, C. Stehning, and B. Gleich. Spatially selective remote magnetic actuation of identical helical micromachines. Science Robotics, 2(3):2845, 2017. doi: 10.1126/scirobotics. aal2845.

[9] M. Graeser, T. Knopp, P. Szwargulski, T. Friedrich, A. von Gladiss, M. Kaul, K. M. Krishnan, G. Adam, H. Ittrich, and T. M. Buzug. Towards Picogram Detection of Superparamagnetic Iron-Oxid Particles Using a Gradiometric Receive Coil, Scientific Reports, 7(6872), 2017, doi: 10.1038/s41598-017-06992-5.

Percutaneous transluminal angioplasty (PTA): MPI vs. X-ray guidance

S. Herz [a*], P. Vogel [b], T. Kampf [c], P. Dietrich [a], M. A. Rückert [ ], [ ]

[a] Department of Diagnostic and Interventional Radiology, University [ ] Germany
[b] Department of Experimental Physics 5, University of Würzburg, 970[ ]
[c] Department of Diagnostic and Interventional Neur[ ] Germany
[*] Corresponding author, email: herz_s@[ ]

Abstract: Percutaneous transluminal angioplasty (PTA) is an [ ] visualization of the vasculature a fluoroscopy technique, digital [ ] subtracted from following images to minimize background inter[ ] and sensitive tomographic imaging modality that uses magnet[ ] An inherent advantage of MPI is the background-free and radi[ ] compare the potential of [ ]

I. Introduction

Cardiovascular disea[ ] mortality and major [ ] based interventions a[ ] therapy for many [ ]

inflating the PTA-balloon with diluted Ferucarbotran using a syringe.

III. Results

Labeled guidewires and balloon catheters allowed for precise visualization of the position of endovascular instruments. Visualization of stenosis phantoms and MPI-guidance of interventional instruments in near real-time was possible due to an online reconstruction algorithm.

In the experimental setup of this study both the MPI and the conventional x-ray fluoroscopy approach enabled successful treatment of artificial stenoses. In all rounds no residual stenosis was revealed post-interventionally. No major differences concerning duration of the treatment or handling of the endovascular instruments was observed. The spatial resolution of conventional fluoroscopes, however, was distinctly higher than in MPI. Frame rates were comparable between both imaging modalities (X-rays: Angiogram 2 frames/s, fluoroscopy 7.5 frames/s. MPI: 4 frames/s for all procedures.).

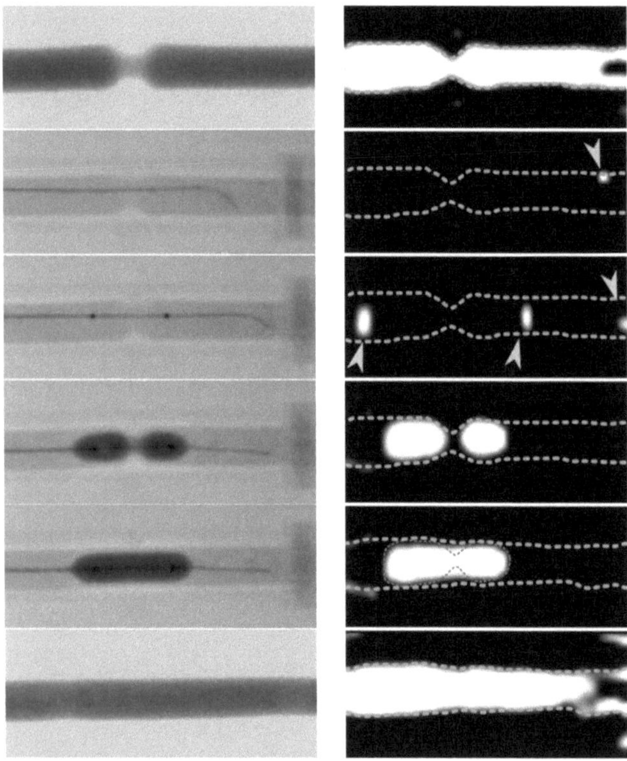

Figure 1: *The left column sketches a conventional x-ray guided PTA, the right column an MPI guided PTA.*
Top row to bottom row: 1) Angiography revealing a 50% stenosis. The inner boundaries of the stenosis phantom are automatically contoured (green dotted line) and serve as road map for MPI guided interventions. 2 + 3) Passing the guidewire and the balloon catheter over the stenosis. Grey dots in the MPI images represent the MPI visible markers of the endovascular instruments. 4 + 5) Dilation of the stenosis. The red dotted line contours the semi-inflated balloon and was added afterwards for reasons of comprehensibility. 6) Angiogram after intervention.

IV. Discussion

The TWMPI scanner in combination with an advanced online reconstruction algorithm enabled near real-time MPI guidance of interventional procedures in the setting of a phantom study. The spatial resolution of MPI is still distinctly lower than the submillimeter resolution of clinical X-ray fluoroscopes. Improved scanner hardware and tailored SPIOs bear potential for significant advancements such as a spatial resolution far below 1 mm. However, advances in scanner design need to consider limitations in specific absorption rate (SAR) and peripheral nerve stimulation (PNS).

V. Conclusions

This study demonstrates the feasibility of near real-time MPI-guided PTA in a phantom model. In the experimental setting of this study MPI guided PTA was similar to the conventional x-ray based approach concerning handling and visualization speed. Slight deficits of MPI concerning spatial and temporal resolution are likely to be overcome in the future. Further improvements in scanner hardware and SPIO design are needed to introduce MPI as competitive method in cardiovascular interventions.

ACKNOWLEDGEMENTS

The authors especially thank Mrs. Ruth Schimann for technical assistance.

AUTHOR'S STATEMENT

Research funding: The project underlying this report was partially funded by the German Research Foundation (BE-5293/1-1). Conflict of interest: Authors state no conflict of interest. Informed consent and ethical approval: This article does not contain any studies with human participants or animals performed by any of the authors.

REFERENCES

[1] B. Gleich and J. Weizenecker. Tomographic imaging using the nonlinear response of magnetic particles. *Nature*, 435(7046):1217-1217, 2005. doi: 10.1038/nature03808.

[2] T. Knopp and T. M. Buzug. *Magnetic Particle Imaging: An Introduction to Imaging Principles and Scanner Instrumentation.* Springer, Berlin/Heidelberg, 2012. doi: 10.1007/978-3-642-04199-0.

[3] P. Vogel, et al., Traveling Wave Magnetic Particle Imaging, *IEEE TMI*, vol. 33(2), pp. 400-7, 2014. Doi:10.1109/TMI.2013.2285472.

[4] P. Vogel et al., Dynamic Linear Gradient Array for Traveling Wave Magnetic Particle Imaging, *IEEE Trans. Magn.*, 2018. doi: 10.1109/TMAG.2017.2764440

[5] P. Vogel, et al., Flexible and Dynamic Patch Reconstruction for Traveling Wave MPI, *IJMPI*, vol. 2(2):1611001, 2017. doi: 10.18416/ijmpi.2016.1611001

Session 06: Synthesis and Spectroscopy

Aqueous micromixer synthesis to gain reproducible, high performance MPI tracers

A. Baki[a], N. Löwa[b], C. Knopke[c], S. G. Diamond[c,d], O. Kosch, F. Wiekhorst[b], R. Bleul[a*]

[a] Fraunhofer IMM, Mainz, Germany
[b] Physikalisch-Technische Bundesanstalt, Berlin, Germany
[c] Lodestone Biomedical LLC, Lebanon, Hanover, New Hampshire, USA
[d] Thayer School of Engineering at Dartmouth, Hanover, New Hampshire, USA
* Corresponding author, email: regina.bleul@imm.fraunhofer.de

Abstract: A series of single-core iron oxide nanoparticle samples have been produced as potential tracer for magnetic particle imaging (MPI) by an aqueous micromixer based synthesis route. Magnetic particle spectroscopy (MPS) reveal the general capability of the produced nanoparticles as MPI tracer, since the MPS spectral amplitudes of most samples are significantly higher than of the MPI gold standard Resovist®. Preliminary MPI investigations using a preclinical field-free-point scanner device confirm the performance enhancement compared to Resovist. The presented synthesis approach stands out due to its high reproducibility as well as cost, time and yield efficiency.

I. Introduction

Magnetic Particle Imaging (MPI) is an exciting new imaging technique using magnetic nanoparticles as tracer. Though it promises great potential for clinical application in cardiovascular disease diagnosis, it so far only reached the preclinical level and still requires significant improvements in both the highly complex scanner instrumentation, and the development of MNP tracer with enhanced dynamic magnetic properties as well as peculiar biological properties like higher blood half-life time and stability in physiological media. Resovist®, a former contrast agent for magnetic resonance imaging (MRI), is still commonly used as gold standard for MPI. Resovist® consists of iron oxide nanoparticle clusters, which do by far not perform optimal for MPI. According to theoretical models [1] single-core iron oxide nanoparticles with a distinct size of about 30 nm core diameter would be more beneficial tracer. Those single-core particles in this size range are not easily accessible and generally require highly sophisticated and time-consuming synthesis strategies. These include thermal decomposition in organic solvents at high temperatures followed by phase transfer to aqueous media [3] or biotechnological biomineralization with microorganisms [4] suffering from process-related highly immunogenic microbiological impurities. The here presented micromixer based synthesis approach addresses these issues and aims on a cost-efficient, safe and reproducible production method to obtain single-core iron oxide nanoparticles in the required size range.

In this work, we analyzed the performance of a set of MPI tracer produced by aqueous micromixer synthesis by Magnetic Particle Spectroscopy (MPS) to demonstrate the great potential of the synthesis approach.

II. Material and Methods

II.I. Aqueous Micromixer Nanoparticle Synthesis

The continuous synthesis of iron oxide nanoparticles was performed by precipitation from aqueous, alkaline solutions of iron salts in a micromixer set-up as previously reported [4]. The microfluidic mixing device consists of HPLC pumps (Knauer, Germany), Caterpillar micromixer (Fraunhofer IMM, Germany) and various reaction loops of different volumes. Size of magnetic nanoparticles can be adjusted in the range 10 to 50 nm by selecting process parameters as e.g. temperature, mixing ratios and the residence time.

II.II. Characterizing the Nanoparticles

Magnetic nanoparticle geometry was analyzed by imaging with Transmission Electron Microscopy (TEM). Measurements were performed at a Zeiss Libra 120 on carbon coated copper grids at 120 kV acceleration voltage, images were taken with a CCD camera. Particle dispersions in aqueous media were additionally measured by analytical centrifugation (Differential Centrifugal Sedimentation, DCS) as ensemble method. Centrifugation experiments were performed with a device from CPS, Instruments, Inc. at 24000 rpm with a calibration polyvinyl chloride standard (239 nm).

The iron concentration of the particle samples was determined using the Phenanthroline protocol. First, the MNP were dissolved in concentrated hydrochloride acid and subsequently mixed with hydroxylamine. Formed ferroin complexes were measured photometrically at $\lambda=510$ nm and iron concentrations of the samples were estimated employing a calibration curve of iron oxide standard solutions.

Magnetic Particle Spectroscopy measurements were performed to assess the MPI performance of the nanoparticles using a commercial Magnetic Particle Spectrometer (MPS-3) (Bruker, Germany) detecting the non-linear magnetic response of magnetic nanoparticles exposed to an oscillating field (frequency 25 kHz, amplitude 25 mT) All measurements were performed at 37°C applying 30 μL of undiluted MNP samples. We used the amplitude of the third harmonic A_3 normalized to the iron amount (A_3^* in units of Am^2/kg(Fe)) and the ratio of fifth to third harmonic A_5/A_3 (in units of %) to assess the MPI tracer performance compared to Resovist (A_3^*=11.0(5) Am^2/kg(Fe) and A_5/A_3=38(1) %).

Additionally, low frequency analyses of the particle samples were carried out using a custom-built spectrometer (NCS2, Lodestone Biomedical LLC). Low frequency AC measurements below 10 kHz can be a valuable addition to standard 25 kHz AC characterization methods as low frequencies are often more sensitive to the binding state of the particle. Low frequency characterization can therefore help to identify high performance particles for biomarker and drug targeting applications.

NCS2 measurements were performed at an applied AC field at a frequency of 1 kHz and a 20 mT (RMS) amplitude, while keeping the sample at a temperature of 25°C. Readouts were taken with a digital implementation of a lock-in amplifier with in-phase and quadrature reference tones at 3 kHz. The reported magnitudes are proportional 3rd harmonic A_3 of the sample magnetic moment.

III. Results and Discussion

A series of experiments was performed to investigate the influence of the average particle core size on the MPI performance. By just varying the residence time in the micromixer set up single core nanoparticles of different average core size in the relevant range between 20 and 30 nm were obtained.

Fig. 1 shows a TEM micrograph of one promising tracer candidate. The average core diameter of the sample was with 28 nm at the higher end of the investigated size range. The particles are relatively homogenous in shape and size.

These samples were characterized by MPS in both devices. Fig. 2 shows the results of measurements at 1 kHz with the NCS2 device, Lodestone Biomedical LLC. With one exception exhibited all samples the same or even higher signal amplitudes up to a factor two as Resovist®. These promising results were confirmed MPS by measurements with the commercial MPS-3 (Bruker) at 25 kHz as well as preliminary by MPI imaging investigations using the preclinical Bruker device (MPI 25/20 FF).

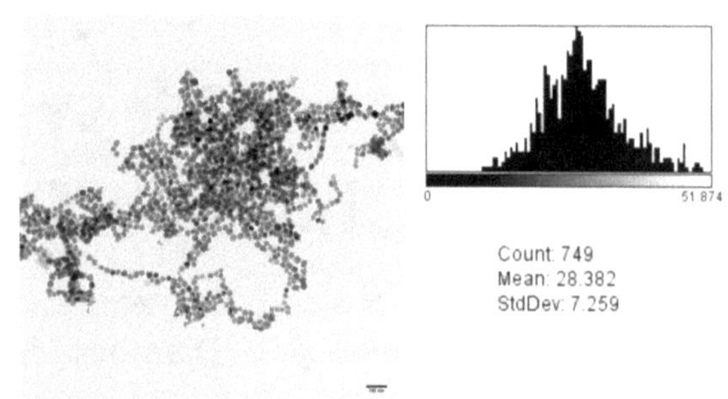

Figure 1: *TEM image including automatic size analysis of one the best tracer candidates from the continuous micromixer synthesis*

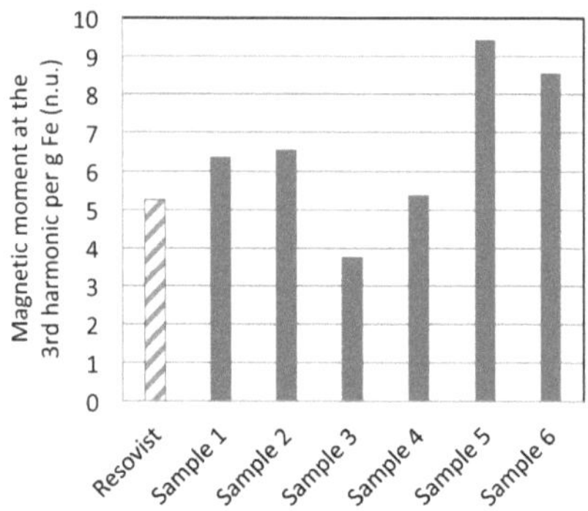

Figure 2: *NCS2 measurements of a series of liquid micromixer nanoparticle samples*

IV. Conclusions

The aqueous micromixer-based synthesis strategy provides the tunable production of single-core magnetic nanoparticles of different sizes as MPI tracer. The analyzed samples showed promising MPS as well as first MPI performance.

ACKNOWLEDGEMENTS
We gratefully acknowledge financial support from the European Regional Development Fund (EFRE). R.B. thanks the Fraunhofer-Gesellschaft for the support within the Fraunhofer TALENTA program.

REFERENCES
[1] B. Gleich and J. Weizenecker. Tomographic imaging using the nonlinear response of magnetic particles. *Nature*, 435(7046):1217-1217, 2005. doi: 10.1038/nature03808.
[2] R. Hufschmid, H. Arami, R. M. Ferguson, M. Gonzales, E. Teeman, L. N. Brush, N. D. Browning, and K. M. Krishnan. Synthesis of phase-pure and monodisperse iron oxide nanoparticles by thermal decomposition. *Nanoscale*, 7(25):11142–11154, 2015. doi:10.1039/C5NR01651G.
[3] A. Kraupner, D. Eberbeck, D. Heinke, R. Uebe, D. Schüler and A. Briel. Bacterial magnetosomes – nature's powerful contribution to MPI tracer research. Nanoscale, 9, 5788-5793, 2017. doi: 10.1039/c7nr01530e.
[4] A. Baki, N. Löwa, R. Thiermann, C. Bantz, M. Maskos, F. Wiekhorst, R. Bleul. Continuous synthesis of single core iron oxide nanoparticles for MPI tracer development. IWMPI Book of Abstracts 2017, ISBN 978-3-945954-34-8.

Suspensions of sub-micron microfabricated magnetic discs

Leon Abelmann [a,b,c], André-René Blaudszun [a], Henk van Wolferen [b], Kees Ma [b], Per A. Löthman[c]

[a] KIST Europe, Saarbrücken, Germany
[b] University of Twente, Enschede, Netherlands
[c] Saarland University, Saarbrücken, Germany
* Corresponding author, email: l.abelmann@kist-europe.de

In this contribution, we demonstrate a mass production method for suspensions of nanofabricated magnetic Au/NiFe/Au discs with diameters below 200 nm. We analyze the magnetic response of the microfabricated discs by magnetometry when they are still on the carrier wafer and in suspension. Compared to micron-sized elements, the coercivity and remanence of 180 nm discs is strongly reduced. The etching procedure used in the manufacturing process results in a magnetic redeposition layer, which adds to the magnetic signal. The metal discs are easily dispersed in acetone. For transfer to aqueous solutions, surface modification with PEG and PLL has been attempted. It appears the redeposition layer prevents full coverage of the discs.

I. Introduction

Suspensions of microfabricated magnetic metal elements offer a promising alternative to colloidal suspensions of iron-oxide particles in the application of magnetic particle imaging. The ability to tailor the hysteresis loop by means of material composition, shape and film thickness, opens up avenues to increase the energy in the higher harmonic response of the dispersion to the drive field.

Up to now, these microfabricated elements have diameters in the order of 1-3 μm [1-3]. These discs are mainly captured in small capillary blood vessels, such as the lung [1]. For longer circulation times, smaller particles are required. However, conventional contact mask lithography is not capable of producing discs below the diffraction limit of the light source used in the exposure tool. In most research environments, this limits the resolution of contact lithography to about 1 μm. Since the patterns required are however highly repetitive (arrays of discs), one can successfully apply laser holography. In this contribution, we demonstrate the use of laser interference lithography (LIL) [4]. With this method disc diameters below 200 nm can be realized over a 10x10 cm² area, with exposure times below two minutes.

II. Material and Methods

The base layer for the discs is an Au(20 nm)/Ni$_{80}$Fe$_{20}$(20)/Au(20) stack sputter deposited on a silicon wafer with a silicon oxide layer and anti-reflection coating. This bottom anti-reflection coating serves primarily as a sacrificial layer. For lithography, a top anti-reflection layer and an AR-N-7520-11 resist layer are spin coated. The resist film is exposed in a laser lithography setup with a Lloyd

mirror configuration at an angle of 26°, leading to a grating periodicity of 300 nm. The discs are etched in a process identical to the 2 μm discs of our earlier work [3]. Since the bottom anti-reflection coating is resistant to acetone, the wafer was first etched in Microstrip 5010 at 80 °C for 30 min, after which the discs were collected in acetone using the standard procedure. PEG coating was performed by means of a FL-PEG-SH (Nanocs) agent in ethanol.

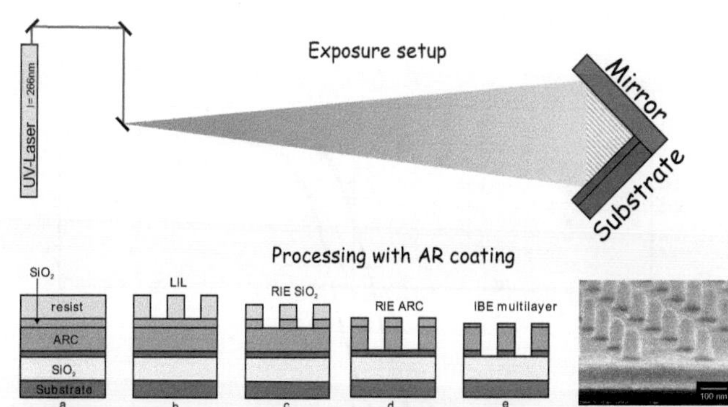

Figure 1: *Laser interference lithography. Top: By means of a mirror, a standing wave grating is created in a photoresist film. Bottom: By double exposure an array of resist pillar is realized, which is etched into a Au/NiFe/Au film by means of ion beam etching.*

III. Results and discussion

Figure 3 shows discs with a diameter of 180 nm, after drying the suspension in acetone on a silicon wafer. On close inspection, a redeposition layer can be observed on one side of the discs. Large flakes of redeposition layer can also be found in the dispersion, indicating that the redeposition layer is most likely magnetic.

After PEG coating, we observe that also only one face of the discs has a PEG coating. We speculate it is the face opposing the redeposition layer. Further investigation is currently in progress.

The VSM hysteresis loops (figure 3) of the discs on the carrier wafer show clearly that the remanence and coercivity decrease dramatically when compared to 2 μm discs. The saturation field on the other hand is very low, so suspensions of these particles are expected to give the same high signal as the 2 μm discs, and outperform Resovist [3]

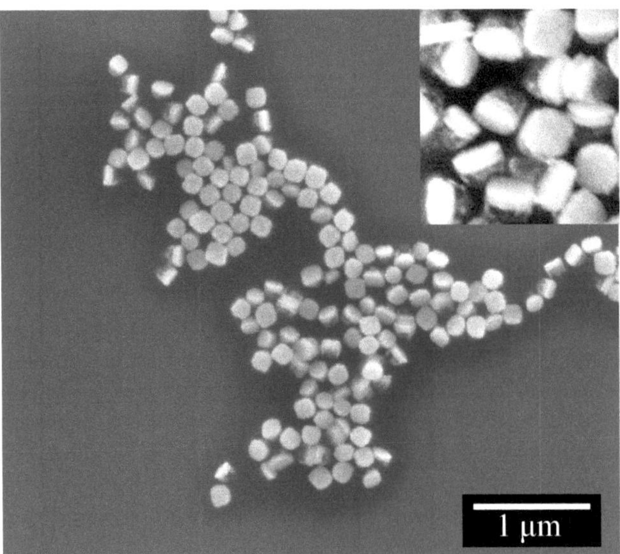

Figure 2: *180 nm diameter Au/NiFe/Au discs after drying on a silicon wafer. The insert shows a redeposition layer on one face. There are strong indications this layer is magnetic.*

IV. Conclusions

We prepared dispersions of Au(20 nm)/NiFe(20)/Au(20) discs of 180 nm diameter by laser interference lithography. The discs on the fabrication wafer have no remanence and coercivity. The etching procedure used in the manufacturing process results in a magnetic redeposition layer, which adds to the magnetic signal. This redeposition layer prevents full coverage of the discs by a PEG coating, which prevents transfer of the discs to aqueous solution.

REFERENCES

[1] Nikitin, M.; Orlov, A.; Sokolov, I.; Minakov, A.; Nikitin, P.; Ding, J.; Bader, S.; Rozhkova, E. & Novosad, V. Ultrasensitive detection enabled by nonlinear magnetization of nanomagnetic labels *Nanoscale, Royal Society of Chemistry,* **2018**, *10*, 11642-11650

[2] Mansell, R.; Vemulkar, T.; Petit, D.; Cheng, Y.; Murphy, J.; Lesniak, M. & Cowburn, R.Magnetic particles with perpendicular anisotropy for mechanical cancer cell destruction *Scientific Reports,* **2017**, *7*, 4257

[3] Löthman, P.; Janson, T.; Klein, Y.; Blaudszun, A.-R.; Ledwig, M. & Abelmann, L. Magnetic Particle Spectrometry of Microfabricated Magnetic Particles *International Journal on Magnetic Particle Imaging,* **2017**, *3*

[4] Wolferen van, H. A. G. M. & Abelmann, Laser Interference Lithography
in L. Hennessy, T. *(Ed.) Lithography: Principles, Processes and Materials, Nova Publishers,* **2011**, 133-148

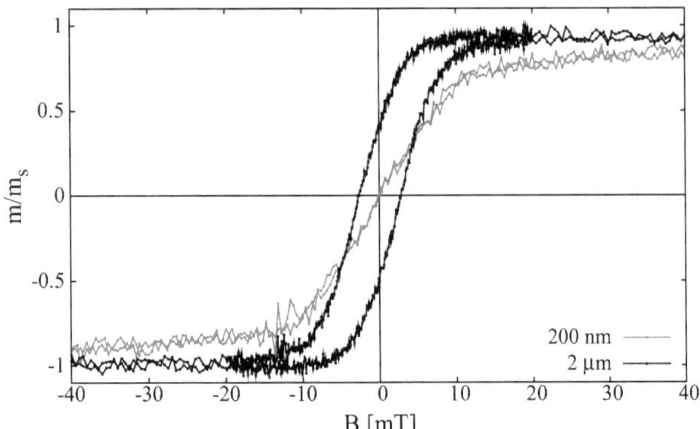

Figure 3: *Vibrating Sample Magnetometry of an array of Au/NiFe/Au discs when still on the carrier wafer. When the disc diameter is reduced from 2 μm to 200 nm, the coercivity strongly decreases. The saturation field however remains low.*

Since we clearly have a magnetic redeposition layer, there is concern that the magnetic signal is a combination of the response of the discs and the redeposition layer. The total magnetic moment, however, agrees with the amount of NiFe in the discs only, so we assume the contribution is minor.

Effect of dextran on the nucleation and growth of nanostructures with an In-situ Magnetic Particle Spectrometer (INSPECT)

A. Malhotra[a*], A. von Gladiss[a], T. M. Buzug[a], and K. Lüdtke-Buzug[a]

[a] *Institute of Medical Engineering, University of Lübeck, Lübeck, Germany*
[*] *Corresponding author, email: {malhotra,luedtke-buzug}@imt.uni-luebeck.de*

Magnetic nanostructures form the backbone of magnetic particle imaging (MPI). Therefore, it is very vital to understand the nucleation and growth of the nanostructures for synthesizing tailored nanostructures for both imaging as well as therapy. State of the art magnetic particle spectrometers (MPS) can only characterize the nanostructures retrospectively, i.e. after the completion of the synthesis process. In this research, a novel in-situ magnetic particle spectrometer (INSPECT) is presented, which can be used to characterize the complete synthesis process. INSPECT is a powerful tool to track the nucleation and growth of the nanostructures in real time. This research gives a brief hardware introduction to INSPECT as well as illustrates the effect of the quantity of dextran in an alkaline-based co-precipitation synthesis process.

I. Introduction

Synthesizing nanostructures for imaging modalities such as magnetic particle imaging (MPI), magnetic resonance imaging (MRI) and other therapeutic modalities such as magnetic fluid hyperthermia (MFH) is a challenging task [1-2]. Currently, various techniques and devices are available for characterizing the nanostructures such as VSM (vibrating sample magnetometer, measures the static magnetization), AC magnetometers (alternating current magnetometers, measures the magnetic susceptibility) and various magnetic particle spectrometers such as 1D and multidimensional MPS [3-6]. All these devices provide physical and geometrical information about the nanostructures but after the completion of the synthesis process. Therefore, most of the critical information regarding the nucleation and growth of the nanostructures is unobserved. Furthermore, x-ray scattering and transmission electron microscopy (TEM) is used for real-time monitoring of the nanostructure's growth, but the primary drawback with these devices is a tedious setup and a small measurement chamber [7-8]. This makes these devices inept for the use in normal chemistry laboratory where multiple syntheses are being performed on a day-to-day basis. The aim of this research is to develop a spectrometer for real-time monitoring of nanostructures, which can be used in a chemistry laboratory and can be directly integrated into the synthesis process. To achieve this, an in-situ magnetic particle spectrometer (INSPECT) is introduced, and assessment regarding the role of the coating material (Dextran T70) at different flow rates involved in the alkaline co-precipitation is presented.

II. Material and Methods

II.I. In-situ magnetic particle spectrometer (INSPECT)

In this section, the hardware realization of INSPECT is described. The diameter of the reaction chamber is approximately 72 mm and can easily fit a standard 100 ml flask. The block diagram of INSPECT is shown in Fig. 1.

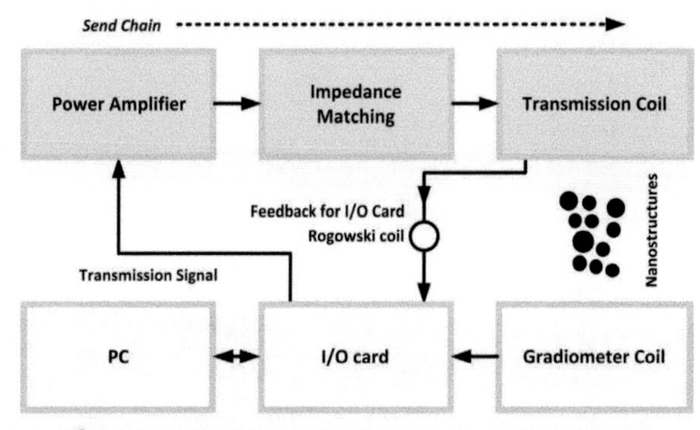

Figure 1: *The block diagram of INSPECT consisting of various components for both the send chain and receive chain.*

For the generation of the transmission signal (T_x) and for the acquisition of the receive signal (R_x) an X3-25M (Innovative Integration, USA) is used. The generated sinusoidal signal T_x has a frequency of 23 kHz and after amplification provides the necessary magnetic field up to 10 mT. For the receive chain, a gradiometer coil is used for acquiring the signals from the nanostructures. The total measurement time for one measurement is one second for acquiring 10 periods with

2300 averages. The measurements for an MPS usually consist of amplitude and phase spectra but with the help of the INSPECT, the change in the magnetic moment of the particles can be tracked throughout the synthesis process.

II.II. Nanostructure synthesis and measurement protocol

Alkaline co-precipitation in water is used for the synthesis of nanostructures. The details of the experiment as well as the synthesis process are explained by Lüdtke-Buzug [9]. For this particular research, the flask containing a mixture of iron salts, dextran, and demineralized water is placed in INSPECT. Then, at a constant flow rate ammonia (NH_3) is added under ultrasonic control (45 kHz). Before starting the synthesis process, an empty measurement is acquired, which is subtracted from the subsequent measurements to correct for background noise. The measurements are acquired every 5 min over the entire duration of the synthesis process. For this research, the effect of the quantity of dextran is studied and all other parameters are kept constant (see Table 1).

Table 1: *Parameters for the synthesis of nanostructures with different quantities of dextran.*

Probe	Amount/g	Flow Rate/ ml/h
Sample 1	$FeCl_3$ $6H_2O$: 1.32 ± 0.01 $FeCl_2$ $4H_2O$: 0.50 ± 0.01 Dextran: 1.32 ± 0.01	10
Sample 2	$FeCl_3$ $6H_2O$: 1.32 ± 0.01 $FeCl_2$ $4H_2O$: 0.51 ± 0.01 Dextran: 0.33 ± 0.01	10
Sample 3	$FeCl_3$ $6H_2O$: 1.32 ± 0.01 $FeCl_2$ $4H_2O$: 0.51 ± 0.01 Dextran: 1.32 ± 0.01	20
Sample 4	$FeCl_3$ $6H_2O$: 1.32 ± 0.01 $FeCl_2$ $4H_2O$: 0.51 ± 0.01 Dextran: 0.99 ± 0.01	20

III. Results

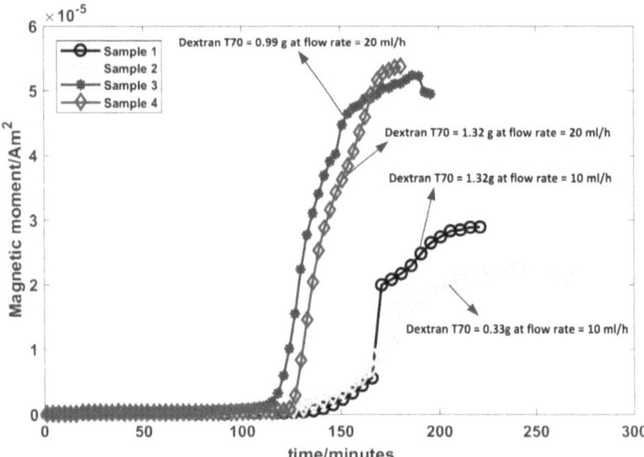

Figure 2: *Change in the magnetic moment of the third harmonic versus time for the complete synthesis process.*

Fig. 2 visualizes the magnitude of the third harmonic versus time for all the samples. It provides information regarding the change in the magnetic moment versus time for the complete synthesis process.

IV. Discussion and Conclusions

The amount of dextran plays a critical role in the growth phase of the nanostructures. The initialization of the growth corresponds to the amount of dextran in the chemical synthesis. At a lower flow rate of 10 ml/h, it holds that the smaller the amount of dextran, the earlier the magnetic moment increases. This corresponds to the fact that the core of the nanostructures is growing faster. On the other hand, a higher amount of dextran leads to a more rapid and uniform growth and even causes a delay in the saturation effect. This can be clearly seen in Fig. 2 as Sample 1 with dextran T70 = 1.32 ± 0.01 g has a steeper slope as compared to Sample 2 with dextran T70 = 0.33 ± 0.01 g. At a higher flow rate of 20 ml/h, the same inference can be drawn that the higher the amount of dextran, the later the nanostructures start growing. In Sample 3 (T70 = 0.99 ± 0.01 g) this effect can be seen at a time step of around 100 mins and for Sample 4 (T70 = 1.32 ± 0.01 g) the growth starts occurring around 50 mins. Therefore, the amount of dextran directly corresponds to the size of the core of the nanostructures. The lower the amount of dextran, the higher the core size of the nanostructures is in co-precipitation based chemical synthesis. It can also be seen that with higher flow rates the nucleation and growth is more rapid and uniform as seen in Sample 3 and Sample 4 versus Sample 1 and Sample 2.

ACKNOWLEDGMENTS

We gratefully acknowledge the financial support from the Federal Ministry of Education and Research, Germany (BMBF, grant numbers 13GW0069A and 13GW0230B).

AUTHOR'S STATEMENT

The authors state no conflict of interest.

REFERENCES

[1] Gleich, B. & Weizenecker, J. (2005), *'Tomographic imaging using the nonlinear response of magnetic particles'*, nature 435, 1214-1217. doi: 10.1038/nature03808.

[2] Lópeza, M., AntonioTeijeiro and Rivasa, J. (2013), *'Magnetic nanoparticle-based hyperthermia for cancer treatment'*, Reports of Practical Oncology & Radiotherapy 18(6), 397-400. doi:10.1016/ j.rpor.2013.09.011

[3] Biederer, S. et al. *Magnetization response spectroscopy of superparamagnetic nanoparticles for magnetic particle imaging.* J. Phys. D: Appl. Phys. 42 (2009).doi:10.1088/0022-3727/42/20/205007.

[4] Graeser, M., von Gladiss, A., Weber, M. & Buzug, T. M. *Two dimensional magnetic particle spectrometry.* Phys. Medicine & Biol. 62 (2017).

[5] Tay, Z. W. et al. *A high-throughput, arbitrary-waveform, MPI spectrometer and relaxometer for comprehensive magnetic particle optimization and characterization.* Sci. Reports 6 (2016) doi:10.1038/srep34180.

[6] Chen, Xin et al. *First Measurement and SNR Results of a 3D Magnetic Particle Spectrometer. International Journal on Magnetic Particle Imaging*, [S.l.], v. 4, n. 1, oct. 2018. ISSN 2365-9033.

[7] Liao, H.-G., Cui, L., Whitelam, S. & Zheng, H. *Real-time imaging of pt3fe nanorod growth in solution.* Sci. 336, 1011–1014 (2012). doi: 10.1126/science.1219185.

[8] Renaud, G. *Real-time monitoring of growing nanoparticles.* Sci. 300, 1416–1419 (2003). doi:10.1126/science.1082146.

[9] Lüdtke-Buzug, K. (2012), *'Magnetische Nanopartikel'*, Chemie in unserer Zeit 46(1), 32-39. doi: 10.1002/ciuz.201200558

Intracellular dynamics of superparamagnetic iron oxide nanoparticles for MPI

E. Teeman[a], C. Shasha[b], J. E. Evans[c], and K. M. Krishnan[a,b,*]

[a] *Department of Materials Science & Engineering, University of Washington, Seattle, WA*
[b] *Department of Physics, University of Washington, Seattle, WA*
[c] *Environmental Molecular Sciences Laboratory, Pacific Northwest National Laboratory, Richland, WA, USA*
[*] *Corresponding author, email: kannanmk@uw.edu*

Abstract: Superparamagnetic iron oxide nanoparticles (SPIONs) are central to Magnetic Particle Imaging (MPI) and their performance can be optimized for specific applications through tailored synthesis and coating methods. In vitro and in vivo, SPIONs are subject to a variety of environments with structurally confined spaces and a heterogenous mixture of species whose presence affect the mechanisms through which SPIONs align with an applied magnetic field. This work highlights the dominant factor in decreased MPS performance, magnetostatic interactions, after cellular internalization of SPIONs.

I. Introduction

MPI[1] is a promising and developing technique for a wide variety of applications including, but not limited to, acute stroke detection[2], cancer detection[3], stem-cell tracking[4], and blood-pool imaging[5]. The continued development of MPI is dependent on tailoring SPION performance in environments expected in in vitro and in vivo applications. These environments include high concentrations of various salts, proteins, and enzymes which adhere to the surface of foreign materials as well as affect solution viscosity. Further, SPIONs can be encapsulated within vesicles that can hold their contents in closer proximity than would otherwise be normal allowing for enhanced magnetostatic interactions between them. These environments have the possibility to affect the mechanisms, Brownian and Néel, by which SPIONs respond to an applied alternating magnetic field. In this study, we directly observe the intracellular localization and state of SPIONs to confirm the expected environments to which they will be exposed. Additionally, we determine the degree to which each relaxation mechanism is affected by these environmental conditions which will inform future use and optimization of SPIONs for applications of MPI.

II. Material and Methods

SPIONs used in this work were prepared by thermolysis of iron oleate in the presence of 1-octadence and oleic acid.[6] Hydrophobic SPIONs were dispersed in aqueous solution through coating with amphiphilic polymer. Characterization included transmission electron microscopy (TEM) for core size, size distribution, and SPION localization and size post-internalization in cells, dynamic light scattering (DLS) for hydrodynamic size and zeta potential, inductively coupled plasma - optical emission spectrometry (ICP-OES) for concentration, and magnetic particle spectroscopy (MPS) for magnetic and imaging performance. Mixtures of glycerol in water and mannitol in water were prepared and a consistent mass and volume of SPIONs were added. Mannitol-water SPION dispersions were lyophilized until fully dry. Samples were then characterized by MPS. Simulation of SPIONs in varying environments were carried out using previously validated Monte Carlo simulations of SPION nonlinear dynamics[7–10]. SPION properties and conditions were controlled for direct comparison to experimental results.

III. Results

SPIONs with core diameters and size distributions of 21.9, 25.3, and 27.7 nm and 0.04, 0.08, and 0.07, respectively, were synthesized and phase transferred to water. They were then internalized in cells and observed to show ~15% decrease in the fifth-to-third harmonic ratio, A_5/A_3. SPIONs were also directly imaged by TEM and their localization in the cells was confirmed to be largely within endosomes and lysosomes (Fig. 1A). Further image analysis, data not shown here, indicates no change in SPION core size or crystallographic structure and provides an estimate of the interparticle separations which range from 35 to 80 nm.

Mixtures of glycerol and water were mixed with SPIONs and their MPS performance observed, as defined by the change in the fifth-to-third harmonic ratio, $\Delta\ A_5/A_3$. No change was observed over the range of measured viscosities both in experiment and in simulation (Fig. 1B) . Lyophilized SPIONs and mannitol mixtures were also characterized by MPS and a varying decrease in A_5/A_3 was observed. Increasing core size from 21.9 to 25.3 to 27.7 nm showed increasing drop in A_5/A_3 seen in Fig. 1C. This is again supported by Monte Carlo simulations with comparisons between experimental and simulated results shown in Fig. 1D. Here we can see that little to no change in A_5/A_3 occurs above ~60 nm of center-to-center interparticle separation.

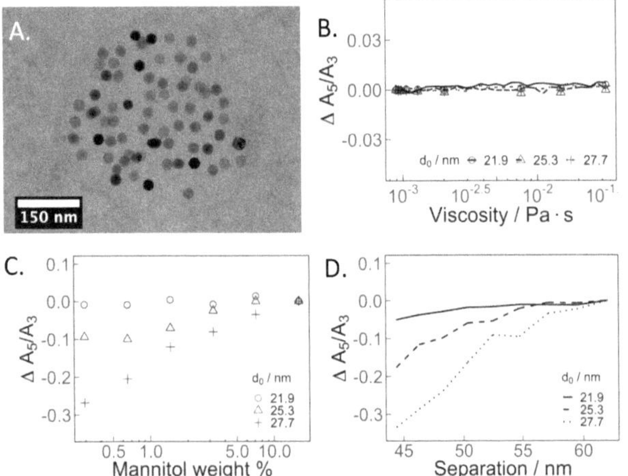

Figure 1: *A. Representative image of cell-internalized SPIONs encapsulated in a vesicle. B. No change in A5/A3 as a function of viscosity. Here a direct comparison, due to known glycerol-water solution characteristics, of exp. and sim. cases shows agreement. Significant decrease in the experimental A5/A3 as core size increases and, C., as a function of decreasing mannitol weight % (exp.-points) and, D., decreasing interparticle separation (sim.-lines).*

IV. Discussion

MPS studies of SPIONs in controlled environments allow for interpretation of their intracellular magnetic performance. It is observed that SPIONs are encapsulated in vesicles, endosomes and lysosomes, after internalization. As SPIONs in these locations do not show degradation or changing physical properties, decreases in MPS signal intensity must be caused by other environmental factors. In these localizations inside cells, SPIONs experience increased viscosities and are held in closer proximity as compared to their freely dispersed counterparts. It is thus important to determine if either or both of these conditions affects performance of SPIONs in the size range relevant to MPI. Here, three core sizes with small size distributions have been exposed to two controlled environments comparable to the intracellular conditions. Viscosity is controlled by varying the ratio of highly viscous glycerol and water in a mixture of the two. Experimental and simulated results, shown in Fig. 1B, indicate no change in performance and suggest that for these sizes the Brownian component of SPION relaxation is not significantly impacted by increased viscosity.

If viscosity can be ruled out as a significant factor in SPION MPS performance, then the effect of their being held in the close confines of intracellular vesicles must be examined. SPIONs held close enough together will experience increased magnetostatic interactions with decreased interparticle separation and increased core size of the SPIONs contributing most to the energy of this interaction. Here the interparticle separation of SPIONs has been controlled by adding more or less physical material thereby holding them further or closer together. It is observed that when decreasing the amount of

physical material, mannitol in this instance, the A_5/A_3 and thus performance of SPIONs is decreased. This effect is amplified by the core size with larger cores being more strongly affected than smaller ones. This result is supported by simulations where the interparticle separation of SPIONs can be directly controlled by available parameters and the range of separations is selected based on direct observation by TEM of interparticle separations after internalization in cells.

V. Conclusions

In pursuing a variety of in vivo imaging and cell tracking applications using MPI, it is crucial to understand SPION performance under different environmental conditions. This is necessary to ensure SPIONs continue to perform as expected when they enter in vitro and in vivo environments. Here, we have shown that the most important factor to consider in cellular environments is the extent to which SPIONs' interparticle separation is affected and how magnetostatic interactions decrease performance, especially of larger SPIONs. In addition, these results suggest that it may be advantageous to use smaller core sizes of SPIONs than otherwise would be optimal for some applications to prevent significant loss of magnetic performance and thus retaining the ability to image them in MPI.

ACKNOWLEDGEMENTS

This work was supported by NIH Grant No. 5R03EB024819-02. The TEM work, supported by the Department of Energy, Office of Biological and Environmental Research, Molecules to Mesoscale Bioimaging project no. 66382, was performed using Environmental Molecular Sciences Laboratory, a national scientific user facility sponsored by the DOE – OBER and located at Pacific Northwest National Laboratory. C. S. was supported by NSF Grant no. DGE-1256082.

AUTHOR'S STATEMENT

Authors state no conflict of interest.

REFERENCES

1. Gleich, B. & Weizenecker, J. Tomographic imaging using the nonlinear response of magnetic particles. *Nature* **435**, 1214–1217 (2005).
2. Ludewig, P. *et al.* Magnetic Particle Imaging for Real-Time Perfusion Imaging in Acute Stroke. *ACS Nano* **11**, 10480–10488 (2017).
3. Yu, E. Y. *et al.* Magnetic Particle Imaging: A Novel in Vivo Imaging Platform for Cancer Detection. *Nano Lett.* **17**, 1648–1654 (2017).
4. Bulte, J. W. M. *et al.* Quantitative "Hot-Spot" Imaging of Transplanted Stem Cells Using Superparamagnetic Tracers and Magnetic Particle Imaging. *Tomography* **1**, 91–97 (2015).
5. Khandhar, A. P. *et al.* Evaluation of PEG-coated iron oxide nanoparticles as blood pool tracers for preclinical magnetic particle imaging. *Nanoscale* **9**, 1299–1306 (2017).
6. Kemp, S. J., Ferguson, R. M., Khandhar, A. P. & Krishnan, K. M. Monodisperse magnetite nanoparticles with nearly ideal saturation magnetization. *RSC Adv.* **6**, 77452–77464 (2016).
7. Shasha, C., Teeman, E. & Krishnan, K. M. Harmonic Simulation Study of Simultaneous Nanoparticle Size and Viscosity Differentiation. *IEEE Magn. Lett.* **8**, 1–5 (2017).
8. Engelmann, U. M., Shasha, C., Teeman, E., Slabu, I. & Krishnan, K. M. Predicting size-dependent heating efficiency of magnetic nanoparticles from experiment and stochastic Néel-Brown Langevin simulation. *J. Magn. Magn. Mater.* **471**, 450–456 (2019).
9. Shah, S. A., Reeves, D. B., Ferguson, R. M., Weaver, J. B. & Krishnan, K. M. Mixed Brownian alignment and Néel rotations in superparamagnetic iron oxide nanoparticle suspensions driven by an ac field. *Phys. Rev. B* **92**, 094438 (2015).
10. Gardiner, C. *Stochastic Methods: A Handbook for the Natural and Social Sciences.* (Springer, 1985).

Magnetic nanoparticles based binding imaging with a scanning magnetic particle spectrometer

J. Zhong[a]*, M. Schilling[a], and F. Ludwig[a]

[a] *Institut für Elektrische Messtechnik und Grundlagen der Elektrotechnik, Technische Universität Braunschweig, Braunschweig, Germany*
* *Corresponding author, email: j.zhong@tu-braunschweig.de*

Abstract: This study investigates the imaging of magnetic nanoparticles (MNPs) bound with biomolecules via a custom-built scanning magnetic particle spectrometer (SMPS). The spatial distributions of the 1st and 3rd harmonics of MNPs are measured with the SMPS while the harmonic ratio of the 3rd to the 1st – due to its independence of MNP concentration – is used to determine the binding status of the MNPs. Experimental results indicate that the SMPS can distinguish the MNPs with and without coated streptavidin due to their different hydrodynamic sizes. It demonstrates the feasibility of further investigation on imaging biomolecules bound onto the MNPs coated with streptavidin.

I. Introduction

The determination of the biomolecular binding behavior onto the surface of magnetic nanoparticles (MNPs) is of great interest and importance to biomedical and biological applications. Homogeneous binding sensing based on a change of the Brownian relaxation time of MNPs upon binding was studied by a number of groups [1,2]. Visualizing the spatial distribution of biomolecular binding behavior is of great interest and significance to nanotheranostics, e.g. breast cancer detection, which, however, has not yet been realized to date.

Magnetic particle imaging (MPI) is a new imaging modality to measure the spatial distribution of MNPs [3]. In addition to electrical scanning, a mechanically scanning magnetic particle spectrometer (SMPS) was developed to simultaneously image the spatial distributions of MNP concentration and temperature [4]. This study investigates the feasibility of the SMPS for imaging the binding behavior of biomolecules onto the surface of MNPs, e.g. the binding behavior between IgG with biotin and streptavidin. For the proof-of-concept, MNPs coated with and without streptavidin are investigated by measuring the spatial distributions of the 1st (M_1) and 3rd (M_3) harmonics with the SMPS.

II. Material and Methods

The experimental samples are plain and streptavidin-coated BNF-Starch particles with iron concentrations of 5 mg/ml and 2.3 mg/ml dispersed in water and in phosphate buffered saline with pH of 7.4 and 0.02% sodium azide, respectively. An ac susceptometer is used to measure the ac susceptibility of the experimental BNF particles to estimate the hydrodynamic size. A phantom with two lines is filled with the BNF particles coated with and without streptavidin while the SMPS is used to measure the spatial distributions of the 1st and 3rd harmonics for binding imaging.

III. Results

Fig. 1 shows the imaginary parts of the ac susceptibility of BNF particles without (plain) and with streptavidin. The peak frequency of the imaginary part of streptavidin-functionalized BNF particles at about 300 Hz is lower than that of plain BNF particles at about 500 Hz. These characteristic frequencies correspond to hydrodynamic sizes of 110 nm for the streptavidin-coated BNF particles and of 98 nm for the plain BNF particles.

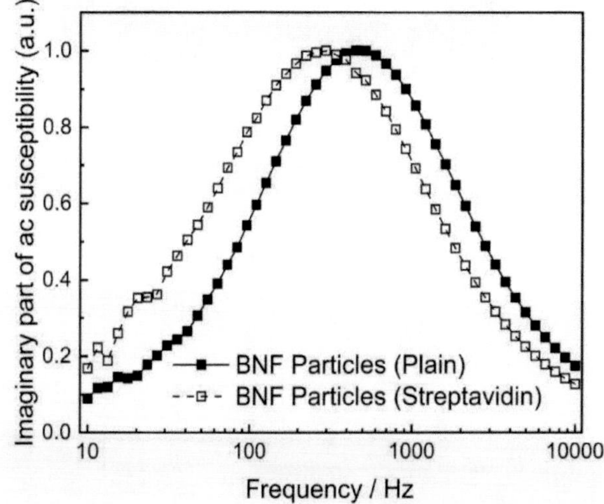

Figure 1: *Imaginary parts of ac susceptibility vs. frequency of the BNF particles (closed symbols: streptavidin, open symbols: plain).*

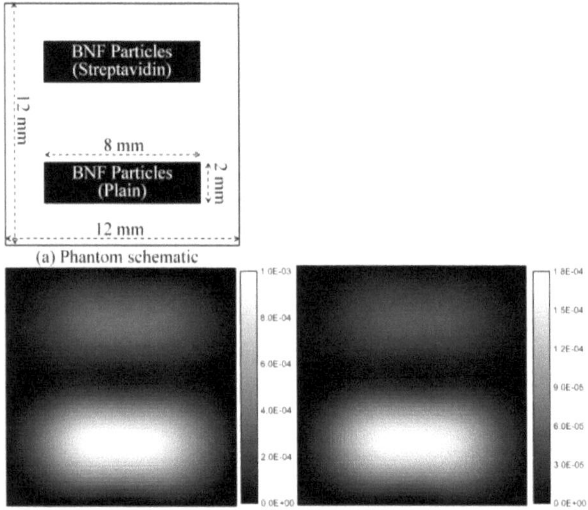

Figure 2: (a) Schematic of phantom, (b) measured spatial distribution of the 1st harmonics, and (c) measured spatial distribution of the 3rd harmonics. An ac magnetic field with frequency of 1033 Hz and amplitude of 10 mT is applied.

Fig. 2a shows the schematic of the phantom with two lines filled with plain and streptavidin-coated BNF particles, respectively. The scanning field-of-view is 12 mm × 12 mm with a step resolution of 0.2 mm. Figs. 2b and 2c show the measured spatial distributions of the 1st and 3rd harmonics.

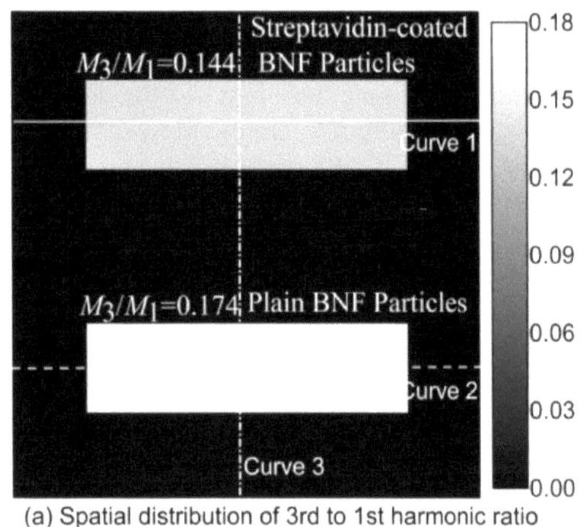

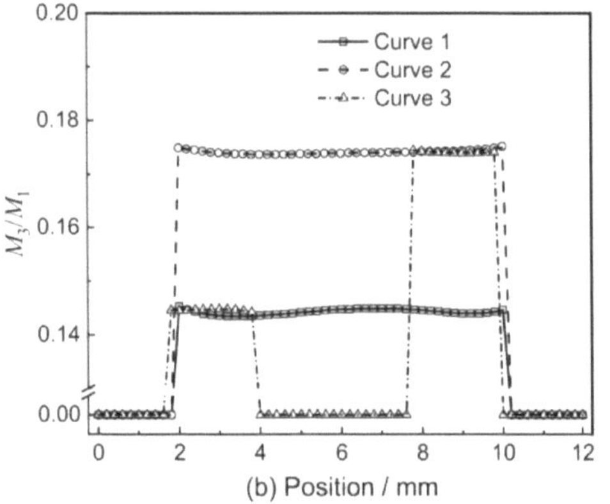

Figure 3: (a) Spatial distribution of the 3rd to 1st harmonic ratio, (b) 1D curves of the harmonic ratio at three different positions.

Fig. 3a depicts the 2D spatial distribution of the harmonic ratio M_3/M_1 whereas Fig. 3b shows the corresponding 1D curves at three different positions located at the curves shown in Fig. 3a.

IV. Discussion

The amplitude of each harmonic (M_1 and M_3) is dependent both on the MNP concentration and hydrodynamic size whereas the harmonic ratio M_3/M_1 is only dependent on the hydrodynamic size. Fig. 3 shows that M_3/M_1 for MNPs with streptavidin amounts to about 0.145 whereas that for MNPs without streptavidin is about 0.175. With a larger hydrodynamic size, the MNPs can rotate slower to follow the excitation ac magnetic field, which decreases the strength of the harmonic amplitude. This phenomenon is more crucial for higher harmonics, e.g. the 3rd harmonic. Therefore, the harmonic ratio of the MNPs with streptavidin is smaller than that of MNPs without streptavidin. Our experimental results demonstrate the feasibility of the SMPS for imaging binding behavior, which can be further extended to study the binding behavior between biotin and streptavidin.

V. Conclusions

This study aims at imaging the binding behavior of biomolecules onto the surface of MNPs via a custom-built magnetic particle spectrometer. Specific binding of analytes enlarges the hydrodynamic size of MNPs, causing significant changes in the MNP signal. Our SMPS allows one to measure the spatial distribution of the 1st and 3rd harmonics for binding imaging. The experimental results demonstrate the feasibility of the SMPS to distinguish MNPs with different hydrodynamic size, which can be further extended to image the binding behavior between biotin and streptavidin.

ACKNOWLEDGEMENTS

Financial support from German Research Foundation (DFG) (ZH 782/1-1) is acknowledged.

AUTHOR'S STATEMENT

Conflict of interest: Authors state no conflict of interest. Informed consent: Informed consent has been obtained from all individuals included in this study. Ethical approval: The experiments are not related to any experiments on animals or humans.

REFERENCES

[1] J. Dieckhoff, A. Lak, M. Schilling and F. Ludwig. Protein detection with magnetic nanoparticles in a rotating magnetic field. *Journal of Applied Physics*, 115, 024701, 2014. doi: 10.1063/1.4861032.

[2] S. Schrittwieser, B. Pelaz, W. J. Parak, S. Lentijo-Mozo, K. Soulantica, J. Dieckhoff, F. Ludwig, A. Guenther, A. Tschoepe and J. Schotter, Homogeneous biosensing based on magnetic particle labels, *Sensors*, 16: 828, 2016. doi: 10.3390/s16060828.

[3] B. Gleich and J. Weizenecker. Tomographic imaging using the nonlinear response of magnetic particles. *Nature*, 435(7046):1217-1217, 2005. doi: 10.1038/nature03808.

[4] J. Zhong, M. Schilling and F. Ludwig. Magnetic nanoparticle temperature imaging with a scanning magnetic particle spectrometer. *Measurement Science and Technology*, 29: 115903, 2018. doi: 10.1088/1361-6501/aae3bd.

One-Dimensional Multi-Frequency Spectrometer

C. Knopke[a], B.W. Ficko[a], and S. G. Diamond[a,b*]

[a] *Lodestone Biomedical LLC, Lebanon, Hanover, New Hampshire, USA*
[b] *Thayer School of Engineering at Dartmouth, Hanover, New Hampshire, USA*
[*] *Corresponding author, email: Solomon.G.Diamond@Dartmouth.edu*

Magnetic Particle Spectroscopy (MPS) is an important measurement method to characterize the non-linear behavior of magnetic nanoparticles (MNPs). MPS systems provide valuable data for developing efficient magnetic particle imaging (MPI) methods and optimizing MNP contrast agents [1]. We developed a multi-excitation-coil spectrometer to recreate complex AC field patterns that are otherwise only found in 3D MPI systems. The here presented Nanoparticle Characterization System (NCS) is capable of creating gradient fields and multi-frequency excitation fields as well as AC field-free-points. With its integrated sample mover, the NCS enables investigations into the effects of these field patterns on a 100 μl sample along one dimension.

I. Introduction

I.I. Spectrometer

In this paper we present a custom built MNP spectrometer that distinguishes itself from its commercially available counterparts through a unique set of features. At the core of the measurement system sits a recirculating liquid cooled five coil configuration (Fig. 1 C). There are two independently-controlled excitation coils and the three pick-up coils that can be read out independently with gradiometer compensation performed digitally in real-time processing. The signal generation and data readouts are achieved via high-end audio studio equipment and customized commercial digital audio workstation software.

Independent control of the two excitation coils enables the measurement system to generate a variety of AC field conditions. By using a linear actuator that moves the sample along the central axis of gradiometer, the spectrometer can be used to study complex field conditions that are otherwise only found in 3D imaging systems. The system settings can be configured to generate a single or multi-frequency AC-signal. Currently, the main frequency can be set from 400 Hz to 2500 Hz. Additional frequencies can be added at frequencies up to 10000 Hz. The phase and gain of each frequency can be adjusted individually.

When the two drive coils are set with opposing phase, an AC field-free-point can be generated. Additionally, if the drive coils are set to different amplitudes, an AC gradient field can be created. With the audio power amplifier, magnetic fields up to 30 millitesla can be applied.

I.II. Frequency Sweep and linear positioning

The features of the presented spectrometer can support a broad variety of applications. In this paper, we experimentally demonstrate two features of the NCS: Frequency sweep and linear positioning.

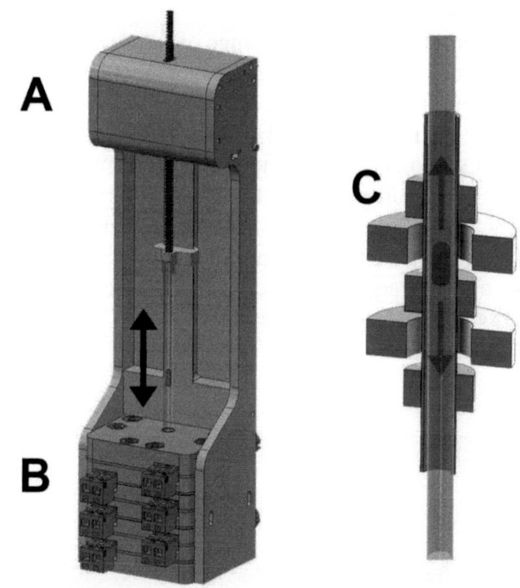

Figure 1: *Illustration of 1-dimensional sample mover (A) with encased spectrometer (B). C) Cross-section of the five coil configuration with sample-straw (⌀=5.7 mm) in center.*

II. Material and Methods

II.I. Spectrometer

The drive and detection coils were purchased from Jantzen Audio (Praestoe, Denmark). The temperature of the gradiometer is held constant with a P310 rack-mounted chiller from TermoTek AG (Baden-Baden/Germany).

The AC signal generation and real-time processing is carried out with the REAPER digital audio workstation software and amplified with a Benchmark Media Systems AHB2 power amplifier (Syracuse, USA). The system's digital-to-analog converter and an analog-to-digital converter are also from Benchmark Media Systems (DAC3 DX; ADC16). The sample movement is performed with a non-captive NEMA 11 stepper motor from Koco Motion US LLC (Morgan Hill, USA) that is controlled by a FP-Sigma programmable logic controller from Panasonic. The motor movement control was integrated into the REAPER audio software using a MIDI to CV converter (Pro SOLO MkII, KENTON). Analogously, the motor positioning feedback was integrated with a Pro CV to MIDI converter from KENTON (London, UK). The sample mover has a minimum step size of 0.05 mm and a stroke length of 32 mm.

II.II. Nanoparticles

We obtained streptavidin-coated iron oxide MNP from Ocean Nanotech (San Diego, USA): SHS-30-01; SHS-20-01, and microMod Partikeltechnologie GmbH (Rostock, Germany): BNF-Starch (10-19-102). Each sample contains 10 µl of undiluted MNP.

III. Results & Discussion

III.I. Frequency Sweep

To demonstrate the operating range of the system, a series of MNP measurements was carried out. Three particle samples with different iron oxide core sizes were measured at 500 Hz, 1000 Hz and 1500 Hz. The amplitude of the drive field was set to 20 mT for each measurement. Displayed in Fig. 2 are the harmonic spectra of the samples at different frequencies. The amplitude of the harmonic spectrum reflects the non-linear magnetic response of a particle system and is frequency dependent. For each measurement an empty measurement is subtracted.

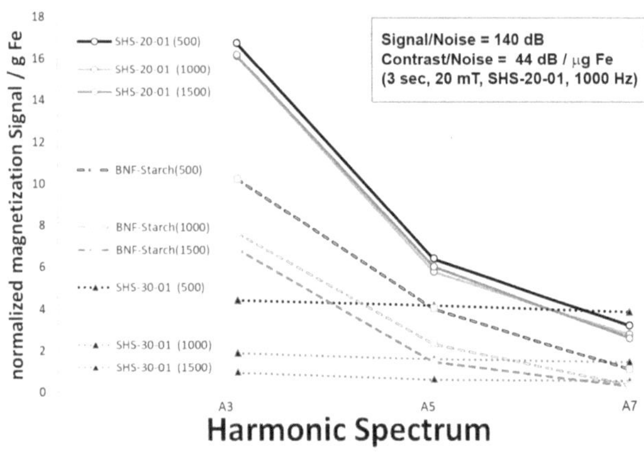

Figure 2: *Harmonic signal per gram iron of three different particle samples at 500 Hz, 1000 Hz and 1500 Hz.*

Fig. 2 illustrates the difference in signal strength per gram iron for each particle type. The results show that SHS-20-01 particles had overall the strongest signal per gram iron. Depending on the frequency and the investigated harmonic, SHS-30-01 and Mircomod's BNF-starch particles have a weaker signal. The ratio of the third to fifth harmonic (A3/A5), which is another indicator for the particles characteristic non-linear behavior, varies with the particle type, but not with the tested frequencies. The frequency sweep revealed that the signal amplitude of the SHS-30-01 and the Micromod BNF-Starch particles are highly frequency dependent, whereas SHS-20-01 where less affected by the frequency change.

III.II. Linear positioning

In the second experiment we demonstrate the effects of an AC gradient field along one dimension with the help of the linear sample mover. With a linear positioning sweep over 25.2 mm carried out by the sample mover in 63 steps, the location of the magnetic field-free point (FFP) can be visualized (Fig. 3). The gradient at the central FFP is 1.6 mT/mm. Two additional FFPs that can be seen in the measurements arise from the gradiometer subtractions.

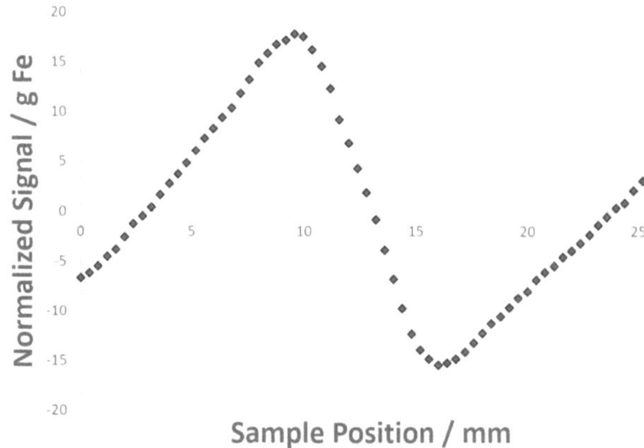

Figure 3: *Magnetic Signal (3rd Harmonic) of 20 µl liquid SHS-20-01 sample at 63 positions in an AC gradient field.*

Through the positioning sweep, the MNP responses in complex magnetic field patterns such as in AC field gradients can be studied in one dimension. The sample mover can also be used to study and improve the characteristics of the spectrometer. In the present results, the positioning sweep revealed that the magnetic AC signal of the two excitation coils is not perfectly symmetric due to slight variations in the coil placement.

V. Conclusions

The frequency sweep offers a valuable investigation tool to determine the potential of MNP contrast agents for low-frequency imaging modalities. A system expansion to higher and lower frequencies would provide additional functionality. A fully integrated sample mover is a helpful addition for performing automated sample sweeps to map MNP responses in complex magnetic field patterns.

REFERENCES

[1] Biederer, S., et al. "Magnetization response spectroscopy of superparamagnetic nanoparticles for magnetic particle imaging." Journal of Physics D: Applied Physics 42.20 (2009): 205007.

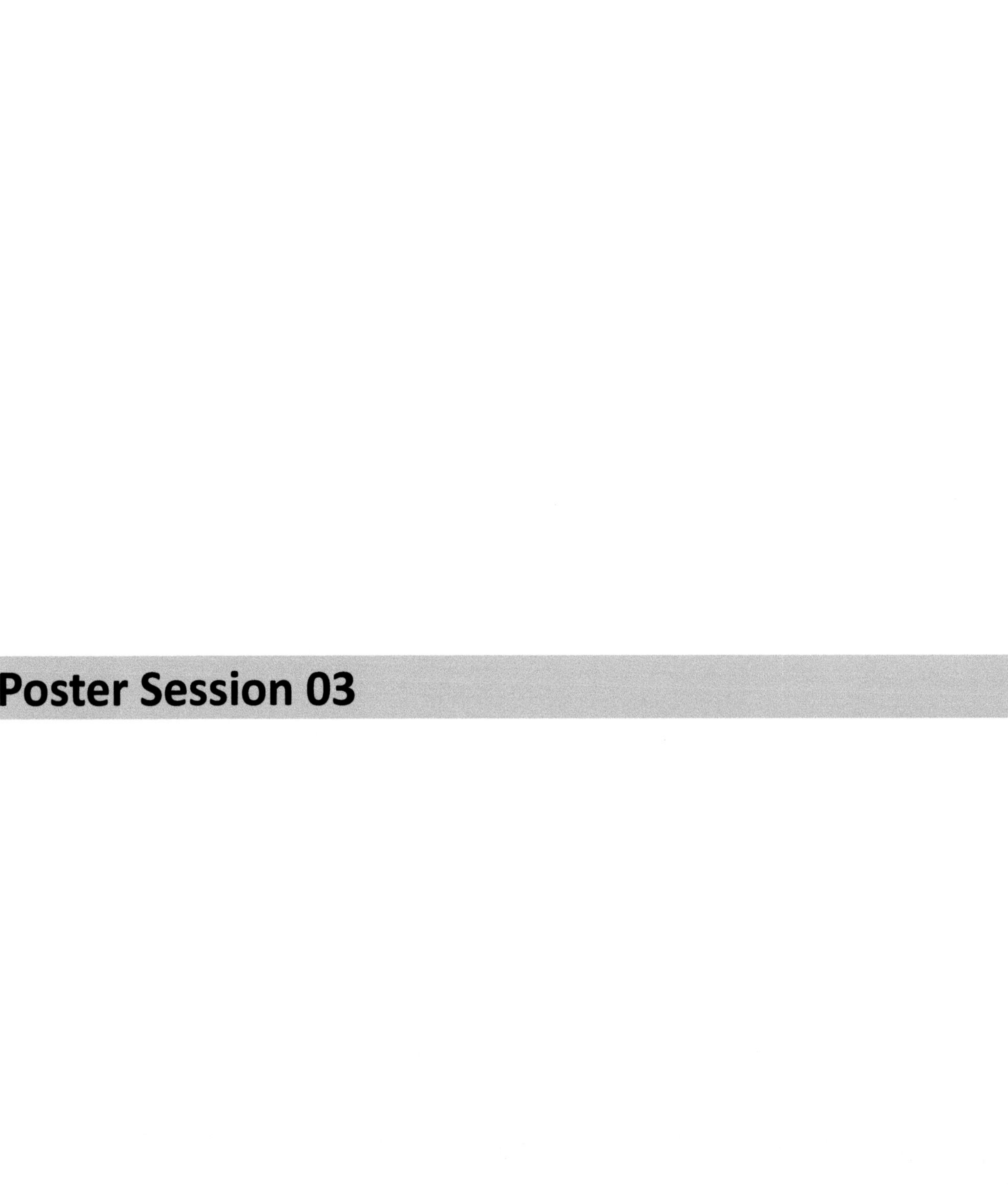

Poster Session 03

An Inline Reconstruction Technique for MPI

A. Cordes[a]*, and T. M. Buzug [a]*

[a] *Institute of Medical Engineering, Universität zu Lübeck, Lübeck, Germany*
* *Corresponding author, email: {cordes,buzug}@imt.uni-luebeck.de*

Recent developments in magnetic particle imaging (MPI) have revolutionized the ability to visualize the spatial distribution of superparamagnetic nanoparticles with high raw data acquisition rates. To exploit the full potential of MPI in interventional applications, efficient reconstruction algorithms that allow for real-time imaging are mandatory. In this work, we introduce an inline reconstruction technique that is fast enough to handle the incoming raw data. Based on precomputed deconvolution kernels, the method allows updating the image continuously during the measurement without large computational effort. Simulation experiments demonstrate that even an accurate reconstruction of moving objects is possible.

I. Introduction

The main requirements for interventional applications in magnetic particle imaging (MPI) are a good spatial resolution and a reduced reconstruction time. Besides system matrix based approaches [1], recent developments in MPI demonstrate that the x-space reconstruction method shows promising results for cartesian trajectories and offers the potential to meet these requirements [2]. For such trajectories magnetic particle imaging (MPI) can be modeled as a linear shift-invariant system with a well-defined point spread function (PSF) [3,4]. Therefore, an image can be reconstructed by gridding the voltage signal to the known location of the field free point (FPP). In a postprocessing step, the system blur can be reduced by applying a deconvolution [5]. Finally, a combination of two orthogonal collinear scans allows for isotropic spatial resolution [6]. But while this method shows good results for MPI systems based on cartesian trajectories, it is much more challenging for non-linear trajectories [7]. For Lissajous-based data acquisition schemes the PSF varies for each spatio-temporal position. Consequently, an exact reconstruction requires time-dependent deconvolution kernels [7]. In this contribution, we demonstrate that such precomputed deconvolution kernels allow for an efficient image reconstruction for non-linear trajectories. By updating the image continuously during the measurement without a renewed system matrix inversion, the proposed method is fast enough to handle the incoming raw data. Simulation experiments demonstrate that even a fast and accurate reconstruction of moving objects is possible.

II. Material and Methods

II.I. Deconvolution Kernels

In order to compute time-dependent deconvolution kernels the system response $s_{mn} := s_n(t_m)$ has to be known for each position $r_n, n = 1, ..., N$ of the sampled field of view (FOV) and for each discrete time point $t_m, m = 1, ..., M$. By inversion of the resulting system matrix $S = [s_{mn}]_{n=1,...,N, m=1,...,M}$ using the singular value decomposition $S = U\Sigma V^T$ the deconvolution kernel $d_m(r_n) \in \mathbb{R}^{N \times 1}$ corresponding to the time point t_m is finally given by the mth column of $S^{-1} = V\Sigma^{-1}U^T \in \mathbb{R}^{N \times M}$. Based on $d_m(r_n)$ an image $f(r_n)$ can be calculated as follows

$$f(r_n) = \sum_{m=1}^{M} u(t_m)d_m(r_n), \qquad (1)$$

where $u(t_m)$ is the measured voltage signal at time point t_m. However, it should be noted that the matrix S is ill-conditioned. A well-known method for dealing with such ill-posed problems is the truncated singular value decomposition (TSVD). In the case of TSVD, regularization is achieved by neglecting components of the solution corresponding to small singular values.

II.II. Inline Image Reconstruction

As visualized in Fig. 1, the deconvolution kernels $d_m(r_n)$ allow for a continuous image reconstruction during the measurement. By adding the contribution of the value measured at the current FFP position and subtracting the corresponding value of the previous trajectory repetition, the reconstructed image can be updated as follows

$$f_m^i(\vec{r}_n) = f_{m-1}^i(\vec{r}_n) + \left(u(t_m^i) - u(t_m^{i-1}) \right) d_m(\vec{r}_n), \qquad (2)$$

where $f_m^i(\vec{r})$ denotes the image obtained after the acquisition of the m-th value during trajectory repetition i.

II.III. Simulation Experiment

In order to demonstrate that the proposed method offers the potential for an efficient reconstruction of moving objects, simulation experiments based on a rotated L-phantom and ideal magnetic fields are performed. The particle characteristics are modeled via Langevin theory assuming a particle diameter of 30 nm. With a 4° rotation per repetition of the Lissajous trajectory and a repetition time t_R of 1.2 ms, the angular velocity amounts to approximately 58 rad/s. The applied selection field gradient amounts to $1.25 \text{ Tm}^{-1}\mu_0^{-1}$ in x- and y-direction and the FOV with a size of 2.5 cm $\times$ 2.5 cm is discretized into 71×71 pixels. The 2D Lissajous trajectory of the FFP is generated with drive field frequencies $f_x = 26.881$ kHz and $f_y = 26.041$ kHz. Based on the precomputed deconvolution kernels and the simulated noise-free voltage signal the moving phantom is reconstructed according to equation (2).

III. Results and Discussion

Reconstructed images of the rotated L-phantom for different rotation angels α are shown in Fig. 2. Despite data inconsistencies, the images demonstrate that it is possible to clearly detect the phantom without an unacceptable loss in image quality. The movement of the phantom can be visualized without strong motion artifacts. Only slight distortions at the edges and a mild blurring are visible.

V. Conclusions

Independent of the applied FFP trajectory, the proposed method offers the potential to reconstruct the particle distribution with high spatial and temporal resolution. Since the deconvolution kernels are computed prior to the actual measurement, no computationally expensive steps are required during the intervention. This way, a fast reconstruction of moving objects is possible. An application of the proposed method to measured data remains for future work.

Author's statement
Funding by the Federal Ministry of Education and Research via the Project SAMBA-PATI (FKZ: 13GW0069A) is gratefully acknowledged. Authors state no conflict of interest.

References
[1] T. Knopp and M. Hofmann. *Phys. Med. Biol.*, 61:11. N257-N267, 2016. doi: 10.1088/0031-9155/61/11/N257.
[2] P.W. Goodwill, K. Lu, B. Zheng and S. M. Conolly. *Rev. Sci. Intrum*, 83:033708,2012. doi: 10.1063/1.3694534.
[3] P.W. Goodwill and S. M. Conolly. *IEEE Trans Med Imaging*, 30(9):1581-90,2011. doi: 10.1109/TMI.2011.2125982.
[4] P.W. Goodwill and S. M. Conolly. *IEEE Trans Med Imaging*, 30(9):1581-90,2011. doi: 10.1109/TMI.2011.2125982.
[5] A. Cordes and T.M. Buzug, *International Workshop on Magnetic Particle Imaging*, 49, 2018.
[6] K. Lu, P. Goodwill, B. Zheng and S. Conolly. *IEEE Trans Med Imaging*, 37(9):1989-97,2018. doi: 10.1109/TMI.2017.2787500.
[7] A. Cordes and T.M. Buzug, *International Workshop on Magnetic Particle Imaging*, 128, 2016.

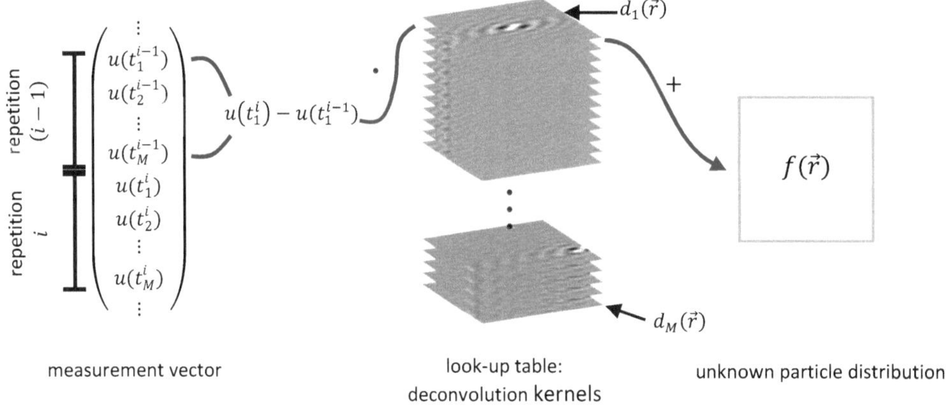

Figure 1: By adding the contribution of the value measured at time point t_m^i and subtracting the corresponding value of the previous trajectory repetition, the reconstructed image $f(\vec{r})$ can be updated continuously during the measurement.

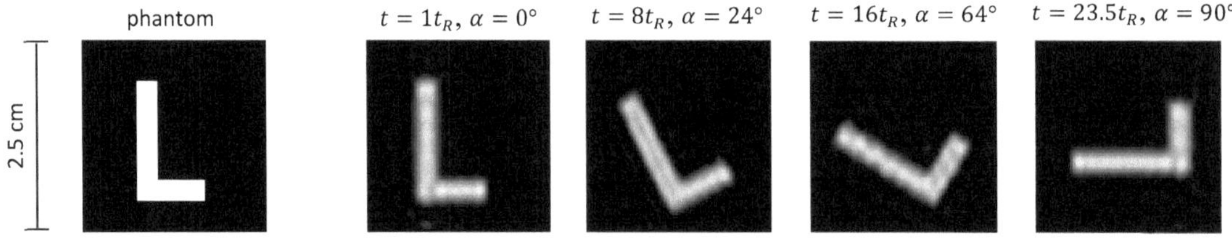

Figure 2: Left: L-phantom which is rotated around the center of the FOV. Right: Reconstructed images for different rotation angles α. Simulation parameters are chosen according to section II.III.

MPI using sub-voxel focus field offsets

M. Herbst[a]*, H. Lehr[a], and J. Franke[a,b]

[a] *Bruker BioSpin MRI GmbH, Ettlingen, Germany*
[b] *Physics of Molecular Imaging Systems, RTWH Aachen, Germany*
* *Corresponding author, email: michael.herbst@bruker.com*

Abstract: To reconstruct MPI data using a system function (SF) approach, this function needs to be acquired prior to the reconstruction and determines the matrix of the resulting image. Signal from locations which were not sampled during the acquisition of SF, will be distributed to voxels with the most similar signal, i.e. neighboring voxels. In this work, sub-voxel focus field offsets are used to precisely display the location of objects, which are placed between the grid of the SF. The method can reconstruct sub-voxel position differences, incorporating data from multiple focus-field steps and interpolated system function into one extended reconstruction.

I. Introduction

I.I. MPI Reconstruction and Resolution

MPI data reconstructed using a system function approach [1] is clearly bound to the grid of this system matrix. This becomes obvious looking at the signal equation, where each point of the reconstructed image $c(r)$ (polar coordinates r) is related to the signal $u(f)$ (frequencies f) via its representation in the system function $SF(f,r)$:

$$u(f) = SF(f,r) \cdot c(r)$$

By inverting this equation and solving it in a least square sense, the image can be reconstructed. Assuming an object, which is placed on the sampling grid of the SF, an exact correspondence of its signal can be found, and its position (and concentration) is correctly reconstructed (Fig.1a). However, if this object is shifted from the SF-grid by half a voxel, each of the neighboring SF voxels shows a signal equally similar to the one from the object (Fig.1b) and therefore contains a portion of the total concentration.

Focus fields (FF) add an additional offset to the magnetic field and can therefore be applied to introduce a virtual sub-voxel shift between SF and object. In the example shown, the object can be shifted to fit the SF-grid and can be correctly reconstructed (Fig.1c).

In this work, data acquired at different FF positions are combined in one extended reconstruction, which is performed on an interpolated SF-grid.

II. Material and Methods

II.I. Theory

As shown in Fig.1, the systems focus fields can be used to apply accurate sub-voxel shifts. Assuming that the object remained unchanged during the field shift (1b and 1c), information from different FF-steps can be incorporated in one reconstruction.

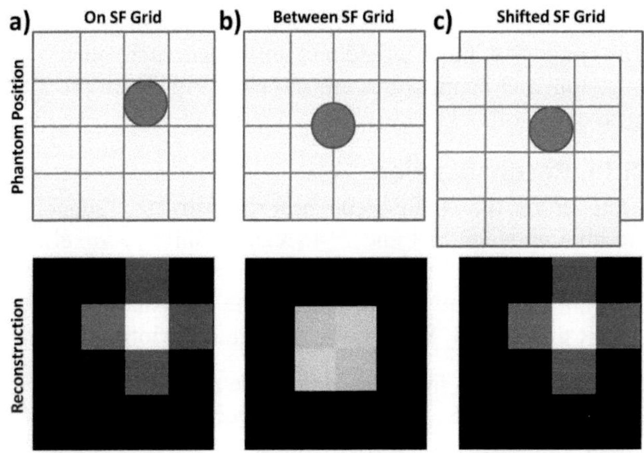

Figure 1: *An 8 μl probe was measured using a 3D Lissajous trajectory. Reconstructed data from two phantom positions are shown: a) on the grid of the system matrix used for reconstruction. b) shifted by half a voxel in x and y. c) focus fields are used to virtually shift the SF grid relative to the object.*

To compensate for such sub-voxel shift during reconstruction, the SF needs to be interpolated to a finer grid. Therefore, the acquired SF is interpolated using spline interpolation (SF_{IP}). To avoid keeping SF_{IP} in memory, this interpolation is performed during reconstruction for each point and frequency. The image equation becomes:

$$[u_1, u_2, \ldots, u_N] = SF_{IP}(f', r') \cdot c_{IP}(r')$$

This combines signal from different FF-steps u_n ($n \in 1{:}N$) and allows solving the equation for a concentration c_{IP} on a finer imaging grid r'. The signal vector includes now a multiple of the original frequencies. Therefore, the frequency index of SF_{IP} becomes f', which can be directly mapped to the original frequencies.

The approach is similar to the one described in [2], but instead of using several FF-steps to reconstruct an enlarged imaging volume, the information from the FF-steps is combined in the same volume.

II.II. Acquisition

All experiments were performed on an MPI-Scanner (MPI25/20FF, Bruker BioSpin MRI GmbH, Ettlingen). A 3D Lissajous trajectory with drive field strength of 12 mT in each dimension and a selection field gradient of 2 T/m were used. Two 3D SFs were acquired: one on a 2 mm grid (SF-LR, matrix 16×16×8, 8 µl Resovist, Bayer AG) and one on a 1mm grid (SF-HR, matrix 32×32×16, 1 µl Resovist).

The acquisition was performed with 4 FF-steps, each shifted in plane by ¼ of a voxel compared to the previous one. At each FF-position, 20 averages were acquired.

Object data were acquired with an 8 µl probe of Resovist, which was positioned at different points using the systems robot. Each position was acquired with 4 FF-steps, each shifted by ¼ of a voxel in plane compared to the previous one. At each FF-step, 20 averages were acquired. Signals from different positions were added up to build a virtual phantom, assuming that particles from different point probes (distance $\geq$ 4 mm) would not influence each other. This phantom and its measures are shown in Fig. 2e on the 2 mm grid of SF-LR.

II.III. Reconstruction

Data from the 4 FF-steps are reconstructed separately, combining steps 1+3 and 2+4 (relative shift: ½ voxel), and including all four steps. The reconstructions were performed in ParaVision with SF-LR, using the Kaczmarz algorithm (SNR threshold 4, 8 iterations, no regularization).

For comparison, the same data were reconstructed on a 1 mm grid using SF-HR. Due to lower SNR in the SF the algorithm was adapted (SNR threshold 2, 20 iterations, rel. regularization 10^{-8}, denoising of the SF [3]).

III. Results

In Figure 2 results of different reconstructions are shown:

a) Data from the four FF-steps are reconstructed independently using SF-LR. It can be seen that the ability to locate signal depends on its position relative to the grid of SF-LR.

b) Datasets, which were acquired with a relative FF-shift of ½ voxel, are combined and reconstructed on a grid with twice the resolution. Since the shift between the four steps was ¼ voxel, datasets 1 and 3 are combined as well as 2 and 4. It can be seen that both images show the same features, independent of the position of the objects points.

c) All four datasets are incorporated into one reconstruction on a grid four times the resolution of the original one.

d) The data from the four FF-steps are reconstructed separately using the system function SF-HR with twice the resolution of SF-LR.

e) The phantom is shown with measures. Distances between points are 5 mm in the upper half and 4 mm in the lower half.

For better visualization, only the central part of each volume (region of interest in one slice) is shown.

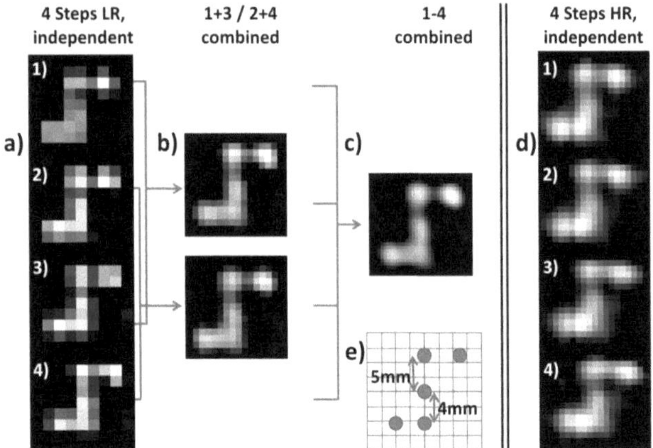

Figure 2: *Signal from five well-defined positions acquired at four different focus-field steps, shifted by ¼ of a voxel in the x- and y-direction. A sketch of the phantom is shown in (e).*
Images shown in a-c were reconstructed using SF-LR. a) the four steps are reconstructed separately. b) two steps are combined to form an image. c) all 4 datasets are used to reconstruct one image. d) The four steps are reconstructed using SF-HR.

IV. Discussion

It was shown that MPI data with small FF-offsets can be incorporated into an extended image equation. This was used to reconstruct four times the number of imaging voxels per dimension. While this improved localization of the probes, it has to be kept in mind that this will not necessarily improve the ability to differentiate between objects. The influence on the actual image resolution needs to be investigated in further detail.

At the current state, the method is implemented for 2D interpolation. An extension to the third dimension would be feasible, but would further increase the time requirements for reconstruction, which scales with the number of voxels.

V. Conclusions

In this work, the incorporation of data with sub-voxel FF-offsets in an extended reconstruction was successfully shown. This reconstruction lead to a more robust object localization and might be used to increase image resolution in system function based MPI.

ACKNOWLEDGEMENTS

The authors acknowledge the financial support from the German Federal Ministry of Education and Research, FKZ 13GW0069D.

REFERENCES

[1] B. Gleich and J. Weizenecker. Tomographic imaging using the nonlinear response of magnetic particles. *Nature*, 435(7046):1217-1217, 2005. doi: 10.1038/nature03808.

[2] P. Szwargulski et al. Efficient Joint Image Reconstruction of Multi-Patch Data reusing a Single System Matrix in Magnetic Particle Imaging. *IEEE,2018*. doi: 10.1109/TMI.2018.2875829.

[3] A. Weber et al. Reconstruction Enhancement by Denoising the Magnetic Particle Imaging System Matrix Using Frequency Domain Filter. *IEEE Transactions on Magnetics, vol. 51, no. 2, feb 2015.*

Multi-parametric image reconstruction in Magnetic Particle Imaging

N. C. Holle[a]*, D. Pantke[a], S. Reinartz[a], A. Mogarkar[a], and V. Schulz[a]

[a] Department of Physics of Molecular Imaging, Institute for Experimental Molecular Imaging, RWTH Aachen University, Aachen, Germany
** Corresponding author, email: nils.holle@rwth-aachen.de*

Abstract: This work outlines a deduction of an analytic expression for the MPI system matrix in frequency space for arbitrary scanner dimensionalities, including a simple particle relaxation model, and a versatile fitting approach to the reconstruction of functional parameters from MPI measurements. The basic idea is the variation of functional model parameters in order to minimize a loss function, based on the previously derived expression for the system matrix. Simulation studies and first parameter reconstructions from measurements acquired using a multi-frequency MPI setup have been performed successfully.

I. Introduction

Since its invention, Magnetic Particle Imaging has mainly been focused on the visualization of the super-parametric iron oxide particle (SPIO) distribution by exploiting the particles' non-linear magnetization response. A presumably very useful extension of the current particle distribution-only imaging is the in-vivo measurement of (local) functional parameters such as the temperature or the tracer binding status, encoded in the particle relaxation times, with a variety of possible target applications, including tumor cell labeling, atherosclerosis and inflammation, the distinction between intra and extra cellular sites and the evaluation of the physical and chemical surrounding of the particles. The main goal of the present work is the establishment of a versatile foundation for the extraction of such functional parameters from MPI measurements. The MPI setup used for simulation studies as well as an experimental prove-of-concept is the multi-frequency device currently developed at RWTH Aachen [1]. It features a combined passive and active compensation approach, which allows for the first harmonic to be used during reconstruction.

II. Material and Methods

II.I. Derivation of the system function in x-space

The first part of this derivation is based on [2]. An expression for the MPI system function with an arbitrary number of dimensions may be derived using Faraday's law of induction and a Langevin model for the magnetization response of the SPIOs at position $\vec{x}$ and time t, $\vec{M}(\vec{x},t) = \rho(\vec{x})m\mathcal{L}\left(\frac{|\vec{H}(\vec{x},t)|}{H_{\text{sat}}}\right)\frac{\vec{H}(\vec{x},t)}{|\vec{H}(\vec{x},t)|}$, with $\mathcal{L}(x)$ the Langevin function, $\rho(\vec{x})$ the local particle concentration, m the magnetic moment of a single particle. $\vec{H}(\vec{x},t)$ the magnetic field at position $\vec{x}$ and time t, and $H_{\text{sat}} = k_{\text{B}}T/\left(\mu_0 M_{\text{sat}}\frac{\pi}{6}d^3\right)$ the saturation parameter, where k_{B} is Boltzmann's constant, T the particle temperature, μ_0 the vacuum permeability, M_{sat} the saturation magnetization, and d the particle diameter. The magnetic field is the sum of a (static) selection field $\vec{H}_{\text{S}}(\vec{x})$ and a temporally varying drive field $\vec{H}_{\text{D}}(\vec{x},t)$; the position $\vec{r}(t)$ of the field-free point (FFP) is defined by the property $\vec{H}_{\text{D}}(\vec{r}(t),t) + \vec{H}_{\text{S}}(\vec{r}(t)) = 0$. In time space, this leads to a system function $\vec{s}(t) = \mu_0 m\mathbf{R}\frac{d}{dt}\int \rho(\vec{x})\vec{\mathcal{L}}(\vec{r}(t) - \vec{x})d^d x$, with the (approximately constant) sensitivity pattern of the receive coils $\mathbf{R}$, and $\vec{\mathcal{L}}(\vec{x}) = \mathcal{L}\left(\frac{|G\vec{x}|}{H_{\text{sat}}}\right)\frac{G\vec{x}}{|G\vec{x}|}$, with the selection field gradient G. This expression may be simplified by applying a Fourier transform $\mathcal{F}$, which yields $\hat{\vec{s}}(\omega) = i\omega\mu_0 m\mathbf{R}\mathcal{F}\left[\int \rho(\vec{x})\vec{\mathcal{L}}(\vec{r}(t) - \vec{x})d^d x\right](\omega)$. A discretization of space $\rho(\vec{x}) = \frac{V}{N}\sum_i \delta(\vec{x} - \vec{x_i})\rho_i$ divides the volume V of the field of view (FOV) into N equally sized line sections, pixels or voxels and leads to an expression for the MPI system matrix, which is $S_{ij} = i\omega_i\mu_0 m\mathbf{R}\frac{V}{N}\mathcal{F}\left[\vec{\mathcal{L}}(\vec{r}(t) - \vec{x_j})\right](\omega_i)$. This expression may now be extended using a simple relaxation model, which is the convolution with a relaxation function $\Gamma(t)$, an exponentially decaying function for times greater than zero with an effective relaxation time of τ. In frequency space, this corresponds to a function $\hat{\Gamma}(\omega) = \frac{1}{1+i\tau\omega}$, which leads to $S_{ij} = S_{ij}^{\text{rf}} \times \hat{\Gamma}(\omega_i)$. The relaxation model may be extended to more than one relaxation time (to incorporate both Brownian and Néel relaxation) or locally varying relaxation properties, for example to determine the local tracer binding status.

II.II. Parameter fitting

The expression for the system matrix in frequency space may now be used for a reconstruction of functional parameters such as H_{sat} and τ from MPI measurements. Common to all reconstructions is the underlying fitting scheme; assuming a measured spectrum $\{\hat{s}_i\}$ and a known particle distribution

$\rho(\vec{x})$, the free model parameters such as the saturation parameter and the (global) particle relaxation time are varied to minimize a loss function. The measurement setup considered here is only one dimensional, although the model as well as the fitting method work for two- and three-dimensional setups as well. All frequency components besides the harmonics of the excitation signal are omitted in the following. The influence of the send chain of the MPI setup must be included into the fitting process, as it determines the phase shift between generated and emitted excitation signal, which leads to an excitation frequency dependent phase shift in the FFP trajectory $\vec{r}(t)$. The calculated spectrum is then forward corrected using the receive chain characteristics. This includes the addition of artificial noise to the spectrum, which may be estimated from measurements. The application of the frequency dependence of the receive chain and artificial noise is implemented as a linear transformation $\hat{s}_i \rightarrow c_i \hat{s}_i + \eta_i$, with $c_i \in C$ the receive chain correction of frequency component i and $\eta_i \in C$ the noise of that component. A logarithmic version of the sum of squares, namely $L_{\log}(\{p_k\}) = \sum_i \ln |c_i \sum_j S_{ij}(\{p_k\})\rho_j + \eta_i - \widetilde{s_i^{\text{meas}}}|$, is used as a loss function, which showed to be more robust against an insufficient compensation of the drive-field feed-through than the usual sum of squares, as higher harmonics have more weight using the latter loss function. Differential evolution [3], a global optimization meta-heuristic, with a population size of 15 is used for minimizing the loss function. As was already mentioned, the particle distribution must be known prior to the parameter reconstruction, which is because wrong estimations of functional parameters are always counterbalanced by wrong estimations of the particle distribution in standard system matrix-based reconstruction methods such as the Kaczmarz algorithm. Thus, a single measurement is not sufficient to reconstruct both particle distribution and functional parameters; a sequence of measurements is needed, the exact composition of this sequence depends on the parameters of interest.

III. Results

Fig. 1 shows an exemplary reconstruction result for the saturation parameter and a single (effective) relaxation time from a measured spectrum using a known particle distribution, namely a delta sample at the center of the FOV. The fitted parameters are then used to reconstruct a second particle distribution (Fig. 2) to demonstrate that the derived expression for the MPI system matrix can be used for model-based reconstructions.

IV. Discussion

The result of the fit for the effective relaxation time τ corresponds well to previously reported values [4]. The value for H_{sat} is of the same order of magnitude, but larger than it was expected to be [2], which is most likely due to a low magnetic moment m of a single particle. Using the fitted parameters, the model derived here is successfully able to reconstruct a more complex phantom.

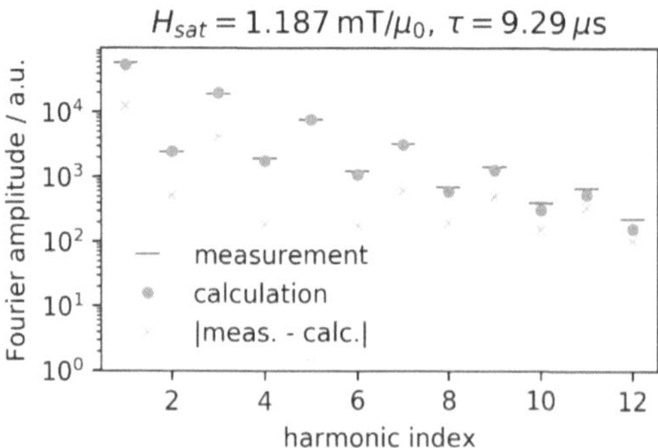

Figure 1: *Parameter fitting example for a voltage trace acquired using a delta sample of Perimag® particles and the multi-frequency MPI device with a gradient of 0.7016 T/m, a drive field amplitude of 9 mT/μ_0, a sinusoidal excitation at 10 kHz, a sampling rate of 1 MHz, and 50000 data points.*

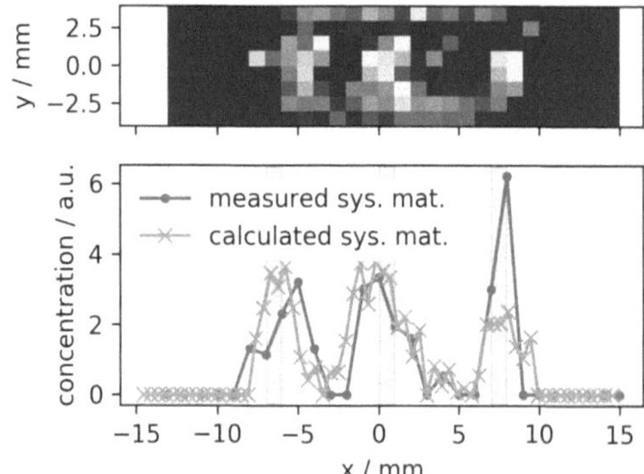

Figure 2: *Particle distribution reconstruction for a phantom of Perimag® particles, measured using a drive field amplitude of 8.5 mT/μ_0 and all other settings as in Fig. 1. The upper plot shows the distribution reconstructed using a measured 2D system matrix, the crosses in the lower plot use the model presented in this work, with the fitted values of Fig. 1. The dotted curve in the lower plot indicates the particle distribution from the upper plot at $y = 0^-$ mm. Both reconstructions were conducted using the Kaczmarz algorithm with 50 iterations and no regularization. The real distribution is indicated by the green semi-transparent area.*

V. Conclusions

A simple expression for the MPI system function and matrix with an arbitrary number of dimensions was derived, including a simple model for the particle relaxation. This expression may easily be extended to locally varying relaxation times and saturation parameters. The model was then used for a first fitting-based reconstruction of the functional parameters H_{sat} and τ. To conclude, the approach presented here provides a solid basis for further research on the reconstruction of (local) functional parameters.

REFERENCES

[1] D. Pantke *et al.* "1D Multi-Frequency MPI by passive and active Drive Field Feed-Through Compensation", IWMPI 2019.

[2] T. März and A. Weinmann, Model-Based Reconstruction for Magnetic Particle Imaging in 2D and 3D, arXiv:1605.08095 [math], May 2016.

[3] R. Storn and K. Price. "Differential Evolution – A Simple and Efficient Heuristic for global Optimization over Continuous Spaces", Journal of Global Optimization , vol. 11, no. 4, pp. 341–359, Dec. 1997.

[4] R. J. Deissler *et al.* "Dependence of Brownian and Néel relaxation times on magnetic field strength", Medical Physics , vol. 41, no. 1, p. 012 301, Jan. 2014.

Selection-Field-Induced Warping in X-Space MPI

Ecrin Yagiz[a,b*], Mustafa Ütkür[a,b], Orhun Caner Eren[a], Emine Ulku Saritas[a,b,c]

[a] *Department of Electrical and Electronics Engineering, Bilkent University, Ankara, Turkey*
[b] *National Magnetic Resonance Research Center (UMRAM), Bilkent University, Ankara, Turkey*
[c] *Neuroscience Program, Sabuncu Brain Research Center, Bilkent University, Ankara, Turkey*
[*] *Corresponding author, email: ecrin@ee.bilkent.edu.tr*

Abstract: In magnetic particle imaging (MPI) scanners, the selection field becomes non-linear in regions away from the center of the MPI scanner. This work demonstrates that, with basic x-space reconstruction approach, unaccounted non-linearity of the selection field causes warping in the reconstructed image. We also show that simple unwarping algorithms can be applied to effectively address this issue, once the displacement map acting on the reconstructed image is determined.

I. Introduction

In x-space model of magnetic particle imaging (MPI), the ideal signal is defined via the response of the nanoparticles to an oscillating drive field. [1], [2]. A typical assumption of x-space MPI is that the selection field gradient is constant in the imaging field-of-view (FOV). While such highly linear gradient fields are achievable using large magnets and/or additional shim coils, practical trade-offs (e.g., the total cost of the system) may limit this approach. For the case of system function reconstruction, the field non-linearity is implicitly taken into account and corrected, following a lengthy calibration procedure. For basic x-space reconstruction, geometric warping effects are expected to occur if the FOV extends beyond the linear region [2]. Similar problems have been investigated in magnetic resonance imaging (MRI), as the non-linearity of the magnetic field gradients cause what is called "gradient warping" [3],[4]. Here, we perform a simulation-based investigation of selection-field-induced warping for basic x-space reconstruction. We show that the warping effects are relatively benign and can be effectively addressed to achieve a geometrically accurate representation of the underlying nanoparticle distribution.

II. Material and Methods

Simulations were performed in four stages: 1) Magnetic fields were simulated for both the ideal and non-ideal selection field cases. The simulation parameters were based on our in-house FFP MPI scanner that features (2.4, 2.4, -4.8) T/m selection field gradients [5]. 2) Imaging simulations were performed using either the ideal or non-ideal selection fields, followed by x-space MPI reconstruction [6]. 3) The selection-field-induced warping of the MPI image was quantified for each pixel via a displacement map. 4) A potential solution of the warping artifact was investigated. These stages are described in detail below.

II.I. Magnetic Field Simulations

Magnetic field values, $\vec{B} = (B_x, B_y, B_z)$, were calculated for the dimensions of our FFP MPI scanner. This scanner has two permanent disk magnets with 7-cm radius and 2-cm thickness. The separation of the two magnets is 8 cm, with North poles facing each other. For the ideal selection field simulations, the following is used,

$$\vec{B} = G\vec{x} \tag{2}$$

Here, $\vec{x}$ is position and G is the gradient matrix. For the ideal case, G is diagonal and trace(G)=0. Taking our FFP MPI scanner as reference, (G_{xx}, G_{yy}, G_{zz})=(2.4, 2.4, -4.8) T/m was used. The selection field was numerically calculated at all points in the FOV, considering the geometry of the permanent magnets [7].

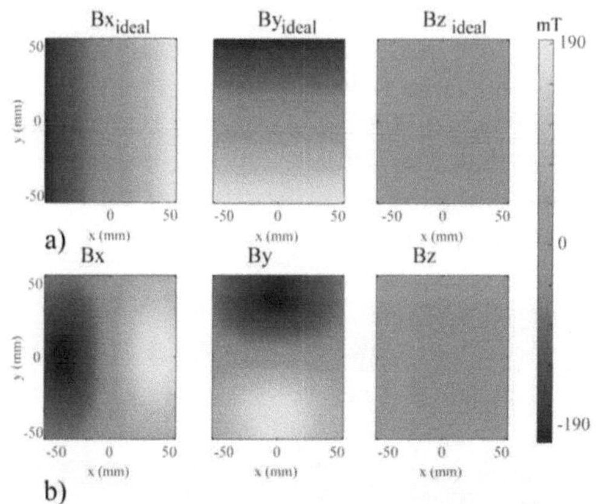

Figure 1: *Selection fields in x-, y-, and z-directions at z=0 for a) the ideal case, and b) our FFP scanner. For the ideal case, constant G_{xx}, G_{yy}, and G_{zz} were assumed.*

The simulated magnetic fields in x-, y-, and z-directions are shown in Fig. 1, together with the corresponding ideal cases, at z=0 plane. The nonlinearity of the selection field away from the scanner center can be clearly seen.

II.II. Imaging Simulations

Imaging simulations were performed using an in-house MPI simulation toolbox in MATLAB (Mathworks, Natick, MA). The phantom consisted of point source SPIOs that are placed uniformly in the FOV with 10 mm separation, as seen in Fig 2a. The following drive field parameters were utilized: 20 mT at 25 kHz along the x-direction (corresponding to a theoretical partial FOV (pFOV) size of 16.7 mm). 25 nm nanoparticle diameter was assumed and relaxation effects were ignored. The overall FOV was 4 cm × 4 cm at z=0 plane. The discretization was Δx = 0.01 mm and Δy = 1mm along the x- and y-directions, respectively. After filtering out the fundamental harmonic, images were obtained using pFOV-based x-space reconstruction [6].

II.III. Simulations for Displacement Map Calculation

A point source SPIO was placed at a single position on a predetermined 1 mm × 1 mm grid in the FOV. The displacements in both x- and y-directions were quantified using the resulting image from the realistic fields. These steps were repeated by moving the point source to another grid point.

II.IV. Correction via Displacement Map

The displacement map obtained in Section II.III was spline interpolated to calculate a finer map for every pixel in the realistic image. This interpolated displacement map was then utilized to correct the image from realistic selection fields using MATLAB's built-in "*imwarp*" function, using geometric transformation.

III. Results & Discussion

Figure 2 shows the result of the imaging simulations from the ideal and the realistic selection fields. In the realistic case, the selection-field-induced warping is visible, especially in regions far away from the center of the FOV. The SPIOs that are actually at the boundaries of the phantom are pushed towards the center of the FOV (see the red arrows in Fig. 2c).

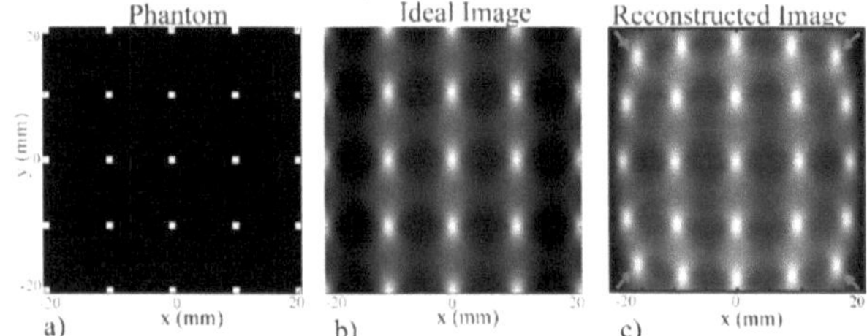

Figure 2: *Phantom with point source SPIOs placed at 10 mm separations. X-space reconstructed MPI image for the case of b) ideal selection field, and c) realistic selection field. The discretization for these simulations was Δx=0.01 mm along the scanning direction and Δy = 1mm along the y-direction.*

Figure 3a and 3b show the displacement map and the corrected image. The SPIOs that were pushed towards the center are pushed back to the edges of the FOV, with some loss of resolution.

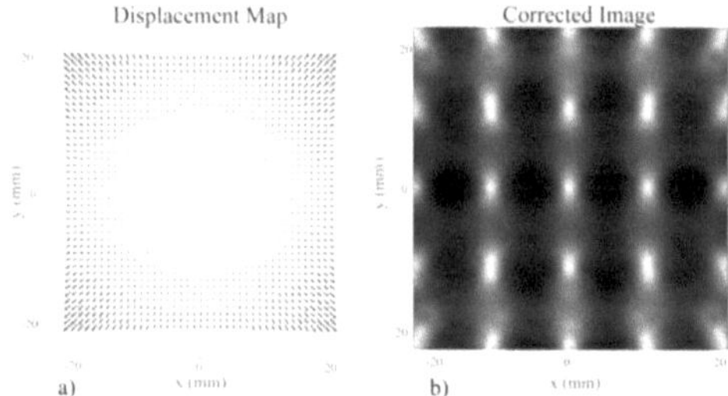

Figure 3: *a) Calculated displacement map, showing the warping of the MPI image in the case of a realistic selection field. b) The corrected version of the image in Fig. 2c. Here, the correction was performed using the displacement map.*

Note that these results did not take into account the drive field and focus field imperfections. Non-idealities in those fields may also cause distortions in x-space MPI images.

IV. Conclusion

In this study, selection-field-induced warping in x-space MPI is demonstrated via simulations. This warping can take place when the FOV is enlarged, such that the gradient of the selection field is no longer constant. This situation arises if the system is not specifically designed for high fidelity linearity in a large volume. The resulting distortion is relatively benign and a corrected image can be obtained using simple image unwarping algorithms.

AUTHOR'S STATEMENT

Research funding: This work was supported by the Scientific and Technological Research Council of Turkey (TUBITAK 217S069). Conflict of interest: Authors state no conflict of interest.

REFERENCES

[1] B. Gleich and J. Weizenecker. Tomographic imaging using the nonlinear response of magnetic particles. Nature, 435(7046):1217-1217, 2005. doi: 10.1038/nature03808.

[2] P. W. Goodwill and S. M. Conolly, "The X-Space Formulation of the Magnetic Particle Imaging Process: 1-D Signal, Resolution, Bandwidth, SNR, SAR, and Magnetostimulation," IEEE Transactions on Medical Imaging, vol. 29, no. 11, pp. 1851–1859, 2010. doi: 10.1109/tmi.2010.2052284

[3] S. J. Doran, L. Charles-Edwards, S. A. Reinsberg, and M. O. Leach, "A complete distortion correction for MR images: I. Gradient warp correction," Physics in Medicine and Biology, vol. 50, no. 7, pp. 1343–1361, 2005. doi: 10.1088/0031-9155/50/7/001

[4] Kybic, P. Thevenaz, A. Nirkko and M. Unser, "Unwarping of unidirectionally distorted EPI images", IEEE Transactions on Medical Imaging, vol. 19, no. 2, pp. 80-93, 2000. doi: 10.1109/42.836368

[5] M. Utkur, Y. Muslu, and E. U. Saritas, "A 4.8 T/m Magnetic Particle Imaging Scanner Design and Construction," 21st National Biomedical Engineering Meeting (BIYOMUT), Istanbul, Turkey, 2017. doi: 10.1109/biyomut.2017.8479214

[6] K. Lu, P. W. Goodwill, E. U. Saritas, B. Zheng, and S. M. Conolly, "Linearity and Shift Invariance for Quantitative Magnetic Particle Imaging," IEEE Transactions on Medical Imaging, vol. 32, no. 9, pp. 1565–1575, 2013. doi: 10.1109/tmi.2013.2257177

[7] S. I. Babic and C. Akyel, "Improvement in the analytical calculation of the magnetic field produced by permanent magnet rings," Progress In Electromagnetics Research C, vol. 5, no. 71, pp. 71–81, 2008.

A novelty 2-D temperature imaging method by scanning magnetic nanoparticles thermometer

Yi Sun [a], Zhongzhou Du [a*], Dandan Wang [a], and Rijian Su [a]

[a] Depqrtment of Computer and Communication Engineering, Zhengzhou University of Light Industry, China
** Corresponding author, email: duzhongzhou@zzuli.edu.cn*

I. Introduction

White light-emitting diodes (LEDs), are extensively used in industrial applications, transportation, and in settings that are part of normal daily life. The thermal management of LED is becoming increasingly problematic because increasingly powerful LED and LED array are being developed [1]. The heat accumulation will cause the junction temperature to rise, thereby reducing the lifetime and luminous efficiency of the LED, and seriously affecting the stability of the LED arrays work. The precise measurement of temperature distribution is key to improve the multi-chip power LED's lifetime and reliability by heat management. It is difficult to provide a perfect solution using traditional temperature measurement methods under extreme conditions, such as the internal of organism, high-power integrated electronic components and so on. Therefore, noninvasive and accurate temperature distribution measurement is of great significance to biomedical, and industrial applications.

A magnetic nanoparticle (MNP) thermometer [2-4] is a noncontact and precise tool for measuring the internal temperature of objects. Currently, the MNP thermometer that has been reported can obtain average temperature of a single point. In studying the influence of magnetic nanoparticle relaxation time on temperature measurement accuracy, Ludwing et al [5] found that the phase lag of magnetic nanoparticles' magnetization is almost negligible under quasi-static magnetic field, and the harmonics of magnetic nanoparticles' magnetization at different position satisfy the superposition principle. It provides an idea for the study of 2-D temperature imaging.

In this paper we present a 2-D temperature imaging method - with scanning MNPs thermometer. In experiments, the internal temperature distribution of multi-chip power LEDs was successfully measured.

II. Material and Methods

Superparamagnetic nanoparticles are sensitive to temperature and can be used to measure the temperature under extreme conditions. The nonlinearity of the Langevin function means that the magnetization induced by an applied magnetic field composes of harmonic components. For a rectangle covered with MNPs, the relationship between total harmonic amplitude at given spatial position (x, y, z_0), $C_i(x, y, \phi, T)$, with 2-D harmonic distribution, $A_i(x, y, \phi, T)$, can be expressed in

$$C_i(x, y, \phi, T) = G(x, y) * A_i(x, y, \phi, T), \tag{1}$$

where $G(x, y)$ is a weighting function.

A deconvolution method enables one to measure the ith harmonics of the magnetization generate by local MNPs at position $P(x, y)$, expressed as

$$A_i(x, y, \phi, T) = F^{-1}\left(\frac{F\left[C_i(x, y, \phi, T) \right]}{F\left[G(x, y) \right]} \right) \tag{2}$$

The harmonic amplitudes at ω and 3ω are functions of concentration ϕ and temperature T. And then, the local temperature of MNPs at position $P(x, y)$ can be calculated by Equation (3)

$$\begin{cases} A_1 = \phi M_s \left(\dfrac{\xi}{3} - \dfrac{\xi^3}{60} + \dfrac{\xi^5}{756} - \dfrac{\xi^7}{8640} + \dfrac{\xi^9}{95040} \right) \\ A_3 = \phi M_s \left(\dfrac{\xi^3}{180} - \dfrac{\xi^5}{1512} + \dfrac{\xi^7}{14400} - \dfrac{\xi^9}{142560} \right) \end{cases} \tag{3}$$

where $\xi = M_s V H_0 / k_B T$, A_1 and A_3 are the amplitudes of fundamental 1th and 3rd harmonics. Solving Equation (3) allows the temperature to be measured using the Levenberg-Marquardt algorithm. The mechanical device, which consists of the 3-D sliding table, step motor and step motor driver, is employed for scanning the 2-D (x, y) area. After the MNPs samples in the whole 2-D imaging area are scanned, the amplitudes of 1th and 3rd harmonics ($A_1(x, y, \phi, T)$ and $A_3(x, y, \phi, T)$) of the MNPs at each pixel point in the area to image can be calculated by using deconvolution algorithm. Consequently, the local 2-D temperature distribution of MNPs can be determined.

III. Results

The MNPs samples (EMG1400, FerroTec.) were mixed with the silica gel and then are directly coated on the top surface of the LED chip for 3 LED chips on the left column. For 3 LED chips on the right column, the MNPs samples and the phosphor powder particles were embedded into the silica gel and then coated on the LED chips. The LED chips in the first, second and third row were applied with an operating voltage of 5.0 V, 5.1 V and 5.2 V respectively. The magnetization response signals of MNPs will be transformed to voltage signals via detection coil and be collected by the data acquisition card. After the magnetization response of one point is measured, the mechanical device will move the detection coil (the outer diameter is 2 mm, the inner diameter is 1 mm, and the length is 3 mm) to the next point.

Figure 1 shows the temperature distribution of a multi-chip power LEDs at different stages from on to off. Since the temperature of location with no magnetic nanoparticle cannot be measured, the temperature of the position is set at room temperature (298K). Figure 1 (a) shows the temperature distribution of the LED sample when the operating voltage is not applied, when the temperature of the entire measuring area is room temperature. Figure 1 (b) and (c) show the temperature distribution at 400s and 600s during the temperature rise stage, respectively. Figure 1 (d) shows the internal temperature distribution of multi-chip power LED when the temperature tends to be stable; The temperature of the first column chip coated directly with magnetic nanoparticles at operating voltage of 5.0 V, 5.1 V and 5.2 V is 305.1 K, 315.3 K and 328.2 K, respectively; The second column chip with phosphor layer and magnetic nanoparticles at operating voltage of 5.0 V, 5.1 V and 5.2 V is 309 K, 333.5 K and 377.8 K. Under the operating voltage of 5.0 V, 5.1 V and 5.2 V, the temperature of the phosphor layer is 3.9 K, 18.2 K and 49.6 K higher than that of the chip. Figure 1 (e) shows the internal temperature distribution of the multi-chip power LED cooling after the withdrawal of the operating voltage. Figure 1 (f) shows the temperature distribution of multi-chip power LED when it is cooled to room temperature. In general, under different operating voltage, the temperature of the phosphor layer is higher than that of the chip; and the higher the operating voltage, the larger the temperature difference between the two.

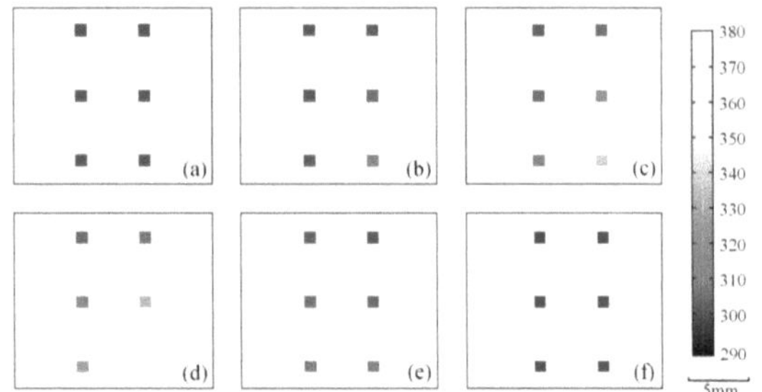

Figure 1: *2-D Temperature distribution of multi-chip power LED in different stages.*

IV. Conclusions

In this study, we reported the 2-D temperature imaging method with scanning magnetic nanoparticles. The method developed is a nondestructive and precise means of measuring the 2-D temperature distribution based on magnetic nanoparticles. We employed the system to

successfully measure the internal temperature distribution of multi-chip power LEDs, thus demonstrating the feasibility of the proposed method for temperature imaging.

ACKNOWLEDGEMENTS

This work was supported by the Natural Science Foundation of China (grant no. 61803346), the Science and Technology Program of Henan, China (grant no. 162102410077), and the Graduate's Scientific Research Foundation of Zhengzhou University of Light Industry (grant no. 2018011).

REFERENCES

[1] Huaiyu, Ye, Sau Koh, Henk van Zeijl, et al. A review of passive thermal management of LED module. *Journal of Semiconductors* 32(1): 014008, 2011 doi: 10.1118/1.3106342

[2] Weaver JB, Rauwerdink AM, Hansen EW. Magnetic nanoparticle temperature estimation. *Medical physics.* 36(5):1822-9, 2009. doi: 10.1118/1.3106342

[3] Zhong, Jing, Wenzhong Liu, Li Kong, et al. A new approach for highly accurate, remote temperature probing using magnetic nanoparticles. *Scientific reports.* 4: 6338, 2014. doi: 10.1038/srep06338

[4] Du, Zhongzhou, Yi Sun, Rijian Su, et al. The phosphor temperature measurement of white light-emitting diodes based on magnetic nanoparticle thermometer. *Review of Scientific Instruments.* 89(9): 094901, 2018 doi: 10.1038/srep06338

[5] Ludwig, Frank, et al. Characterization of magnetic nanoparticle systems with respect to their magnetic particle imaging performance. *Biomedizinische Technik/Biomedical Engineering.* 58(6): 535-545. 2013. doi: 10.1515/bmt-2013-0013

Exploring parameters of magnetic particles in 1D field excitation

Tobias Klemme[a], Thorsten M. Buzug[a], and Alexander Neumann[a]

[a] *Insitute of Medical Engineering, Universität zu Lübeck, Lübeck, Germany*
[*] *Corresponding author, email: {klemme, buzug, neumann}@imt.uni-luebeck.de*

This work explores how different parameters, e.g. magnetic anisotropy, core radius or hydrodynamic radius, influence the signal/spectrum in a one-dimensional excitation field. Simulations are performed using a model considering both the mechanical motion and the magnetization dynamics of the particle.

I. Introduction

The properties of magnetic particles have a great influence on different applications such as magnetic particle imaging (MPI) [1] or magnetic particle hyperthermia [2]. Especially in the field of MPI the magnetization of the particles is often described using Langevin's theory of paramagnetism, where the magnetization only depends on the ratio of magnetic energy to thermal energy. In reality, many other properties of the nanoparticle and the surroundings have to be taken into account [3, 4, 5]. For example, the fact that magnetic particles usually exhibit a magnetic anisotropy which leads to a non-reversible behavior (hysteresis). According to Langevin's theory a bigger core diameter would result in a steeper magnetization curve (the modulus of the particle magnetic moment is given by $|m_p| = M_s V_c$ where M_s is assumed to be constant), whereas in reality, the increasing core diameter would also increase the anisotropy energy $E_A = K V_c$ (assuming uniaxial anisotropy), which leads to an increasing coercive field and remanent magnetization.

As such it is important to study the influence of particle parameters and their influence on the signal using a proper model to describe the magnetization dynamics and motion of the particle within arbitrary fields. Therefore, models and solving methods to describe the behavior of magnetic nanoparticles in magnetic fields are required and have been introduced by various authors [3, 6, 7].

In order to obtain more insight into the influence of particle parameters on the signal/spectrum, the particle behavior in a 1D excitation field has been simulated for different parameters. As an example, this work will focus on the influence of different anisotropy energies on the induced signal dm/dt and its corresponding spectrum.

Additionally, it is studied how the core size and magnetic anisotropy affect the harmonics in interdependence.

II. Material and Methods

The data is acquired by a simulation model introduced by A. Neumann [6], which uses a coupled model of the Landau-Lifschitz-Gilbert-equation (LLG) and Euler's equation, to consider that the magnetic moment of a particle relaxes by a rotation of the magnetization (Néel) and also by a mechanical rotation of the whole particle (Brownian rotation).

Within the simulations the particles saturation magnetization M_s is set to 477464 A/m, and an excitation field strength of 20 mT with a frequency of 25 kHz is chosen. The viscosity of water (1 mPa s) and room temperature (295 K) are used. The simulation time step is set to 5 ps whereby the actual output is oversampled to a time step of 0.2 µs. In all simulations the hydrodynamic diameter is set to 50 nm whereas in simulations, where only the anisotropy has been varied, the magnetic core diameter is set to 24 nm. Each simulation has been performed over 6 periods (240 µs/48Msteps) of the excitation frequency with an ensemble of 2000 particles. (Roughly 20 minutes using 4x Intel E5-4657L v2 CPUs). In the following studies, the first period of the simulation is neglected to avoid initialization artifacts/non-periodic behavior when the magnetic field is applied for the first time, since the magnetic particles are initialized with a random starting orientation and magnetization direction.

III. Results

III.I Influence of different anisotropy constants.

Fig. 1a) shows the normalized magnetic moment for different anisotropy constants and the corresponding normalized excitation signal. The relationship between the time offset and the anisotropy energy is easily recognized and is caused

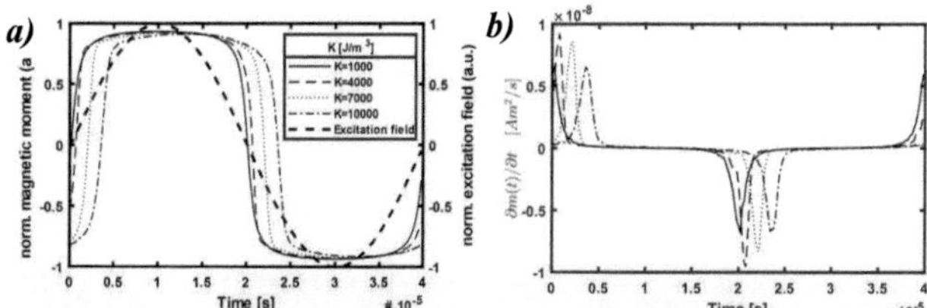

***Figure 1: a)** Plot of the normalized magnetic moment and the associated excitation signal. An increasing anisotropy energy leads to a larger phase-difference; **b)** dm/dt for different anisotropy constants. In addition to the phase difference, different anisotropy energies lead to different signal amplitudes.*

since the magnetic anisotropy exerts an additional torque on the particle magnetic moment which must be overcome to reverse $\vec{m}$ with respect to the easy axis $\vec{n}$. Thus, a larger magnetic field $\vec{H}$ is necessary to reverse the magnetic moment in the direction of the applied field.

Fig. 1b) shows the time derivative of the magnetic moment. It is recognizable that the anisotropy does not only affect the phase between the excitation signal and the magnetic moment, but also influences the magnitude of dm/dt and therefore the switching behavior of the particles magnetic moment with respect to the applied field.

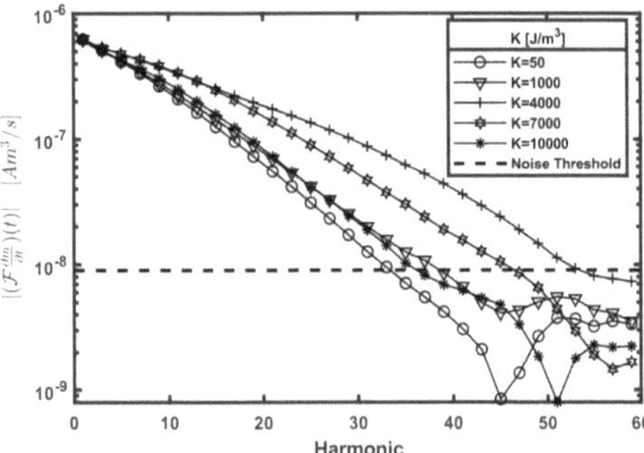

Figure 2: *Magnitude of the harmonics in the spectrum of dm/dt for different anisotropy constants. The highest harmonics occur at K=4 kJ/m³. The noise threshold depends on the number of simulated particles and periods.*

For a system matrix-based reconstruction it is important that the measured spectrum contains many and high harmonics [1]. To demonstrate how different anisotropy constants influence the spectrum of the acquired signal dm/dt, the magnitude of the harmonics is plotted in Fig. 2.

It can be observed that the harmonics are larger for a certain magnetic anisotropy energy KV_c. In case of the different anisotropy constants shown in Fig. 2 and the used other simulation parameters the highest harmonics occur at K = 4 kJ/m³. Both higher and lower anisotropy constants result in lower harmonics.

III.II Interdependence of anisotropy and magnetic radii

To visualize how harmonics are influenced by different core sizes with different anisotropies, Fig. 3 shows a surface plot

of different harmonics for different core radii and anisotropy constantsThe core radius is varied from 5 nm to 25 nm in 2.5 nm steps. K is varied from 1 to 10 kJ/m³ in 1 kJ/m³ steps and additionally simulated with 500 and 100 J/m³. The overall magnetic moments of the different core sizes are normalized by NM_sV_c ($\tilde{m}(t) = m(t)/NM_sV_c$), where N is the number of particles. Additionally, the harmonics of every surface plot are normalized to the largest occurring harmonic within the surface. It can be observed that the optimal anisotropy constant decreases with increasing core radius. Yet even for very big core radii a small anisotropy ($K \leq 1000$ J/m³) leads to slightly higher harmonics, particularly at higher frequencies, whereas the harmonics of particles with large magnetic radii and high anisotropy decreases fast. This fast decrease is most likely to explain with increased Brownian rotation and the resulting friction losses.

IV. Discussion

It has been shown how different anisotropy constants with a fixed magnetic radius or varying magnetic radii and therefore different anisotropy energies can influence the behavior of magnetic particles with a uniaxial anisotropy in a 1D excitation field when Néel- and Brownian rotation are considered. At a specific anisotropy, higher harmonics are observed which might result in a better reconstruction. It must be considered that the simulation has been performed with a 1D excitation field. For other frequencies or 2D/3D excitation the dynamic of a SPION and its magnetic moment is different. Therefore, other particle properties are advantageous or disadvantageous. Nevertheless, it is shown that well chosen particle parameters can improve MPI-performance.

V. Conclusions

Using a varying anisotropy constant and in the second case additionally varying magnetic radii, it is exemplified how particle properties can influence the signals for MPI. Several simulations can be done to gain knowledge how properties like excitation frequency, multidimensional excitation, hydrodynamic radius, viscosity, particle distribution or as described, the magnetic anisotropy affect the acquired signal. This knowledge can help to synthesize good performing SPIONs for application in MPI or magnetic particle hyperthermia.

ACKNOWLEDGEMENTS

Funding by the Federal Ministry of Education and Research via the Project SAMBA-PATI (FKZ: 13GW0069A) is gratefully acknowledged.

REFERENCES

[1] B. Gleich and J. Weizenecker. Nature, 435, 1217 (2005).
[2] S. Dutz and R. Hergt, Nanotechnology 25, 452001 (2014)
[3] D. B. Reeves and J. B. Weaver J. Appl. Phys. 112, 124311 (2012)
[4] J. Weizenecker et al. Phys. Med. Biol. 57 7317 (2012)
[5] S. Biederer et al, ESMRMB Congress 2009, 517 (2009)
[6] A. Neumann and T. M. Buzug. 8th Int. W. on Magn. Part. Imag. 213 (2018)
[7] J. Weizenecker et al. 1st Int. W. on Magn. Part. Imag, 3 (2010)

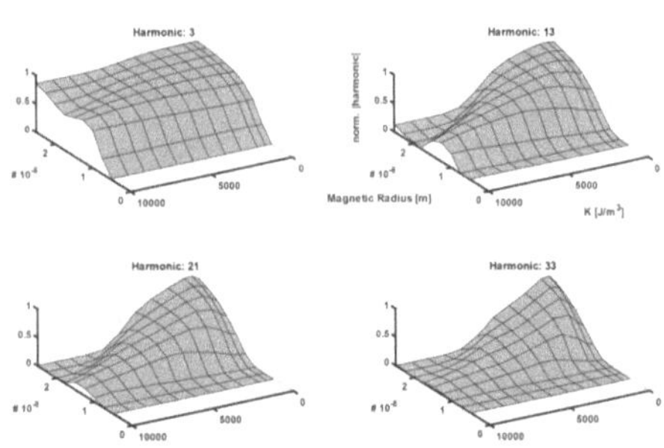

Figure 3: *Normalized harmonics (3,13,21,33) for varying magnetic radii and anisotropy constants*

3D printed magnetic composites as phantoms for Magnetic Particle Imaging

N. Löwa*, H. Paysen, D. Gutkelch, and F. Wiekhorst

Physikalisch-Technische Bundesanstalt, Berlin, Germany
** Corresponding author, email: norbert.loewa@ptb.de*

Abstract: To advance the characterization of MPI scanners long-term stable phantoms with exactly known geometry and magnetic properties are necessary. The technique of 3D-printing employing vat photopolymerization is a fast and cost-effective way to manufacture complex 3D structures out of numerous materials. The aim of our work was to test the feasibility of printing magnetic composites which consist of magnetic nanoparticles embedded in photopolymers. The results of our study clearly demonstrate that 3D printing opens an efficient way to manufacture complex magnetic structures that could resemble body-like parts with defined amounts of magnetic nanoparticles.

I. Introduction

For MPI-research, long-term stable phantoms [1][2] with defined geometry and magnetic nanoparticle (MNP) content are necessary for resolution tests [3][4], for cross-comparison of MPI scanners or as fiducial markers [5] to verify the spatial position of the body under analysis. A fast and cost-effective way to manufacture phantoms is the technique of generative printing, or commonly called 3D-printing. This additive technique allows for manufacturing customized parts with complex shapes out of specific photopolymers solidifying layer by layer under ultraviolet radiation. The aim of our work was to investigate the feasibility of printing composite materials consisting of MNPs embedded in photopolymers for the production of MPI phantoms. To this end, we developed a protocol for systematic quality evaluation of 3D-printed magnetic composites to generate complex, long-term stable MPI phantoms with defined magnetic properties (MNP amount per voxel, signal shape per voxel).

II. Material and Methods

II.I. Magnetic Nanoparticles

We used two commercially available MNP types, Ferucarbotran (Meito Sangyo, JPN) and EFH3 (FerroTec, USA). Ferucarbotran (FCT) is known as the magnetically active part of Resovist® and EFH3 is a light hydrocarbon oil-based ferrofluid usually used for audio speaker applications.

II.II. Photopolymers

Two types of photopolymers were used in our experiments. E-shell 600 clear (ES) and ABS 3SP Tough (ABS) are both light curing resins supplied by EnvisionTEC (Germany). The clear E-Shell was specially designed for applications in the hearing aid industry. The ABS photopolymer is a tough 3D printing material intended for applications where high stress and force resistance is required (e.g. automotive prototypes and consumer goods).

II.III. 3D printing

For 3D printing a commercial 3D printer (Perfactory DSP XL) from EnvisionTEC with an indicated minimal (lateral) xy resolution of 42 µm was used. The z resolution is mainly material dependent and indicated within between 25 µm and 150 µm.

III. Results

III.I. Magnetic properties & long-term stability

Cylinders printed with different concentrations of MNP (0.9 µg/mL up to 3 mg/mL) were measured by means of magnetic particle spectroscopy (MPS). In this way, we determined the capability of 3D printing to generate samples with defined magnetic behavior that are characterized by both a linear scaling of magnetic moment with nominal MNP amount and a constant signal shape (i.e. unchanged properties).

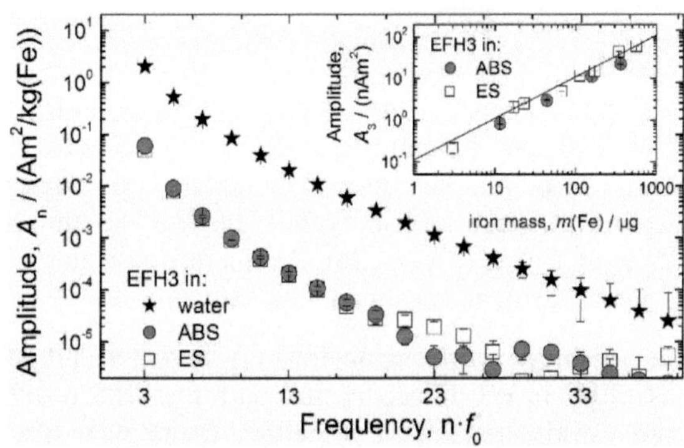

Figure 1: *MPS measurements (B=12 mT) on 3D printed cylinders with embedded MNP (EFH3) in ABS (grey filled symbols) and ES (open symbols) as well as on MNP in liquid suspension (black stars). MPS signals were normalized to the nominal iron amount of each sample (water: 242 µg, ABS: 44 µg, ES: 23 µg). Inset: Linear scaling of third harmonic amplitude A_3 with nominal iron amount m(Fe) in 3D printed samples.*

Finally, we found a linear scaling of the third harmonic amplitude A_3 with nominal iron amount in the printed cylinders (R^2=0.98). Regarding the signal shape, no significant alteration with varying MNP amount was observed for both photopolymers (Fig. 1, grey filled and open symbols). Nevertheless, the signal shape and amplitude changed significantly compared to the initial state of the raw MNP in liquid suspension (Fig. 1, black stars). This can be explained by higher dipolar interactions and reduced mobility present in the solidified material compared to the liquid state. MPS was further used to analyze the long-term stability of the magnetic properties of the samples. Two samples with different MNP concentrations were measured over a period of 48 weeks and the percentage difference compared to the initial state was below 0.5%.

III.II. Processability

The processability of the photopolymers (ES, ABS) without and with MNP (EFH3) was investigated by visual control of a specially developed 3D printed geometric demonstrator. This demonstrator consists of rods arranged at different angles with respect to the printing direction (0°, 30°, 45°, and 90°) each of them with a defined scaling scheme (diameter d=0.1 mm up to 2 mm, length l=10·d). Considering only photopolymers without MNP, the largest range of successfully printed rods was found for ES. Even rods with a diameter of only 0.1 mm were successfully formed whereas for ABS the minimal diameter was five times larger. Interestingly, elements printed in horizontal direction are mostly of a lower quality compared to vertical or tilted orientations for both materials. For ABS, horizontally printed rods were not formed at all. Interestingly, by adding MNP to photopolymers the quality of the rods of the demonstrator improved. A significant improvement was observed for horizontally printed structures, resulting in a wider range of successfully printed elements. Additionally, for ABS, even smaller elements down to 0.25 mm are formed in vertical and tilted orientations after adding MNP.

III.II. MPI

The MPI performance of the 3D printed photopolymers was tested on P-shaped phantoms having an iron concentration of c(Fe)=4.8 mg/mL. The lines of the letters had a thickness and depth of 1.5 mm and an overall length of 12 mm. As a reference, FCT was dispersed in demineralized water, filled in a negative form, and scanned with MPI as well.

Figure 2 displays the lettering for FCT in water and ES as well as EFH3 in ES. In accordance with the MPS results in III.I, the resulting resolution of the light cured phantoms had deteriorated in comparison to FCT in water. However, the structure of the phantom and the orientation of the lines are well visualized. Compared to FCT, the MPI image of the phantom with EFH3 in ES is of slightly lower quality.

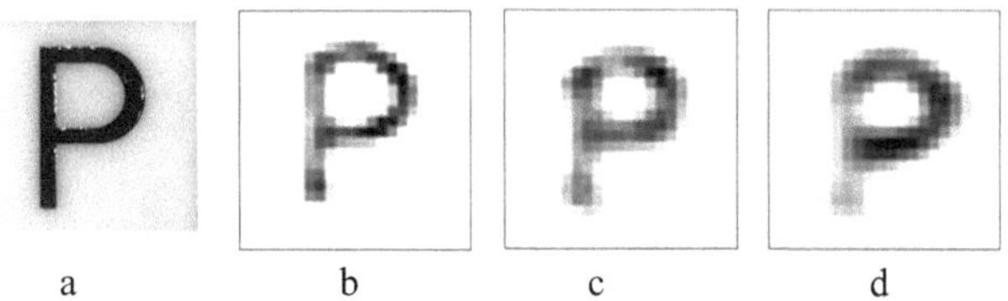

a   b   c   d

Figure 2: *MPI on magnetic phantoms with P-shaped structure. (a) Photo of phantom mask with FCT in demineralized water. (b-d) MPI image of FCT dispersed in demineralized water as well as phantoms with FCT in ES, and EFH3 in ES, respectively.*

IV. Discussion & Conclusion

We printed magnetic composites of different MNP concentrations and found a linear scaling of the magnetic moment with nominal iron amount as well as unchanged signal shapes. This enables to produce MPI phantoms with defined magnetic signaling at different concentrations. As these materials were long term stable (at least) over weeks they are additionally suitable for calibration purposes, quality assurance as well as round robin test phantoms in MPI. Furthermore, rods of different size were 3D printed at different angles with respect to the printing direction to evaluate the processability of magnetic composites. Interestingly, the processability significantly improved for magnetic composites compared to the photopolymer, alone. Finally, the magnetic composites were properly visualized by MPI which qualifies 3D printed magnetic composites for future MPI applications (e.g. as fiducial markers).

3D printing of magnetic composites advances the characterization of MPI scanners by providing defined, long-term stable magnetic phantoms and opens an elegant way to print complex structures that could resemble body-like parts containing defined amounts of MNP.

ACKNOWLEDGEMENTS

This project was supported by the Federal Ministry of Economics and Technology within the TransMeT project "Magnetische Messtechnik für die Größenfraktionierung magnetischer Nanopartikel" and by Deutsche Forschungsgemeinschaft within the research grants "AMPI: Magnetic particle imaging: Development and evaluation of novel methodology for the assessment of the aorta in vivo in a small animal model of aortic aneurysms" (grant SHA 1506/2-1) and "quantMPI: Establishment of quantitative Magnetic Particle Imaging (MPI) application oriented phantoms for preclinical investigations" (grant TR408/9-1).

REFERENCES

[1] A. Mattern et al. Magnetic Nanoparticle-Gel Materials for Development of MPI and MRI Phantoms. *IJMPI*, 4(2): 811001, 2018. doi: 10.18416/IJMPI.2018.1811001.

[2] O. Kosch et al. *Evaluation of a separate-receive coil by magnetic particle imaging of a solid phantom.* JMMM, 471:444-449, 2018. doi: 10.1016/j.jmmm.2018.09.114.

[3] S. Herz et al. Magnetic Particle Imaging for Quantification of Vascular Stenoses: A Phantom Study. IEEE Trans Magn, 37(1):61-67, 2018. doi: 10.1109/TMI.2017.2717958.

[4] J. Franke et al. System Characterization of a Highly Integrated Preclinical Hybrid MPI-MRI Scanner. IEEE Trans Magn, 35(9): 1993-2004, 2016. doi: 10.1109/TMI.2016.2542041.

[5] F. Werner et al. Geometry planning and image registration in magnetic particle imaging using bimodal fiducial markers. Med Phys, 43(6): 2884-2893, 2016. doi: 10.1118/1.4948998.

A Low Cost 3D Printed Magnetic Particle Spectrometer for the Undergraduate Laboratory

J. L. Stafford[a], M. I. Newton[a], and R. H. Morris[a]*

[a] Department of Physics and Mathematics, Nottingham Trent Univertsity, Notingham, NG11 8NS, UK
** Corresponding author, email: rob.morris@ntu.ac.uk*

Abstract: Magnetic Particle Spectroscopy has now secured itself as a valuable technique in both magnetic nanoparticle analysis and a detection technique in its own right. As such, it is increasingly finding its way into university curricula where equipment is mostly too complex, precise or expensive to easily reproduce in an undergraduate setting. In this work we present a low cost (<$250) system which is capable of performing basic magnetic particle spectrometry experiments in the undergraduate lab, comprising of off the shelf components and 3D printed coil bobbins which have intrinsic threads to allow for cancelation coil adjustment. We demonstrate the dependence of the third harmonic at 100Hz fundamental to sample concentration of magnetic nanoparticles (30nm) and find a linear correlation with regression coefficient 0.99.

I. Introduction

Magnetic Particle Spectroscopy (MPS)[1] has rapidly developed over the past decade. As a core technique in both magnetic nanoparticle analysis for Magnetic Particle Imaging[2-4] and a development tool in its own right for general magnetic nanoparticle synthesis, the technique is beginning, at least anecdotally, to secure a place in university curricula for Physics and Chemistry alike. Since undergraduate learning is greatly enhanced with practical experience, there is strong demand for a simple low-cost system. Developments have been seen with regard to the console elements[5] but with less emphasis on the physical hardware. Significant experience or funding is however needed to construct or purchase such a setup. The simplest of systems for MPS from a cost perspective is to utilize a gradiometer coil arrangement to cancel out the drive signal whilst preserving the fundamental in the resulting signal, eliminating the need for filters and reducing the dynamic range requirements for the receiver preamplifier. The location of the cancelation coil with respect to the drive coil has significant impact on the efficiency of this cancellation and therefore the success of the measurement. It is therefore common to include a means by which the coil can be moved by small amounts to achieve the best cancellation[4]. To reduce the burden on the experimental setup, we propose a system in which this adjustment is intrinsic to the coil formers by 3D printing the parts and including a threaded portion.

II. Material and Methods

II.I. Physical Design

The design for the receive and cancellation coil bobbins are produced using 3D CAD (Solidworks 2017, Dassault Systèmes, France) to prepare STL files for printing. A cross sectional view of the design of the three components of the system are shown in Fig. 1. Please note that only the pickup coil and the cancelation coil bobbins are 3D printed using a Stereolithographic 3D printer (Form2, FormLabs, MA, USA). Owing to size limitations of the bed however the drive bobbin is simply a piece of 70mm outer diameter acrylic tubing with end caps.

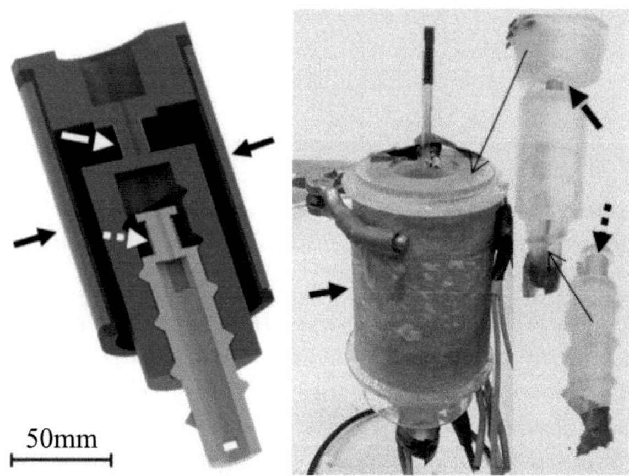

Figure 1: *Cross sectional model (left) and photograph (right) of the coil setup. The cancelation coil (Dashed Arrows) bobbin is screwed into the pickup coil (Broken Arrows) bobbin which is placed inside the 8 layer drive coil (Solid Arrows).*

The parts are printed with standard clear resin (FLGPCL04, FormLabs, MA, USA) since it was found that some black resins contained magnetically active compounds which were not suitable for subsequent measurements. The drive (70mm Ø x 102mm), pickup and cancellation coils (11mm Ø x 14mm) were wound around the formers, all using 81 stranded 46AWG Litz wire (Mike's Electronic Parts, OH, USA). The drive coil comprises 8 layers, connected as 4 parallel pairs of windings secured with epoxy resin (Bostik, WI, USA).

II.II. System Design and Components

The system utilizes amplification elements as proposed by Gehrcke[6] but utilizing low cost microcontrollers to provide the original drive signal and to digitize the resulting signals. A full system diagram is shown in Fig 2.

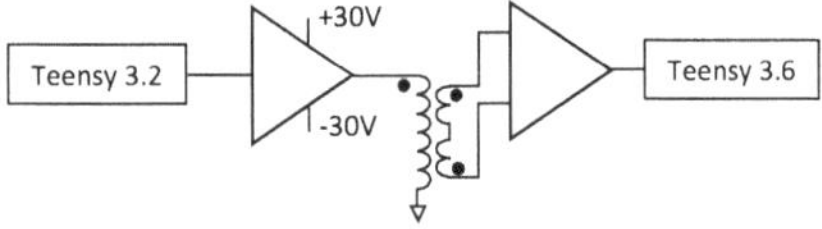

Figure 2: *Schematic of console. Transmit and Receive amplifiers may be off the shelf mains powered or low-cost modules.*

The microcontroller (Teensy 3.2, PJRC, OR, USA) is chosen to provide the drive signal as it yields superior performance to comparable Arduino microcontrollers but utilizes the same programing environment and price point. A faster clock speed microcontroller (Teensy 3.5) is chosen for digitization to allow for the collection of higher order harmonics than is afforded by alternative microcontrollers. The digitized signal is sent over serial to a host PC or stored on the in-built SD card for later processing. In either case, a python GUI is used to display the drive signal, the received (after cancellation) and amplified raw signal and the power spectral density. Example data using off the shelf amplifiers is shown in Fig 3.

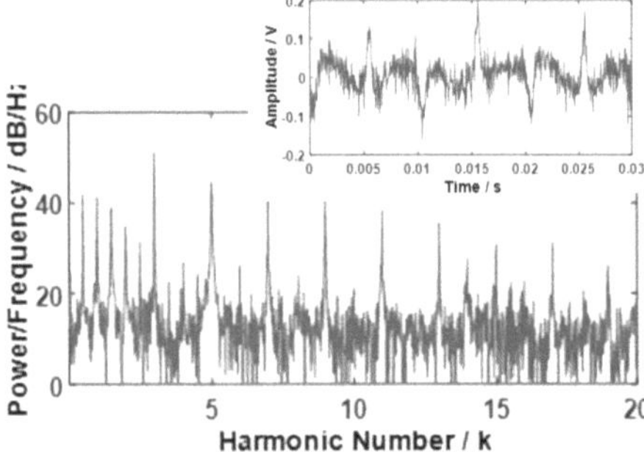

Figure 3: *Inset: The collected signal (after cancellation and amplification) Main: The resulting power spectral density (N.B. the smaller peaks surrounding the fundamental are background noise, present in the absence of a sample).*

The system as described is used to collect the signal from dilutions of commercially available nanoparticles (30 nm, PEG functionalized 1 mg/mL Fe in H_2O, 747408-10ML, Ocean Nanotech LLC, CA, USA via Sigma Aldrich, UK) ranging from 100% (1 mg/ml) to 50% (500 µg/ml) at 100Hz and (51.5±2)mT.

III. Results

The amplitude of the fifth harmonic for the range of concentrations described in section II.II is shown in Fig 4. The data suggests that there is a saturation occurring at the higher concentrations, which is not evident as clipping in the raw signal traces. It is believed that this to be related to the sedimentation of SPIOs at these higher concentrations during the measurement. These higher concentrations are subsequently removed from the fit. The expected dependence of amplitude on concentration is still seen as expected.

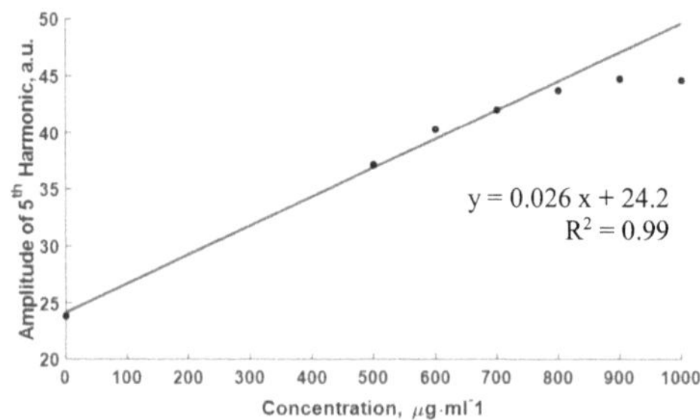

Figure 4: *Plot of 5th harmonic amplitude for varying concentrations of 30nm PEG functionalized SPIOs. The signal in the absence of sample gives the value at 0%.*

III.II. Cost Evaluation

The cost and source of possible low-cost components is detailed in Table 1 to allow the reader to produce an equivalent system.

Table 1: *Cost and source of components. Prices have been converted into USD.*

Element	Source	Quantity	Line Price
3D Printed Parts	Form Labs	<0.3l resin	$55
Acrylic Tube	The Plastics Shop	100mm	$5
81/46 Litz Wire	Mike's Electronics	500ft	$60
Teensy 3.2	PJRC	1	$20
Teensy 3.6	PJRC	1	$30
LM3884 module	Ebay	2	$40
AD604 module	Ebay	1	$15
		Total	$225

IV. Conclusion

We have detailed the construction, and validated the functionality of, a low cost, simple to construct 3D printed magnetic particle spectroscopy system suitable for deployment in the undergraduate laboratory. Full characterisation of this system will determine its suitability for research of unknown nanoparticles being developed for other applications.

ACKNOWLEDGEMENTS

JLS gratefully acknowledges funding from the Nottingham Trent University's Vice Chancellor's PhD Bursary.

AUTHOR'S STATEMENT

Research funding: The authors have received no external funding for this work. Conflict of interest: Authors state no conflict of interest.

REFERENCES

1. Biederer et al. (2009). *Journal of Physics D: Applied Physics*, *42*(20), 205007. 10.1088/0022-3727/42/20/205007
2. Gleich, B., & Weizenecker, J. (2005). *Nature*, *435*(7046), 1214–1217. https://doi.org/10.1038/nature03808
3. Behrends, A. et al. (2015). *Current Directions in Biomedical Engineering*, *1*(1), 249–253. 10.1515/cdbme-2015-0062
4. Tay, Z. W. et al. (2016) Sci. Rep. 6, 34180; 10.1038/srep34180 (2016).5.
5. Rückert MA, Vogel P, Behr VC. Proceedings of the 8th International workshop on magnetic particle imaging; 2018 Mar 22-24; Hamburg, Germany.Lubeck, Germany : Infinite science GmbH; 2018. p. 121-122.
6. Gehrcke, J. (2010). Masters Thesis: https://gehrcke.de/files/stud/gehrcke_MScThesis_magnetic_particle_imaging.pdf. Pp75-76. Accessed 17th November 2018.

MPI Velocity Mapping in a coronary Vessel Phantom

R. Siepmann[*a], **H. Nilius**[a], **F. Mueller**[a], **K. Mueller**[a], **S. M. Dadfar**[c], **V. Schulz**[a] **and S. D. Reinartz**[b]

[a] *Physics of Molecular Imaging Systems, RWTH Aachen University, Aachen, Germany*
[b] *Department of Diagnostic and Interventional Radiology, Uniklinikum Aachen, Aachen, Germany*
[c] *Experimental Molecular Imaging, RWTH Aachen University, Aachen, Germany*
[*] *Corresponding author, email: robert.siepmann@pmi.rwth-aachen.de*

Abstract: Magnetic Particle Imaging (MPI) may have the potential to diagnose early stages of coronary artery disease. In this study, glass tubes of varying inner diameters, simulating coronary vessel diameter, were brought in a circulation phantom. Standardized SPION-boluses were injected at coronary-specific flow rates, representing normal and hyperemic flows, and visualized using MPI. The acquired image data were analyzed using two different algorithms to compute the mean velocity. Both calculated velocity data sets were in good agreement with our analytic model. This shows that MPI might be a strong alternative to clinically established methods in cardiovascular imaging.

I. Introduction

Diagnosis and treatment of Cardiovascular diseases (CVD) occupy large parts of medical resources worldwide. According to estimates, 1.02 million Americans will sustain a coronary event in 2017 alone, from which approximately 36% will die of it [1]. To optimize the outcome for patients, an early diagnosis is crucial. Currently, invasive coronary angiography represents the gold standard to detect pathologic hemodynamics by Fractional Flow Reserve (FFR) measurements. However, coronary angiography as an invasive procedure has serious drawbacks. For a start, there is a high radiation exposure with 8 to 10 mSv per treatment [2]. Additionally, serious complications such as peripheral artery occlusion, arrhythmia, stroke or myocardial infarction may occur even in diagnostic examinations. Magnetic Particle Imaging (MPI) holds certain characteristics that could make it a strong alternative to clinically established methods. High spatial and temporal resolution [3] without using radiation makes it interesting, especially, for cardiovascular imaging. As shown by Karthika et al. [4], stenoses as a risk constellation for cardiac events can be detected by blood flow velocity analysis. A study which supports MPI's utility for this kind of application has recently been performed: Kaul et al. [5] successfully measured blood flow velocities in the inferior vena cava of mice using MPI.

The aim of this study is therefore to evaluate MPI's feasibility for detecting velocities that are present in coronary vessels in physiologic state (20 cm/s) and under hyperemia (40 cm/s) [6]. Based on a recently published experimental setup [7] we introduced a centrifugal pump and an ultrasound flow measurement device for providing steady state water flow [8]. In this study, we measured standardized SPION-boluses in straight glass tubes using MPI and compared different algorithms for velocity computation.

II. Material and Methods

Three glass tubes with an inner diameter of 4, 6 and 10 mm were used as coronary phantoms. They were connected via PVC tubes to a centrifugal pump (MEDOS Deltastream DP3, MEDOS Medizintechnik AG, Stolberg, Germany) to establish a closed water circuit. The respective flow rates were adjusted using an ultrasonic flow meter (BioProTT™ FlowTrack plus, em-tec GmbH, Finning, Germany) in order to obtain velocities inside the glass tube ranging from 0.2 to 0.65 m/s. 0.5 ml SPION-boluses (perimag®, micromod, Berlin, Germany) with an iron content of 25 mg/ml were injected at specific flow rates using a syringe pump (Perfusor fm, Braun®, Melsungen, Germany) and visualized by a preclinical MPI scanner (MPI PreClinical, Bruker, Ettlingen, Germany).

1 mm isotropic 3D MPI datasets with a temporal resolution of 20.8 ms were acquired using drive field amplitudes of (14,14,14) mT in (x,y,z)-direction. This led to a System matrix-FOV of 28x28x14 mm³. Images were reconstructed by using the Kaczmarz algorithm.

Circulation model velocities in the glass tube were calculated by adapting the measured flow rates of the flow meter to the inner diameter of the glass tubes. These velocities were defined as the gold standard.

The reconstructed images were analyzed with a dedicated python script. After the signal intensities of the whole field of view (FOV) were added up for every frame, a Butterworth filter was applied to reduce noise artifacts and, subsequently, the baseline was subtracted. Then, velocities were calculated using two different algorithms.

The first algorithm uses the full width at half maximum (FWHM), which is computed by the number of frames at which at least half of the maximum intensity is present. As the temporal resolution as well as the size of the FOV in flow direction is known, the velocity can be calculated.

The second algorithm refers to the thermodilution method [9]. It follows, that, in this case, the flow rate can be calculated by dividing a correction factor by the area under the signal intensity curve (AUC) at predetermined time points. We defined the AUC as being bounded by the beginning of the peak and the time point at which 33% of the maximum signal intensity is reached during the intensity drop after the peak. The correction factor is constant for measurements of a specific inner diameter and determined by calibrating to gold standard velocities. As the inner diameter is known, the velocity can be determined by using the calculated flow rates. Calculated velocity data sets were then compared to the gold standard using Pearson's correlation coefficient, which was computed for each size of glass tube for both methods.

III. Results

Every bolus injected was distinctly visible in the reconstructed images. The computed velocities using the FWHM and the tracer dilution method in comparison to the gold standard are shown in Fig. 1 for a glass tube with an inner diameter of 0.4 cm, exemplarily. Average Pearson's correlation coefficients for all sizes of glass tubes were r = 0.906 for the FWHM method and r = 0.88 for the tracer dilution method. This indicates good agreement to the gold standard for both methods.

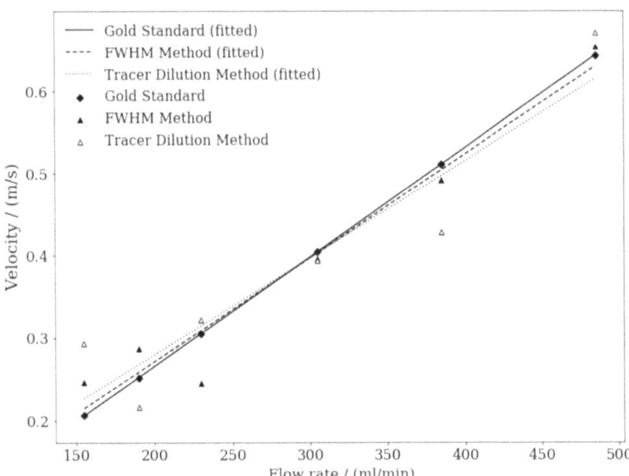

Figure 1: *The plot shows the computed velocities acquired by the FWHM method and the tracer dilution method in comparison to the gold standard data and their respective linear regression fits for the glass tube with an inner diameter of 0.4 cm.*

IV. Discussion

This study aims for quantification of coronary flow by measuring velocities using MPI. We were able to compute velocities from 0.2 m/s up to 0.65 m/s, which cover the ones relevant for coronary artery disease. This is a considerable advantage compared to other non-invasive imaging modalities including CT, MRI and ultrasound. For these, a reliable flow investigation is still not available, especially in patients with implanted stents.

Several studies in this area have already been done. Most of them focused on the visualization of perfusion rather than a characterization of the tracer flow itself. Concerning CVD diagnostics, the combination of both the visualization and the computation of flow parameters might be of great interest and allows to detect stenotic vessels in an early stage.

V. Conclusions

MPI has the ability to non-invasively detect pathologic hemodynamics in coronary blood vessels due to its high spatial and temporal resolution and without using radiation. A valid velocity computation under physiologic as well as pathologic conditions would greatly illustrate MPI's applicability in cardiovascular imaging. Therefore, further studies should address flow quantification including high flow rates in more complex geometries, i.e. stenoses.

ACKNOWLEDGEMENTS

We thank our colleagues from the department of "Physics of Molecular Imaging Systems" who provided knowledge and expertise that greatly assisted the research.

AUTHOR'S STATEMENT

Research funding: The author state no funding involved. Conflict of interest: Authors state no conflict of interest.

REFERENCES

[1] "Heart Disease and Stroke Statistics—2017 Update: A Report From The American Heart Association," p. 461.

[2] T. Kobayashi and J. W. Hirshfeld, "Radiation Exposure in Cardiac Catheterization: Operator Behavior Matters," *Circulation: Cardiovascular Interventions*, vol. 10, no. 8, Aug. 2017.

[3] B. Gleich and J. Weizenecker. Tomographic imaging using the nonlinear response of magnetic particles. *Nature*, 435(7046):1217-1217, 2005. doi: 10.1038/nature03808.

[4] Karthika, A. Kirubha, and Nilkantha, "Identification of stenosis in coronary arteries using velocity and wall shear stress analysis," in *2017 International conference of Electronics, Communication and Aerospace Technology (ICECA)*, Coimbatore, 2017, pp. 547–551.

[5] M. G. Kaul et al., "Magnetic particle imaging for *in vivo* blood flow velocity measurements in mice," *Physics in Medicine & Biology*, vol. 63, no. 6, p. 064001, Mar. 2018.

[6] H. V. Anderson, M. J. Stokes, M. Leon, S. A. Abu-Halawa, Y. Stuart, and R. L. Kirkeeide, "Coronary artery flow velocity is related to lumen area and regional left ventricular mass," *Circulation*, vol. 102, no. 1, pp. 48–54, Jul. 2000.

[7] R. Siepmann, H. Nilius, M. Straub, S. M. Ali Dadfar, M. Darguzyte, V. Schulz. Towards quantitative Flow Characterization of Fluids using Magnetic Particle Imaging. *International Workshop on Magnetic Particle Imaging (8th IWMPI) 2018.*

[8] P. Adedayo, S. Wang, A. R. Kunselman, and A. Ündar, "Impact of Pulsatile Flow Settings on Hemodynamic Energy Levels Using the Novel Diagonal Medos DP3 Pump in a Simulated Pediatric Extracorporeal Life Support System," *World Journal for Pediatric and Congenital Heart Surgery*, vol. 5, no. 3, pp. 440–448, Jul. 2014.

[9] J. Conway and P. Lund-Johansen, "Thermodilution method for measuring cardiac output," *European Heart Journal*, vol. 11, no. suppl I, pp. 17–20, Jan. 1990.

[10] X. Y. Zhou et al., "First *in vivo* magnetic particle imaging of lung perfusion in rats," *Physics in Medicine and Biology*, vol. 62, no. 9, pp. 3510–3522, May 2017.

Anatomical Rat Phantom for MPI

M. Exner[a,b*], **P. Szwargulski**[a,b*], **P. Ludewig**[c], **T. Knopp**[a,b] and **M. Graeser**[a,b]

[a] *Section for Biomedical Imaging, University Medical Center Eppendorf, Hamburg, Germany*
[b] *Institute for Biomedical Imaging, Technical University Hamburg, Hamburg, Germany*
[c] *Department of Neurology, University Medical Center Eppendorf, Hamburg, Germany*
[*] *Corresponding author, email: miriam.exner@tuhh.de ; p.szwargulski@uke.de*

Abstract: For medical research, a large number of animals are needed every year. The purpose of this work was to design a 3D CAD rat model which can be used to improve experiment planning and thus reduce the number of animals required. It was determined using an anatomy atlas and printed with stereolithography. The result is a model that contains the most important vessels and organs as hollow cavities. In a first MPI measurement, all organs filled with tracer of varying concentration were successfully imaged.

I. Introduction

Medical research requires the use of animals for toxicological studies, pharmaceutical tests, tests of new medical procedures and showing the improvement of imaging technologies within a real case scenario. The total amount of animals used is unknown but estimated to be above 115 million per year worldwide [1]. Animal studies are subject to strict regulations that significantly increase the effort and planning time of an experiment. Additionally, they should follow the 3R rules, replace, reduce, and refine [2]. In magnetic particle imaging (MPI), most technical improvements are tested using phantom geometries. However, these phantoms often lack the complex structure of the anatomy of living subjects, as these are hard to manufacture using subtractive manufacturing techniques. In this work, we present a model of the anatomy of a rat, which might be used for exact planning and design of imaging sequences. By filling its cavities with nanoparticle contrast agent, we evaluated the model using MPI. The model was created in computer-aided design (CAD) based on an anatomy atlas of rats [3] and fabricated with 3D printers. It contains all essential organs and vessels, which are hollow and can be filled with different kind of materials. Due to its anatomy-like structure, static images can be recorded in realistic scenarios and the suitability of an imaging procedure for the medical question can be better assessed. Due to the lack of a complete vascular system, dynamic experiments cannot be performed with the model in its current form. In addition, no physiological questions can be represented. Nevertheless, the number of animals required can be reduced, since an exact planning of the imaging sequence as well as

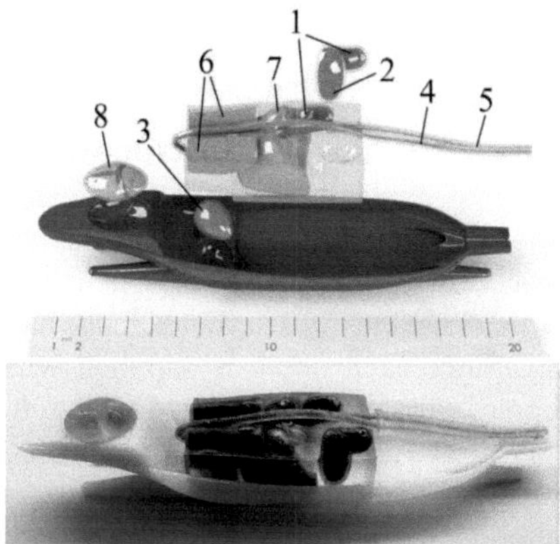

Figure 1: *CAD model and phantom filled with tracer.*

the position planning of the animal in the field of view (FOV) becomes possible. Besides the model itself, the first MPI images of the filled model are presented.

II. Material and Methods

II.I. Model Design

Based on an anatomy atlas containing sagittal, coronal and transverse cut sections of rats [3], an ordinary rat was modeled by measuring the dimensions and the shapes of the main organs and vessels. Furthermore, the shapes of some organs were modified based on MRI images of a mouse to better imitate the lying position of the rat during an experiment. The organs of the model are designed as hollow cavities with a wall thickness of 1 mm. Each organ can be filled individually, to emulate an organ specific perfusion.

Table 1: *Overview of the organs with their volumes, the contained blood volume and the tracer concentrations used for the measurement.*

	1	2	3	4	5	6	7	8
Organ or vessel	Kidney	Spleen	Heart	Aorta	Vena cava	Lungs	Liver	Brain
Organ volume [mm³]	495	318	1488	200	590	3620	14449	1575
Blood volume [mm³] [4]	450	140	490	-	-	660	1660	41
Tracer concentration [µg(Fe) ml⁻¹]	2430	1215	810	810	810	486	270	74

With the printers that were used, it is challenging to fabricate vessels with an inner diameter smaller than 1 mm. For this reason, the caudal parts of the aorta and the vena cava had to be extended. Nevertheless, the model mostly reflects the anatomical data in size and relative position. The entire model measures 203.5 mm × 45 mm × 36 mm and represents an 8-week-old rat of about 200 g. The volumes of the individual organs are listed in Table 1. The CAD model and the printed model filled with tracer are shown in Figure 1. To facilitate the post-processing of the printing procedure, the model was split into several parts. The model was fabricated using the stereolithography printer Form 2 (Formlabs Ltd.), which features a laser spot size of 140 μm and a layer height between 25 and 100 μm. As printing material the non-magnetic Clear resin V4 (Formlabs Ltd.) was used. The model was impregnated with Nano-Seal (JELN GmbH) to prevent the absorption of water. The organs and vessels were filled with perimag (micromod, Rostock, prod. code: 102-00-132, plain surface) at different concentrations (see Table 1). The support skin of the model has the shape of the lower half of the rat's body and guarantees a reproducible positioning of the organs.

II.II. Measurement and Reconstruction

When a tracer is injected into a rat, it is distributed differently throughout the body over time. After the tracer has spread, it accumulates in certain organs [5,6]. We assumed a state in which the particles are evenly distributed in the blood without accumulation. Since each organ is supplied with blood to different degrees, the concentrations of the tracer were determined from the ratio of the blood volume contained in the respective organ to the entire organ volume (see Table 1). The concentration of the heart was also assumed for the vessels. Since these are completely filled with blood in the living animal, a higher concentration should have been used. The measurements were performed using a 3D field free point preclinical MPI scanner (Bruker, Ettlingen). For imaging, an excitation field amplitude of 12 mT in all three directions was applied. Further, a selection field with a gradient strength of $G = \mathrm{diag}(-0.6, -0.6, 1.2)$ Tm^{-1} was used. The resulting FOV was $40 \times 40 \times 20$ mm^3. To cover the entire phantom, we moved it along the x- and z-directions insight the scanner bore. We cover a region of interest (ROI) of $220 \times 40 \times 40$ mm^3 moving the phantom to 21 positions ($7 \times 1 \times 3$). With this approach, we could neglect issues connected to the usage of focus fields like field imperfections. Due to contrast limitations of the reconstruction, the large ratio of the highest to the lowest concentration cannot be reconstructed within one image. To separate the brain and vessels from the kidneys, we divided the reconstruction into three parts along the longitudinal axis of the rat. The first 6, the middle 9 and the last 6 patches were combined and reconstructed jointly [7].

III. Results

Figure 2 presents the reconstruction results as a maximum intensity projection in coronal and sagittal view. The images were normalized to the respective maximum intensity. The

signal values below 10 %, 5 % and 25 % of the signal maximum of the respective part were set to 0. By separating the reconstruction, all organs and vessels could be visualized.

IV. Discussion and Conclusion

The phantom is based on an anatomy atlas and reflects the anatomy of the selected organs and vessels. It can be used to evaluate medical procedures, plan and train experiments and animal handling before *in vivo* experiments and to compare *in vivo* images to phantom images of the same structure. The burden for animal studies can be reduced by using the model to determine the position of the rat and its organs in the FOV prior to an *in vivo* experiment. In addition, experimental procedures, sequences and algorithms can be tested in a realistic setup without the regulatory overhead that is necessary for animal studies. Dynamic experiments and physiological processes cannot be simulated in the current form of the model. The model was evaluated using MPI but could also be used for other imaging modalities.

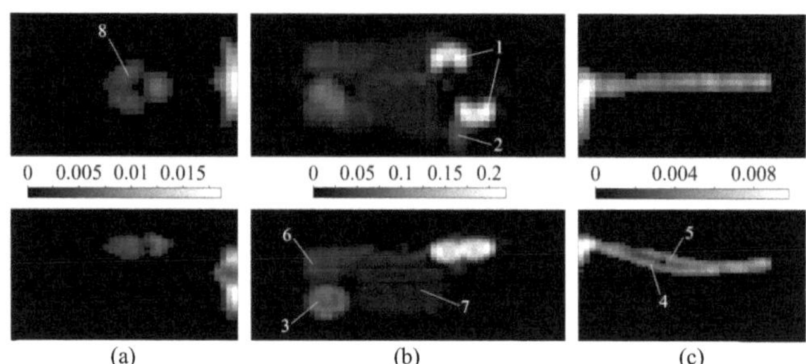

Figure 2: *Reconstruction results in coronal (top) and sagittal (bottom) view. The head region (a), the thoracic and abdominal region (b) and the vessels (c) are shown.*

We demonstrated an anatomical model of a rat that was 3D printed. The phantom has proven to enhance the experiment planning in advance to *in vivo* imaging. Due to the anatomy-like structure, many experiments in rodents can be evaluated in the phantom instead of a living animal. For the future, the model could be extended by a complete vascular system to perform dynamic experiments.

ACKNOWLEDGEMENTS
We thank Dr. Thomas Friedrich, Institute of Medical Engineering (Lübeck), who supported us in the printing process.

AUTHOR'S STATEMENT
Research funding: The authors thankfully acknowledge the financial support by the DFG (grant number KN 1108/2-1) and the BMBF (grant number 05M16GKA).

REFERENCES
[1] K. Taylor et al. *Altern. Lab. Anim.*, 36(3):327-342, 2008.
[2] W. M. S. Russell and R. L. Burch. *The Principles of Humane Experimental Technique*. Methuen, London, 1959.
[3] T. Hayakawa and T. Iwaki. *A Color Atlas of Sectional Anatomy of the Rat*. Adosuri, Tokyo, 2008.
[4] K. Oeff and A. König. *Naunyn Schmiedebergs Arch.*, 1955. doi: 10.1007/BF00246232.
[5] J. Weizenecker et al. *Phys. Med. Biol.*, 2009. doi: 10.1088/0031-9155/54/5/L01.
[6] A. P. Khandhar et al. *Nanoscale*, 2017. doi: 10.1039/c6nr08468k.
[7] P. Szwargulski et al. *IEEE Trans. Med. Imaging*, 2018. doi: 10.1109/TMI.2018.2875829.

Imaging full body biodistribution and signal properties of magnetic nanoflowers.

J.M. Gaudet[a,b*], R. Orendorff[a*], C. Grüttner[c], Y. Zhang[b], M. Wintermark[b], H. Teller[c], P.W. Goodwill[a]

[a] *Magnetic Insight, Alameda, CA, USA*
[b] *Department of Radiology, Stanford, CA, USA*
[c] *micromod Partikeltechnologie GmbH, Rostock, Germany*
[*] *Corresponding author, email: jgaudet@stanford.edu*

Abstract: The imaging performance and utility of Magnetic Particle Imaging (MPI)_is driven by the properties of the magnetic nanoparticle tracer. Some of these properties include the nanoparticle iron oxide core size, crystal structure, and coating. In this study, we investigated the signal properties, blood half-life, and in vivo biodistribution of a novel SPIO „nanoflower" nanoparticle with two different coatings.

I. Introduction

To date, the majority of Magnetic Particle Imaging (MPI) research has been performed with a specific magnetic tracer, ferucarbotran. This is due to a combination of its MPI signal, commercial availability, and clinical status. Also known by the brand name Resovist; ferucarbotran is comprised of multi-core iron oxide nanoparticles with a broad size distribution. Only a small percentage of the nanoparticles are believed to contribute to the resulting MPI signal.[1] Further, ferucarbotran was designed to rapidly accumulate in the Kupffer cells of the liver and performs poorly in situations that benefit from a long-circulating blood pool agent such as functional imaging or cancer imaging.[1]

Recently, magnetic "nanoflower"-shaped iron oxide cores have been of increased interest for application to MPI and Magnetic Hyperthermia Therapy (MHT).[2-4] These nanoflowers contain densely packed iron oxide cores with a larger average particle diameter when compared with ferucarbotran. In this study we compared the MPI signal properties and *in vivo* biodistribution of a commercial iron oxide nanoflower nanoparticle with two different surface coatings.

II. Material and Methods

II.I. *In vitro* characterization

Plain dextran coated and polyethylene glycol (PEG) coated synomag®-D nanoparticles (micromod Partikeltechnologie GmbH, Germany) were evaluated. Phantoms were prepared by diluting stock suspensions with deionized water over a 1-100% range. At each concentration a point source (1 µL) phantom was imaged and the signal measured. Particle stability was also measured under conditions with particles stored at room temperature, at 4°C, and at -20°C.

II.II. *in vivo* imaging

For *in vivo* blood half-life measurements, C57Bl/6 mice were injected in a tail vein with 50 µL diluted tracer (5.5 mg/mL). Two cohorts (n=2) were evaluated comparing the dextran coated and PEG nanoparticles. Projection imaging was performed serially every 4 minutes for 2 hours after which a tomographic image was acquired prior to animal sacrifice. Following MPI, an x-ray computed tomography (CT) (GE Healthcare, Madison, WI, USA) image was acquired for anatomical context. An additional synomag®-D + PEG cohort (n=2) was imaged at 1, 2, 4, 8, 12 and 24 hours after injection.

II.III. MPI imaging and image analysis

Imaging was performed at Stanford University with the MOMENTUM MPI system (Magnetic Insight Inc., CA, USA). The imager produces a 6 T/m x 6 T/m Field Free Line selection field, excites with a 45 kHz drive field, and uses x-space MPI reconstruction.[5] Projection images were acquired (FOV: 12 cm x 6 cm, 4 minute total acquisition and reconstruction time), as well as tomographic images (FOV: 12 cm x 6 cm x 6 cm, 45 minute total acquisition and reconstruction time).

In vitro images were analyzed to measure signal and resolution. A linear regression model from the peak MPI signal at each concentration was used to assess the peak MPI signal per µg of Fe. Full-width at half-maximum resolution was measured using the 1 µL point source. *In vivo* images were analyzed to estimate blood half-life. Blood concentration was measured by placing a region of interest over the heart. All analysis was performed using VivoQuant software (inviCRO, MA, USA).

III. Results

III.I. *In vitro* results

The synomag®-D particles produced ~3.5x more signal per mass of Fe than ferucarbotran with a measured resolution of 900μm (6 T/m selection field gradient). As expected, the synomag®-D nanoparticles demonstrated a linear signal relationship with iron concentration, $R^2 > 0.98$. Storage conditions outside the recommended 4°C was found to influence the particles behavior, with room temperature storage and freezing decreasing the signal by 19% and 23% respectively. No significant differences were observed in the peak signal amplitude and resolution between the plain dextran coated and PEG coated synomag®-D particles.

III.II. *In vivo* results

As expected, following intravenous tail vein injection, dextran-coated synomag®-D particles were rapidly taken up by the liver and spleen ($t_{1/2} < 4$ minutes, see Fig 1B). Surprisingly, low concentrations of iron oxide were also observed in the cranial vasculature after 1 hour. In contrast, the PEG-coated synomag®-D particles were retained within the blood pool for a longer period of time (Fig 1C). After 90 minutes, nanoparticles were observed in the cranial vasculature, pulmonary vasculature, bone marrow, and liver. Measurement of the blood pool signal decreased over the first 45 minutes before stabilizing for the remaining 105 minutes. All animals recovered from injection, imaging, and anesthesia without issue.

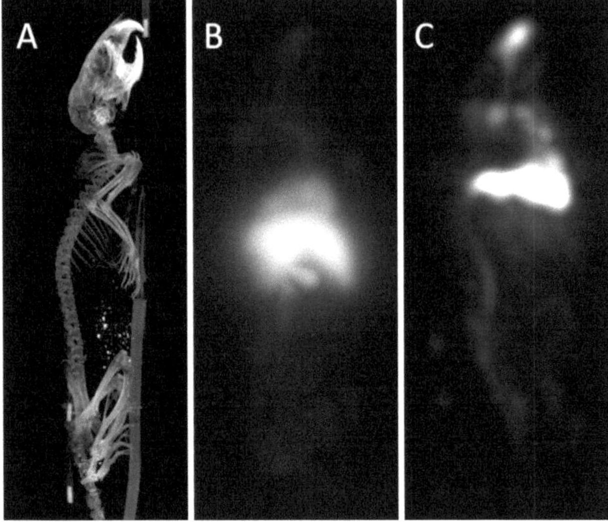

Figure 1: *Sagittal maximum intensity projections showing whole body nanoparticle biodistribution 1 hour after injection. All MPI images have identical windowing and leveling. (A) X-ray CT of representative animal for anatomical context. (B) In < 10 minutes, plain dextran-coated synomag®-D is taken up by the liver and spleen. Small tracer concentrations remain detectable in the lungs and cranial vasculature. (C) In contrast, after 90 minutes synomag®-D+PEG remains detectable in the blood.*

IV. Discussion

This study demonstrates how MPI visualizes nanoparticle biodistribution from different nanoparticle coatings. These coats were shown to influence the physiological behavior without changing the magnetic behavior. The dextran coated nanoparticle (synomag®-D) was rapidly cleared by the liver and spleen, while synomag®-D + PEG nanoparticle remained stable in blood after 45 minutes. We believe that the blood pool signal stabilized after 45 minutes due to saturation of the liver at the injected dosage. Surprisingly, the blood pool signal did not continue to decrease as rapidly, which we believe is the result of saturating the Kupffer cells in the liver. Consequently, we were not able to accurately estimate a blood half-life. In the future work we will inject smaller doses and analyze over a longer time period (24 hours) to determine the blood half-life.

V. Conclusions

Development and assessment of novel SPIO nanoparticles remains an important area of research for the field of MPI. As shown here, synomag®-D particles, with and without PEG coatings, are promising tracers for MPI. By changing the coating, it is possible to both have short and long tracer blood half-life, in addition to changing how the tracer loads cells. Importantly, the change of coating does not change the magnetic behavior of the tracer. We believe that these tracers are ideal for measurements of tissue perfusion, functional tracking, and *in situ* inflammation detection. Ultimately, clinical translation of MPI will depend on the biocompatibility, safety, sensitivity, and batch consistency of SPIO tracers.

AUTHOR'S STATEMENT

Research funding: Research reported in this publication was supported by NIBIB of the NIH under award number R43EB020463. The content is solely the responsibility of the authors and does not necessarily represent the official views of the NIH. Conflict of interest: Authors state the following conflict of interests: JMG, RO, PWG are employees of Magnetic Insight with equity interest. CG and HT are employees of micromod Partikeltechnologie GmbH. Informed consent: Informed consent has been obtained from all individuals included in this study. Ethical approval: The research related to animal use complies with all the relevant regulations and institutional policies and has been approved by the authors' institutional review board.

REFERENCES

[1] Keselman et al. Tracking short-term biodistribution and long-term clearance of SPIO tracers in magnetic particle imaging. *Phys. Med. Biol* 62:3440-3453. 2017. Doi:10.1088/1361-6560/aa5f48

[2] Gavilan et al. Colloidal flower-shaped iron oxide nanoparticles: synthesis strategies and coats. *Part. Part. Syst. Charact.,* 34:1700094. 2017 doi: 10.1002/ppsc.201700094

[3] P. Bender et al. Relating magnetic properties and hyperthermia performance of iron oxide nanoflowers. *J. Phys. Chem.* 122:3068-3077. 2018. Doi: 10.1021/acs.jpcc.7b11255

[4] Kratz et al. Novel magnetic multicore nanoparticles designed for MPI and other biomedical applications: From synthesis to first in vivo studies. *PLOS ONE* 2018 doi: 10.1371/journal.pone.0190214

[5] Goodwill PW, Konkle JJ, Zheng B, Saritas EU, Conolly SM. Projection X-space magnetic particle imaging. *IEEE Trans Med Imaging.* 2012;31(5):1076-1085. doi:10.1109/TMI.2012.2185247.

Magnetically initiated remote controlled drug release from magnetic microspheres

D. Zahn[a], A. Weidner[a], Z. Nosrati[b], K. Saatchi[b], U.O. Häfeli[b], and S. Dutz[a]*

[a] *Institut für Biomedizinische Technik und Informatik, Technische Universität Ilmenau, Germany*
[b] *Faculty of Pharmaceutical Sciences, University of British Columbia, Vancouver, Canada*
* *Corresponding author, email: silvio.dutz@tu-ilmenau.de*

Abstract: In the here presented study, poly(lactic-co-glycolic) acid (PLGA) microspheres for drug delivery were prepared. Magnetic nanoparticles with high magnetic heating performance and the drug camptothecin were embedded into the PLGA matrix, enabling a magnetic targeting of the microspheres and magnetic hyperthermia to induce remote controlled drug release. Resulting microspheres were characterized by means of dynamic light scattering, scanning electron microscopy, magnetometry, magnetic calorimetry, and UV/Vis spectrophotometry for determination of the drug release as a function of time and temperature. The principle of magnetically triggered drug release is demonstrated by magnetic hyperthermia induced release of a drug from the magnetic microspheres.

I. Introduction

Magnetic microspheres (MMS) are essential for magnetic drug targeting and typically consist of a polymeric matrix material loaded with magnetic nanoparticles (MNP) and a drug [1]. MMS can be magnetically guided to a target area where the drug is released either by degradation of the matrix or diffusion. Both release mechanisms can be accelerated by increasing the temperature of the MMS [2]. The needed temperature increase can be achieved by magnetic hyperthermia due to resulting magnetization reversal losses when an alternating magnetic field is applied to the MMS [3]. In order to guarantee optimal magnetic targeting and defined drug release, MMS with uniform and controllable particle sizes, high specific heating rate and known degradation and release kinetics are necessary. To investigate the aspects listed above, poly(lactide-co-glycolide) microspheres (PLGA MS), loaded with the drug camptothecin and magnetic nanoparticles, were prepared and characterized concerning degradation behavior, drug release kinetics, and magnetic properties.

II. Material and Methods

Drug loaded MMS were prepared by an oil/water (o/w) emulsion evaporation method. For that, PLGA, the anti cancer drug camptothecin, and biocompatible bisphosphonate coated MNP prepared as described before [4] were dissolved/ suspended in an organic solvent (o-phase) and emulsified by using a mechanical homogenizer in an aqueous PVA solution (w-phase). The obtained micro droplets were allowed to harden by evaporation of the solvent and collected using centrifugation or magnetic separation. Homogenization velocity was altered and its impact on the MS size was measured via dynamic light scattering (DLS) and scanning electron microscopy (SEM) investigation. Degradation behavior of pure PLGA MS was studied using three types of PLGA with different monomer contents (L/G ratio: 50/50, 65/35, and 75/25) at 20 and 37 °C for 12 weeks. Drug release kinetics of camptothecin was investigated for the same three PLGA types at 20, 37 and 43 °C in water bath to evaluate the influence of different temperatures. Therefore, MS were suspended in phosphate buffered saline and remaining drug concentration in the MS was determined at defined intervals. From these values the released amount of drug was calculated. Drug concentrations were measured by UV/VIS spectroscopy using a standard calibration curve for camptothecin. MMS containing magnetic nanoparticles where investigated by vibrating sample magnetometry (VSM), specific absorption rate (SAR) measurements, and SEM. In a final experiment the magnetically induced drug release is demonstrated. For this, drug loaded MMS were exposed to an alternating magnetic field (f = 410 kHz / H = 24 kA/m) resulting in a temperature increase of the MMS. By tuning the magnetic field amplitude, the temperature of the MMS was kept at 44 °C for one hour. The obtained drug release is compared to the release from MMS stored at 37°C (body temperature) for the same time interval.

III. Results

MMS with perfect spherical shape and tunable mean diameters between 1 and 2 μm were prepared, with an inversely proportional correlation between homogenization velocity and diameter (Figure 1). From scanning electron microscopy images it becomes obvious that, MNP are mainly located at the MMS surface.

Degradation experiments showed significant decomposition of the MS after 5 to 7 weeks at 37 °C, with proportional correlation between glycolide content and degradation velocity. Camptothecin was loaded into the MS with concentrations up to 0.5 wt% (1 wt% intended) and was released in a burst type release profile at 37 and 43 °C within few hours. The release rates increased with increasing temperature (Figure 2).

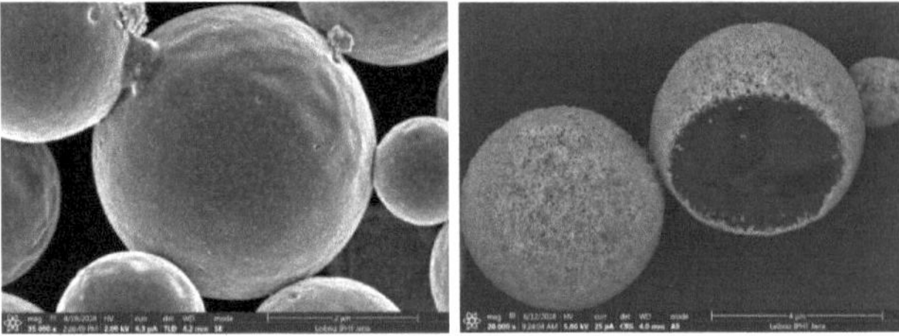

Figure 1: *SEM images of MMS (left) and a cross-section of the MMS (right) prepared by means of a focused ion beam (FIB).*

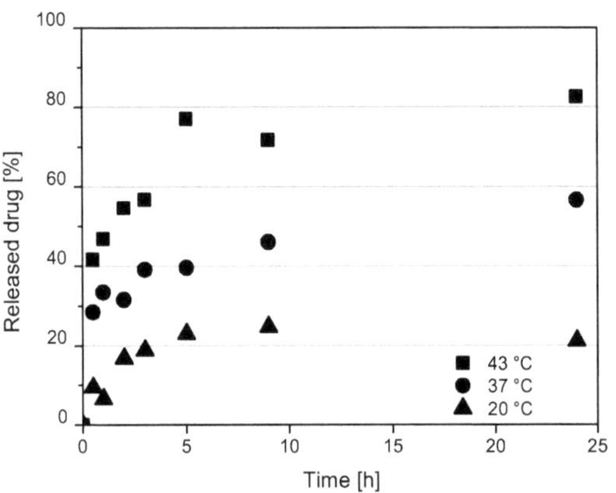

Figure 2: *Drug release profiles for different temperatures confirm the possibility to control the drug release by changing the temperature of the MMS; L/G ratio of PLGA = 65/35.*

During drug release studies no significant differences between the different PLGA types in drug release were measured, which suggests a mainly diffusion-controlled drug release, in which the degradation behavior of the PLGA has only weak influence.

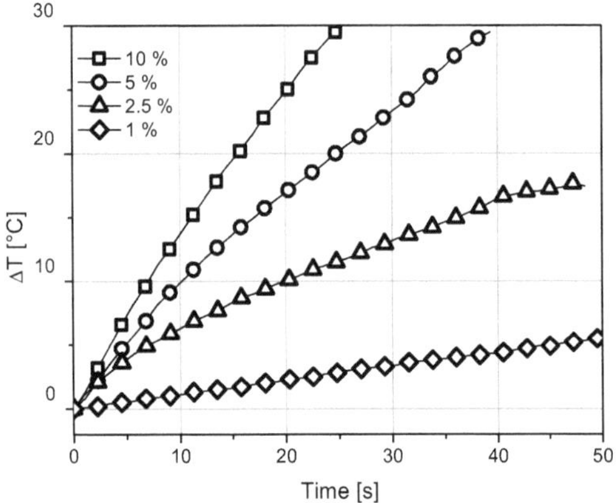

Figure 3: *Total temperature increase during hyperthermia experiments on samples with different MMS concentrations. For a concentration of about 2.5 wt%, which is a realistic value for in-vivo experiments, an increase of about 10 °C is obtained within 20 s.*

Magnetic microspheres show MNP concentrations of about 16 wt% (16 wt% intended) with a saturation magnetization of 12 Am^2/kg, a coercivity of 0.55 kA/m, and a specific heating power of 171 W/g(MMS), suitable for magnetic heating for enforced drug release from the PLGA at a MMS in tissue concentration of 2.5 % by mass (Figure 3).

In the magnetically induced drug release experiments it was found, that magnetic hyperthermia of MMS with temperatures of 44 °C for one hour leads to an increased drug release of about 50% compared to the same particles stored for one hour at 37 °C. This result opens the door for contactless remote controlled drug release initiated by alternating magnetic fields.

IV. Conclusions

Drug loaded magnetic microspheres were prepared by the o/w emulsion evaporation method, whereby the introduction of the drug camptothecin and magnetic nanoparticles did not hinder the generation of spherical shaped particles. Increasing drug release with increasing temperature confirms the approach of loading MNP into the MS to control the drug release by means of magnetic heating. The principle of magnetically triggered drug release is demonstrated by magnetic hyperthermia induced release of a drug from the magnetic microspheres. In ongoing studies, the drug concentrations have to be increased, attempts to distribute MNP more homogenously in the MS will be made and the MPI performance of the MMS will be tested.

ACKNOWLEDGEMENTS

This work was supported by German Academic Exchange Service (DAAD) in the frame of an Alumni Project of Research Mobility (PPP).

AUTHOR'S STATEMENT

Research funding: The author state no funding involved. Conflict of interest: Authors state no conflict of interest. Informed consent: Informed consent has been obtained from all individuals included in this study. Ethical approval: The research related to human use complies with all the relevant national regulations, institutional policies and was performed in accordance with the tenets of the Helsinki Declaration, and has been approved by the authors' institutional review board or equivalent committee.

REFERENCES

[1] Fang, Kun et al. (**2015**): Magnetic field activated drug release system based on magnetic PLGA microspheres for chemo-thermal therapy. Colloids and surfaces. *B, Biointerfaces* 136: 712–720.

[2] Xu, Yihan et al. (**2017**): Polymer degradation and drug delivery in PLGA-based drug–polymer applications. A review of experiments and theories. *Journal of Biomedical Materials Research Part B: Applied Biomaterials* 105/6: 1692–1716.

[3] Dutz, Silvio and Hergt, Rudolf (**2014**): Magnetic Particle Hyperthermia – A promising tumour therapy? *Nanotechnology* 25: 452001.

[4] Dutz, Silvio et al. (**2009**): Ferrofluids of magnetic multicore nanoparticles for biomedical applications. *J. Magn. Magn. Mater.* 321/10: 1501–1504.

Mechanical Design of a Human-Scale Magnetic Particle Imager for Functional Brain Imaging (fMPI)

E. Mattingly [a], E. E. Mason [a,b], C. Z. Cooley [a,c], and L. L. Wald[a,c]

[a] MGH/HST A.A. Martinos Center for Biomedical Imaging, Dept. of Radiology, Massachusetts General Hospital, Boston, MA, USA
[b] Harvard-MIT Health Sciences & Technology, Cambridge, MA, USA
[c] Harvard Medical School, Boston, MA, USA
[*] Corresponding author, email: _EliMattingly22@gmail.com_

Abstract: MPI has the capability for sensitive tracer detection and has detected functional changes in rodent brain hemodynamics but has been limited to pre-clinical platforms. We are extending fMPI to a human-scale FFL based functional brain imaging device and consider here the mechanics required for a mechanically rotating human brain FFL system. Our design employs physically rotating the FFL magnets (~1.5T/m, 500 kg) at 20-30 RPM continuously to form a time-series of functional brain images. Here we present the design process and structural, mechanical, and dynamic considerations along with a preliminary design for the human brain MPI system.

I. Introduction

Magnetic Particle Imaging (MPI), a tracer-based imaging modality first described in 2005 [1], is based on the non-linear response of super paramagnetic iron-oxide nanoparticles (SPIOs) to external oscillating fields. Due to the strong magnetic moment of the SPIOs, and non-existent background signal present in the body, and the fact that SPIO concentration in the brain directly reflects Cerebral Blood Volume (CBV), MPI is a promising modality for functional brain imaging. A pre-clinical trial showed that MPI can detect functional changes in rodent CBV during hypo/hypercapnic modulation [2].

Only a few attempts have been made at scaling up MPI technology for human use. Recently, a design for a clinical scale brain imager has been built for diagnostics of trauma or intracranial hemorrhage in intensive care units [3]. The design used a relative weak FFL gradient, which would likely render the images less useful for neuro-scientific studies. Additionally, fMPI studies will also require a continuously rotating gantry for time-series imaging. Our proposed human brain fMPI device will use an FFL-based MPI system as seen is Figure 1A. The device uses mechanical rotation to simplify electromagnet design and power considerations.

II. Material and Methods

II.I. Design Software

AutoDesk Inventor (AutoDesk, San Rafael, CA) was used for the overall design and finite element analysis of structural components. COMSOL (COMSOL, Inc., Burlington, MA) was utilized for the electromagnetic simulations which provided force estimates between the magnets.

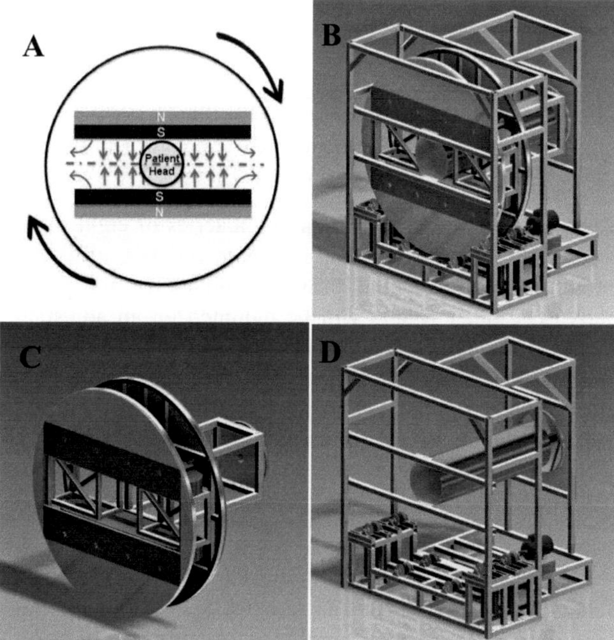

Figure 1. A. Illustration of the functional operation of our design. **B.** Digital rendering of the full assembly. **C.** Rotating "gantry". **D.** Stationary components.

II.II. Mechanical Requirements and Constraints

The rotating structure must support both the mass of the electromagnets (~500 kg for each magnet assembly) as well as the repulsion of the FFL magnets(~5kN) and centripetal forces(~2kN). The base must support the net weight of all gantry elements (~1550 kg). Due to the nature of the design, the physical separation of the FFL magnets determines the gradient strength, and therefore the image resolution and thus we include the capability to move the poles closer when imaging non-human primates. We provide for supporting the magnets at two locations, one with 42cm separation, another with 25cm separation, due to the constraints of the head and internal Tx/Rx hardware. The mass of the gantry was minimized within the constraints of patient safety to reduce motor and braking load as well as reducing weight on the base. The structure is designed to rotate at 20-30 RPM to enable fast time-series imaging (physiological changes in the brain occur on a 3-6 second timeframe) while avoiding PNS and retinal stimulation [4].

III. Results

Figures 1 and 2 show the current state of the design. The device has three sections: 1) the rotating mass, 2) the stationary support for the rotating structure, and 3) a stationary bore tube and patient table, which are mechanically decoupled from the other structures. The rotating component (Fig. 1.C) is supported on rollers on the front and a large bearing in the rear (to handle the thrust-load) and is driven by a large circumferential gear (Fig. 2.A). The gear will be constructed from small brass gear segments to allow for economic manufacturing. The gantry material is welded aluminum, square cross section hollow tubing. This is non-magnetic, sufficiently strong, practical and economical to construct, and satisfies the goal of reducing gantry weight. The outer "rolling" surface of the gantry will be constructed from two precision rolled semi-circles welded together to form a full circle.

This gantry is designed to rotate on a series of eight rollers (Fig. 2C), four on each side. The extra rollers both lighten the individual loads and provide redundancy for patient safety. The outer rollers will be mounted on an adjustable assembly to tune the load sharing ratio of the rollers based on pre-positioned strain gages. To ensure patient safety a series of external shoe brakes which can be remotely actuated is included in the design. Given the moment of inertia of the system is ~500 kg*m^2 and a rotation of 25 RPM the brakes will need to absorb 1.3kJ during stopping.

Each FFL magnet will be attached to the frame by a series of eight 20mm stainless steel bolts. Given a maximum load of 11kN the bolts will have a safety factor of >50 under pure static shear—this is based on the conservative estimate of a 550 MPa for the yield strength of stainless steel. Due to the sensitive nature of the receive chain and the inevitable mechanical vibrations present in the physically rotating system, the non-rotating and rotating components should be mechanically decoupled. This is complicated by the

oscillating moment acting on the drive coil within the homogeneous selection field (which translates the FFL during each projection). Given a drive coil field of 12mTμ_0^{-1} and a selection coil field of 150mT, there will be a 65 Nm moment induced at the drive frequency. The moment induced in the drive coil assembly is mitigated by strongly affixing the drive and receive coil either with epoxy or non-conductive hardware negating relative motion. Additionally, the Tx/Rx hardware will be firmly attached to the copper wrapped fiberglass tube whose rigidity is ensured due to the high moment of inertia and stiffness of the fiberglass tube.

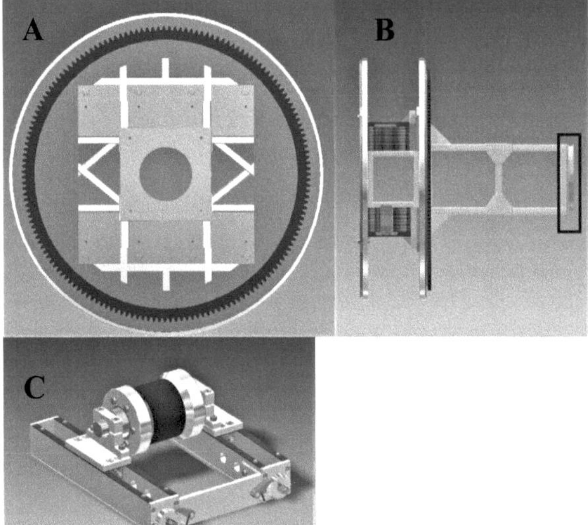

Figure 2. Digital renderings of: **A.** The gantry with the circumferential gear, **B.** Side view of the gantry with the bearing location noted by a rectangular outline, and **C.** roller-location adjustment mechanism.

IV. Discussion

We present a design for a clinical scale MPI system as well as the potential problems associated with the increase of scale such as profoundly greater weight and inertia of the system, and difficulties associated with variable positioning of the FFL magnets. We also discuss design features included to mitigate the consequence of these challenges. Further work includes fatigue and vibrations analysis as well as the construction of the assembly.

Acknowledgements

Thank you to Simon Sigalovsky and Sean Bradley for their work in the construction of preliminary models.

AUTHOR'S STATEMENT
Research funding: The project was funded by National Institutes of Health grant: U01EB025121. Conflict of interest: Authors state no conflict of interest.

REFERENCES
[1] B. Gleich and J. Weizenecker,*Nature*, vol. 435, no. 7046, pp. 1214–7, Jun. 2005.
[2] C. Z. Cooley, et al, *Neuroimage*, vol. 178, pp. 713–720, Sept. 2018.
[3] M. Graeser, et al. "Human-sized Magnetic Particle Imaging for Brain Applications" In Press
[4] E. Mason, et al. *Int J Mag Part Imag,* vol. 3, no. 1, 2017

Evaluation of FFP Performance in Halbach and Radial Permanent Magnet Systems

F. Balcı[a], N. Dogan[b], and A. Bingolbali[a],*

[a] *Department of Bioengineering, Yıldız Technical University, Istanbul, Turkey*
[b] *Department of Physics, Gebze Technical University, Kocaeli, Turkey*
* *Corresponding author, email: ab1353@gmail.com*

I. Introduction

MPI technique has the potential to solve the fundamental problems of medical imaging (e.g., low resolution, long acquisition time, insufficient sensitivity in the diagnosis and relatively high cost). One of the most important principles of MPI theory is the formation of Field Free Point (FFP). The FFP is a small, but the main region in spatial coding in MPI theory [1,2]. In this study, the FFP was generated by using permanent magnets. A permanent magnet system designed with cylindrical shape was used to investigate the FFP performance. High magnetic field strength and uniform gradient are required for the FFP performance. There are several factors that affect the performance of FFP designed with cylindrical permanent magnet system, such as fill factor [3], length and system radius [4], residual induction (B_r) [5], and Halbach and Radial magnetization patterns [3]. In this particular investigation, the effects of residual induction will be discussed with respect to the two different magnetization patterns (Halbach and Radial).

II. Material and Methods

The magnets were designed to be a quadrupole cylinder system. Comsol Multiphysics 5.3a software program [6] was used to simulate Halbach and Radial magnetization patterns (Fig. 1) so to determine their contributions on the FFP point in terms of magnetic flux density and gradient.

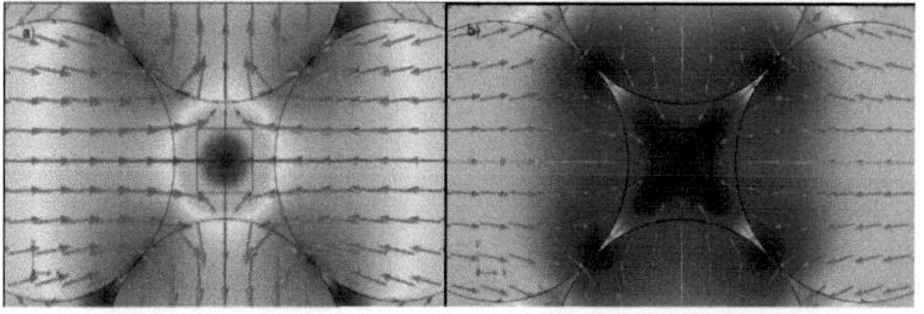

Figure 1: *Two different magnetization patterns were considered in this study: a) Halbach magnetization pattern (selection field shown as vector plots in the x-direction are inward while the vectors in the y-direction are outward), b) Radial magnetization pattern (the selection field vectors are inward in all directions).*

Since NdFeB permanent magnets were considered in the simulation, B_r = 1.05 T for 28UH, B_r = 1.2 T for N35, and B_r = 1.4 T for N48 were taken as the values of residual induction [7].

Each magnet had the same length and diameter. Both values were fixed as 30 cm. The study was performed on both x and z coordinates from -5 cm to 5 cm. Fig. 2 displays the design of the quadrupole magnet system.

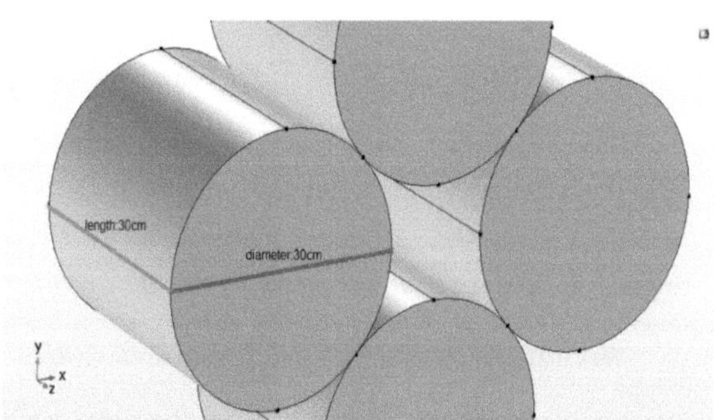

Figure 2: *Design of the quadrupole cylinder magnet system to generate the FFP in 3D. Each magnet length and diameter were equal and 30 cm.*

III. Results and Discussion

Fig. 3 and Fig. 4 show the simulation results by using the B_r values listed above for Halbach and Radial magnetization patterns to obtain magnetic flux (Fig. 3) and gradient (Fig. 4), respectively. Change in the magnetic flux density in the x-axis was 0.16 T at x = ±5 cm once taking the Br values into account for Halbach magnetization pattern (Fig. 3(a)) while it was 0.04 T for Radial magnetization pattern. On the other hand, change in the magnetic flux density in the z-axis was too small (6×10^{-8} T) for Halbach magnetization pattern as shown in Fig. 3(b) while it was 0.047 T at z = ±5 cm for Radial magnetization pattern. Yet, Fig. 5(b) shows that there is negligible magnetic flux density in the z-axis in Halbach. Change in the gradient in the x-axis was 3.24 T/cm (ΔG_x = 3.24 T/cm) once taking the B_r values into account for

Halbach magnetization pattern, as shown in Fig. 4(a), while $\Delta G_x = 0.45$ T/cm in the radial case. Moreover, change in the gradient in the z-axis was zero ($\Delta G_z = 0$) when taking the B_r values into account for Halbach magnetization pattern as shown in Fig. 4(b), while $\Delta G_z = 0.9$ T/cm in Radial magnetization pattern. So, changing B_r factor was more effective in Halbach in the x-axis. Unlike that case, changing B_r factor didn't affect it due to negligible magnetic flux density in the z-axis in Halbach shown Fig. 5(b). Also, the gradients obtained from Halbach magnetization pattern were more stable compared to the radial case as shown in Fig. (4). Yet, G_x in Halbach was stronger than G_x in the radial magnetization pattern at the same B_r value (Fig. 4(a)) whereas $G_z = 0$ in Halbach, but not in Radial (Fig. 4(b)). The FFP performance increased linearly with increasing of B_r value, as expected.

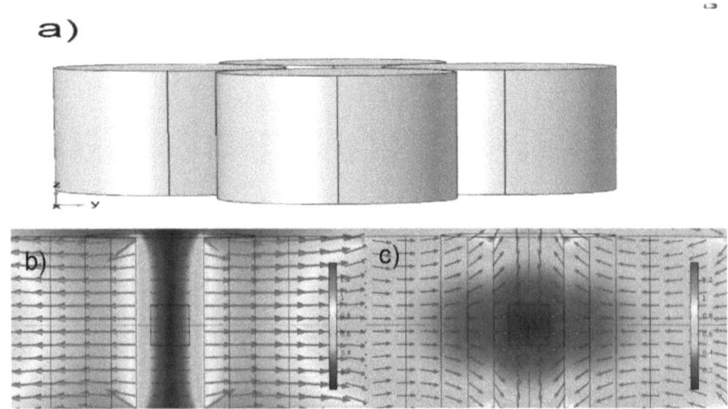

Figure 5: *a) Demonstration of quadruple cylinder system in 3D, b) Halbach, c) Radial.*

IV. Conclusions

The outcomes of this short study can be listed as follows: (1) the gradient in the z-axis was observed more stable than in the x-axis in Radial magnetization pattern, (2) the gradient in the x-axis was observed higher than in the z-axis in Halbach magnetization pattern, (3) Halbach system is superior to Radial system according to the magnetic flux density and gradient results in the x-axis, (4) both magnetic flux density and gradient were more dominant in the Radial system in the z-axis, (5) both magnetic flux density and gradient were negligible and zero, respectively, in Halbach system in the z-axis.

ACKNOWLEDGMENTS

The present work was supported by the TUBITAK (Project number:115E776 & 115E777).

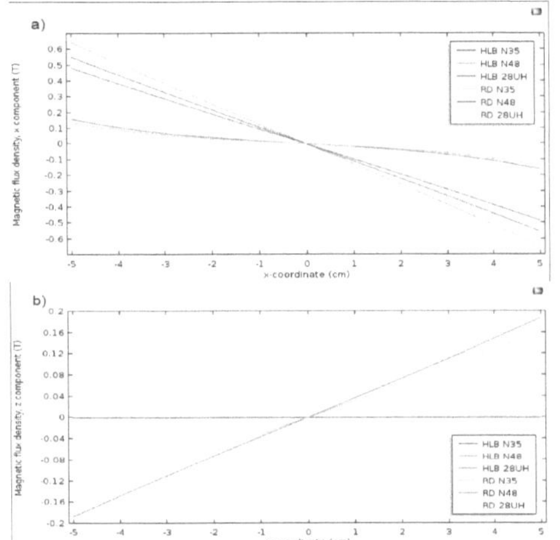

Figure 3: *Effect of Br factor on the FFP in the quadrupole magnet system to yield magnetic flux in the x-axis (a), and in the z-axis (b) for Halbach (HLB), and Radial (RD)*

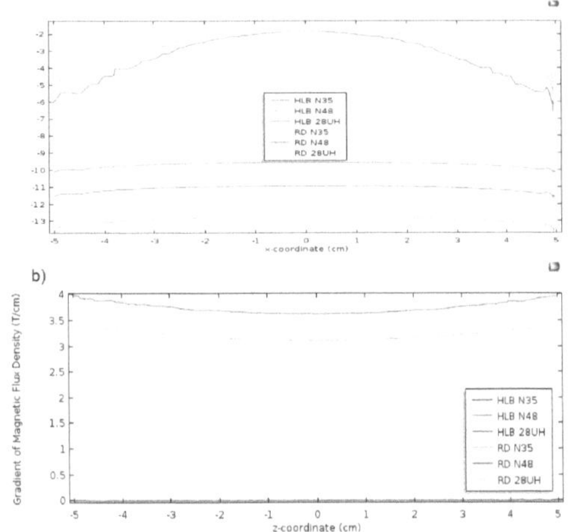

Figure 4: *(a) gradient in the x-axis, (b) gradient in the z-axis for Halbach (HLB), and Radial (RD) magnetization patterns, respectively.*

REFERENCES

[1] B. Gleich and J. Weizenecker. Tomographic imaging using the nonlinear response of magnetic particles, Nature, 435, 1214–1217, 2005. DOI: 10.1038/nature03808

[2] T. Knopp and T. M. Buzug. Magnetic particle imaging: An introduction to imaging principles and scanner instrumentation. Springer, Berlin/Heidelberg, 2012. DOI: 10.1007/978-3-642-04199-0

[3] M. W. Vogel, A. Giorni, V. Vegh, R. Pellicer-Guridi and D. C. Reutens. Rotatable small permanent magnet array for ultra-low field nuclear magnetic resonance instrumentation: A concept study. PLoS ONE, 11, e0157040, 2016. DOI: 10.1371/journal.pone.0157040.

[4] R. Bjørk,a_ C. R. H. Bahl, A. Smith, and N. Pryds, Optimization and improvement of Halbach cylinder design, JOURNAL OF APPLIED PHYSICS 104, 013910 _2008, DOI: 10.1063/1.2952537

[5] S. Sammet, R. M. Koch, F. Aguila, and M. V. Knopp. Residual magnetism in an MRI suite after field-ramp-down: What are the issues and experiences? JMR, 31, 1272–1276, 2010. DOI: 10.1002/jmri.22141

[6] https://www.comsol.com

[7] https://www.hkcm.de/desk.php/

MRI-based field of view selection for precise, real-time targeting in MPI

F. Griese[a,b,*], M. Prieske[a,b], M. Möddel[a,b], R. Werner[c] and T. Knopp[a,b]

[a] *Section for Biomedical Imaging, University Medical Center Hamburg, Hamburg, Germany*
[b] *Institute for Biomedical Imaging, Hamburg University of Technology, Hamburg, Germany*
[c] *Section for Image Processing and Medical Informatics, University Medical Center Hamburg, Hamburg, Germany*
[*] *Corresponding author, email: f.griese@uke.de*

Abstract: Magnetic Particle Imaging visualizes the spatial distribution of superparamagnetic iron oxide nanoparticle but it does not provide anatomical information of the object. In order to use MPI for device tracking or device navigation applications in real-time, it is necessary to register MPI images with imaging modalities that provide an anatomical map e.g. MRI. In this work, we present our extended online reconstruction software tool that performs real-time rigid registration of anatomical MRI background to MPI images.

I. Introduction

Magnetic Particle Imaging (MPI) generates 3D tomographic images [1] with a high temporal resolution by visualizing the spatial distribution of iron oxide nanoparticles (SPIOs). Its high temporal resolution makes MPI a promising candidate for interventional applications such as device tracking, device navigation and device manipulation, which has been demonstrated by Rahmer et al. [3]. For device tracking and device navigation an anatomical map of the target geometry is necessary to navigate a catheter or other medical devices precisely and safely to the desired destination. Therefore, a precise registration of the MRI and MPI imaging volumes performed online and in real-time helps to navigate accurately. Usually, the field of view (FoV) of MPI is limited to only a few centimeters, which makes it challenging to plan the MPI experiment and position the study object optimally, especially if one is interested in measuring a specific part of the object as for example a kidney in a mouse.

In this work, we present our extended online reconstruction software with real-time rigid registration of anatomical MRI background and MPI data. Further, we introduce the combination of long-term stable fiducials, precise positioning of a mouse bed via robot and software to plan and perform MPI experiments based on MRI images.

II. Material and Methods

For fiducial based image registration, we use three spherical bimodal markers [4] in a triangle arrangement [5] as shown in Fig. 1 (left). Each marker has a 2.85 mm diameter core filled with a mixture of one part dental cement and one part perimag in iron concentration 2.8 mg/ml. The silicone shell with a diameter of 5 mm was 3D printed and surrounds the core of each marker. Since silicone is visible in most MRI sequences, the marker shell functions as a fiducial for MRI. Perimag in the marker core generates an MPI signal and performs as a fiducial for MPI. The perimag particles inside the dental cement are immobilized and

induce less signal than mobilized particles but they become resistant to dehydration, and the particles are kept equally distributed throughout the sphere. The three markers are arranged in a way [4] that they are visible from all three perspectives in a maximum intensity projection image.

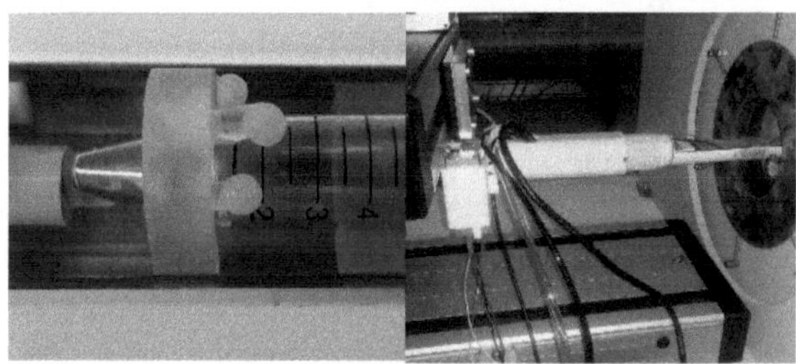

Figure 1: *Three stable spherical fiducials inside mouse bed (left) Robot mount for mouse bed (right).*

A robot mount for the mouse bed as shown in Fig. 1 (right) has been constructed and 3D printed by selective laser sintering (SLS). With the help of the robot mount for the mouse bed, it is possible to move the mouse bed by the robot in all direction x,y and z with a step wide precision of 6.25 μm. Since the mouse bed is attached to the robot, it is possible to reproduce the mouse beds position once the robot is moved in and out several times. This is especially helpful in an experiment where an MPI signal is expected close to the sensitivity limit and the fiducials signal might limit the effective contrast range within the FoV. In this case, the fiducials can be removed while the mouse bed can be positioned at the exact same position determined with the fiducials before. Our online reconstruction software tool [6] has further been extended to perform a manual registration between MRI and MPI live during an MPI measurement. A screenshot with the three spherical markers visible in both modalities is shown in Fig. 3 where both images are real-time overlaid but they are not registered to the correct alignment yet. The chronological order in which a MRI-based live registered MPI measurement is performed are described as follows and depicted in Fig. 2.

1. Initial situation: The MRI image has been acquired with the fiducial markers close to the target geometry.
2. Identifying fiducial markers in MPI: The mouse bed is moved inside the bore until the position and orientation of the markers are identified. The initial registration of the MRI and MPI volume images are performed by aligning both FoV centers. The current robot position P_{rob} is saved.
3. Registration: The manual rigid registration is performed visually by the user by adjusting the rotation matrix R and translation vector T.
4. Selection target FoV: In the UI the user determines the translation T_{target} of the current MPI FoV within the MRI image to the requested MPI FoV overlaying the target in the MRI image. Note that the MPI FoV is usually smaller than the MRI FoV.
5. Moving to selected target FoV: The user can either use the robot to move the mouse bed to the selected target FoV by adding T_{target} to P_{rob} (5.1) or can shift the Focus-fields by T_{target} to place the FoV over the selected part within the mouse bed (5.2). The rigid image registration will use parameters R, $T+T_{target}$.

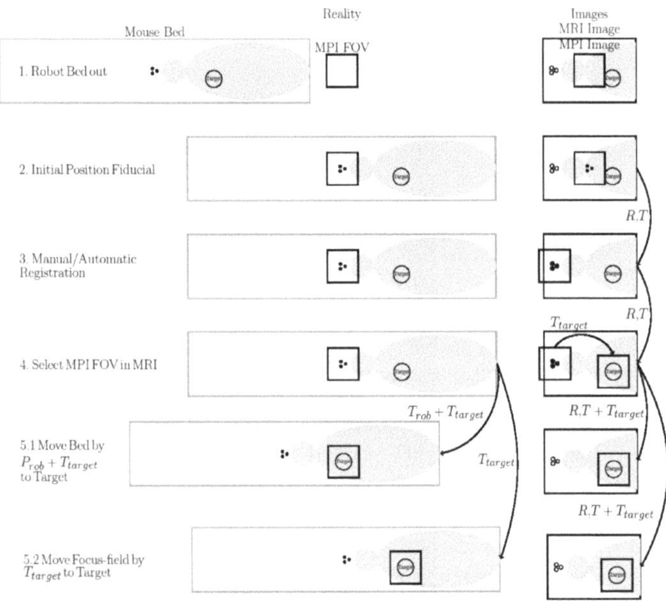

Figure 2: MRI-based FoV selection in MPI live targeting.

III. Results

The described method is used to target the brain of a mouse as shown in Fig. 3 (right) where particles generate a very low signal. In this experiment the fiducials have been removed later because they limit the effective contrast range. The process including interpolation, registration and coloring takes about 0.9 s per frame where the 25x25x25 MPI image has to be interpolated to the 192x192x192 MRI image.

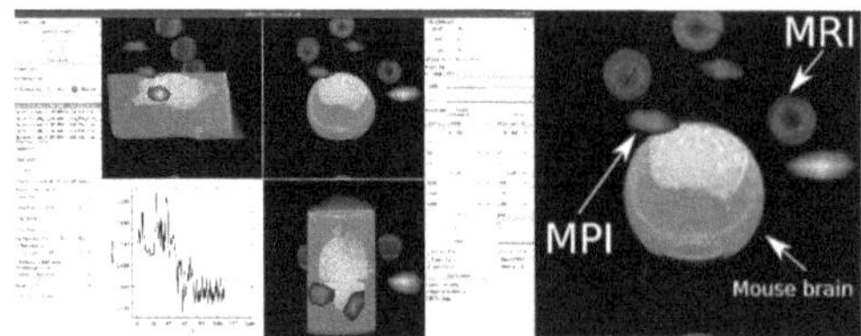

Figure 3: *Software to do a manual registration between MRI and MPI during a live MPI experiment (left) Screenshot xz plain (right).*

IV. Discussion

A method for conducting MPI based on MR image data has been presented. The technique facilitates handling and the development of multi-modal procedure experiments. It enables the user to precisely position the target object inside the MPI FoV, and ensures this position to be reproducible in the case of the fiducials being removed. Our fiducials are a promising long-term stable solution, and form the basis for development of an automatic registration. In this study the registration has been performed manually, but in future studies it should be possible to segment all three spherical positions within both MRI and MPI images and perform an automatic live registration via an iterative closest point algorithm (ICP). Especially in animal experiments this method could improve the workflow and reduce the time effort. The whole process could be optimized by parallel computing strategies.

V. Conclusions

In this study, we present a combination of fiducials, mouse bed robot mount and extended online reconstruction software to plan MPI experiments more precisely based on MRI images. This method makes measurement setups reproducible and disturbing fiducials can be removed. The proposed combination provides groundwork to develop an automatic registration between MRI and MPI images for precise and reliable MPI experiment planning which is based on MRI data.

ACKNOWLEDGEMENTS

F.G., M. P. M.M., R.W., and T.K. thankfully acknowledge the financial support by the German Research Foundation (DFG, KN 1108/2-1) and the Federal Ministry of Education and Research (BMBF, 05M16GKA) and Forschungszentrum Medizintechnik Hamburg (FMTHH, OIfmthh15). Authors state no conflict of interest.

REFERENCES

[1] B. Gleich and J. Weizenecker. Tomographic imaging using the nonlinear response of magnetic particles. *Nature*, 435(7046):1217-1217, 2005. doi: 10.1038/nature03808.

[2] J. Rahmer, C. Stehning, and B. Gleich. "Spatially selective remote magnetic actuation of identical helical micromachines." In: Science Robotics 2.3 (Feb. 15, 2017). doi: 10.1126/scirobotics.aal2845.

[3] F. Werner, C. Jung, M. Hofmann, R. Werner, J. Salamon, D. Säring, M. G. Kaul, K. Them, O. M. Weber, T. Mummert, G. Adam, H. Ittrich and T. Knopp. Geometry planning and image registration in magnetic particle imaging using bimodal fiducial markers. Med. Phys.. 43 2884,2016. doi: 10.1118/1.4948998.

[4] F. Griese, T. Knopp, R. Werner, A. Schlaefer, and M. Möddel. Submillimeter-Accurate Marker Localization within Low Gradient Magnetic Particle Imaging Tomograms. International Journal on Magnetic Particle Imaging, 3(1), 2017.

[5] T. Knopp and M. Hofmann. Online reconstruction of 3D magnetic particle imaging data. Physics in medicine and biology, 61(11):N257, 2016. doi: 10.1088/0031-9155/61/11/N257.

Implementation of a Heating Coil Insert for a Preclinical MPI Scanner Designed Using DEPSO

H. Wei[a]*, A. Behrends[a], Th. Friedrich[a], and T. M. Buzug[a]

[a] Institute of Medical Engineering, University of Lübeck, Lübeck, Germany
** Corresponding author, email: {wei,buzug}@imt.uni-luebeck.de*

Magnetic particle imaging (MPI) is a rapidly developing imaging modality, which determines the spatial distribution of magnetic nanoparticles. Magnetic fluid hyperthermia (MFH) is a promising therapeutic approach where magnetic nanoparticles are used to transform electromagnetic energy into heat. The similarities of MPI and MFH give rise to the potential of integration of MFH and MPI. In this work, the implementation of a heating coil insert designed for a preclinical MPI scanner is presented.

I. Introduction

I.I. MFH and MPI

Magnetic fluid hyperthermia is a method for heating nanoparticles by driving them with an alternating magnetic field. The magnetic nanoparticles (MNPs) are used to couple magnetic energy into the body to heat tissue via hysteresis power loss. MPI is a new imaging modality that makes use of the nonlinear magnetization curve of the MNPs [1]. The physical principle of MFH and MPI are similar, and the magnetic nanoparticles are used for both. Furthermore, in MPI, the gradient fields saturate the nanoparticles everywhere except in the vicinity of a field-free region (FFR). In the saturated regions, the particles are effectively locked in place and only the MNPs in the FFR can respond to an AC excitation field and generate heat, which makes the spatially selective MFH possible. MPI and MFH may be integrated together in a single device for simultaneous MPI–MFH to allow for seamless switching between imaging and therapeutic modes [2].

I.II DEPSO

The great challenge of integrating the heating coil insert into the MPI scanner lies in the minimization of its effect on the MPI receive chain. The voltage induced in the receive coil of the MPI system caused by the insert will damage the low noise amplifier (LNA). Therefore, a compensation unit is needed. A modified version of the algorithm *Differential Evolution Particle Swarm Optimization* (DEPSO) is developed to optimize the compensation coil. Particle swarm optimization is a heuristic optimization algorithm inspired by a social behavior metaphor. It originates from the simulation of the choreography of a bird flock. The candidate solutions, called particles, "fly" through the search space. The velocity is constantly adjusted according to the corresponding particle's experience and the particle's companions' experience [3]. The algorithm is used to minimize the value of a function of several independent variables. DEPSO is a hybrid particle swarm with a differential evolution operator [4]. It introduces random mutations to the particle swarm to increase the population variety, which gives it a better performance than the original *Particle Swarm Optimization* (PSO) algorithm.

II. Material and Methods

II.I. Heating Coil Geometry

The heating coil is a solenoid coil positioned at the center of the scanner bore. It is designed to generate a magnetic field up to 10 mT in amplitude for effective heating of the MNPs. Unserved Litz wire that contains 8000 strands with a diameter of 20 μm each is used. Since it is intended to conduct experiments on the rat brain with the MPI-MFH system, the coil should fit a small size rat and cover the brain area. Therefore, the inner diameter of the coil is chosen to be 66 mm and a length of 30 mm.

II.II. Compensation Coil

The compensation coil is in series with the heating coil but wound in the opposite direction. To minimize the loss in field strength in the center, where the field is supposed to heat up the MNPs, the cancellation coil should be as far away from the heating coil as possible. Taking the space for cooling and the diameter of the Litz wire into consideration, we set the diameter of the cancellation coil to 96 mm. A method similar to [5] is applied to acquire a profile for the induced voltage in a single loop along the bore axis. According to the law of reciprocity, the induced voltage in the coil has a direct linear relation to the induced voltage in the MPI scanner receive coil caused by the field-measuring coil. After that, the DEPSO algorithm is used to optimize the structure of the compensation coil to minimize the induced voltage in the MPI scanner. The flow chart of the DEPSO algorithm is shown in Fig. 1. According to the result given by DEPSO, the compensation coil has 4 turns and should be positioned at -58 mm, -9 mm, 60 mm, 91 mm to the FFP along the bore axis.

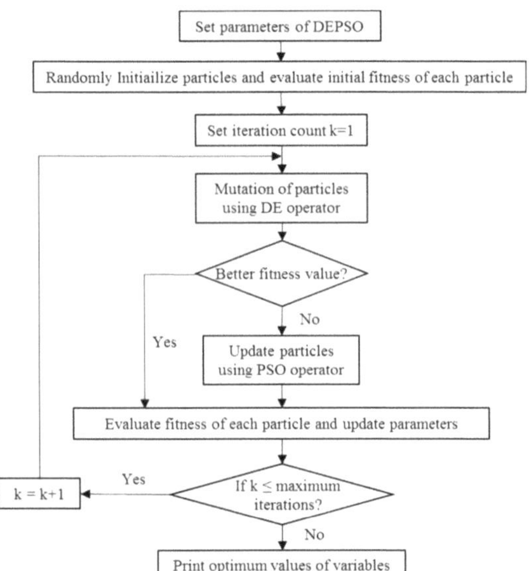

Figure 1: *Flowchart of DEPSO. The term "fitness" refers to a value that evaluates the result found by the algorithm, which is the total induced voltage in this case.*

II.III. Cooling

According to the simulation result of the finite element solver *FEMM* [6], 170 A current is needed to generate 10 mT magnetic field in the center of the coil. Therefore, the insert needs to be cooled. The design of the cooling unit is shown in Fig. 2. The outer diameter is 117 mm to fit the bore size of the MPI scanner; the inner diameter is 61 mm to fit a small rat cassette (59 mm diameter).

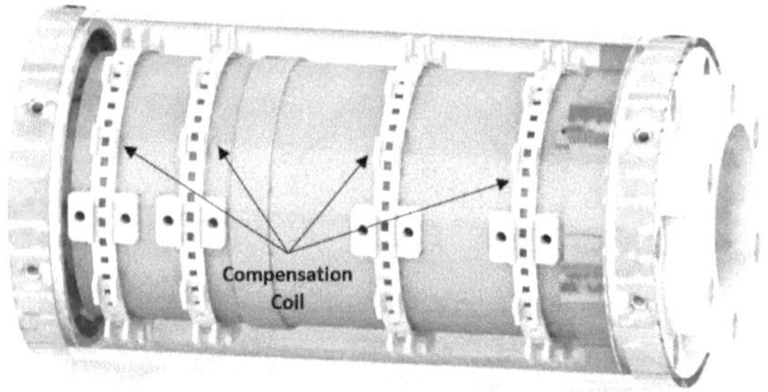

Figure 2: *Cooling unit design of the heating coil insert.*

III. Results

A prototype is manufactured for the field measurement and to test the compensation result. The transmission coefficient from the insert to the LNA output is measured over a frequency range from 100 kHz to 1 MHz by the *Keysight Technologies* E5061B LF-RF Network Analyzer. Since the LNA has a 40 dB amplification, the magnitude of the transfer function should be reduced by 40 dB to remove the amplifying effect of the LNA. Within the range of frequencies from1 kHz to 1 MHz that MFH usually adopts, 700 kHz is chosen to be the working frequency of the heating coil insert for the high attenuation compared to 300 or 500 kHz. At 700 kHz, the magnitude without the LNA amplification is -67 dB, -63 dB and -82 dB for x, y, z channel respectively. The magnetic field generated by the prototype

with 5 A DC signal is measured. The probe of a 3-Channel Gaussmeter (*Gaussmeter 460, Lakeshore Cryotronics, Westerville, USA*) is controlled by a Cartesian Robot from *Isel Automation* to measure the magnetic field strength at the center of the heating coil over an area of 25 mm × 30 mm on the xy plane in steps of 1 mm in each direction. The ideal magnetic field with 170 A current is calculated based on the measured 5 A results. The average field strength is 10.7 mT, with a standard deviation of 8×10^{-4} mT.

IV. Discussion

The transfer function implies that the attenuation of the compensation coil can reduce the voltage induced by the insert coil. Although the compensation result of the compensation coil is remarkable, a filter is still necessary to consume some residual power. The field measurement shows that the insert coil can generate a magnetic field up to 10 mT with the size of a rat brain. The inductance of the coil is 2.45 µH, with 175 A current at 700 kHz, the voltage across the coil will be up to around 2 kV. The high voltage drop needs to be considered when designing and manufacturing the impedance matching and other components of the circuit.

V. Conclusions

Within the scope of this work, a heating coil insert for the preclinical MPI scanner is designed and implemented, which allows generating a high frequency magnetic field suitable for MFH. After the MPI-MFH system is completed, the next step will be to test the compatibility of the insert followed by phantom experiments and the first animal experiments to prove the suitability for therapeutic applications.

ACKNOWLEDGEMENTS

The authors would like to thank D. Steinhagen and R. Schultz for their support in manufacturing the components of the cooling unit.

AUTHOR'S STATEMENT

The authors would like to thank the German Federal Ministry of Education and Research (BMBF) in the framework Health Research (Gesundheitsforschung), contract number 13GW0230B, 13GW0071D and 13GW0069A for financial support.

REFERENCES

[1] B. Gleich and J. Weizenecker. Tomographic imaging using the nonlinear response of magnetic particles. *Nature*, 435(7046):1217-1217, 2005. doi: 10.1038/nature03808.

[2] D. Hensley, Z. W. Tay, et al. Combining magnetic particle imaging and magnetic fluid hyperthermia in a theranostic platform, *Physics in Medicine & Biology*, 62(9), 3483, 2017. doi:10.1088/1361-6560/aa5601

[3] J. Kennedy, R. Eberhart. Particle swarm optimization, *Proc. IEEE Int. Conf. Neural Network*, vol. 4, pp. 1942-1948, 1995. doi: 10.1109/ICNN.1995.488968

[4] R. Storn, K. Price. Differential evolution—a simple and efficient heuristic for global optimization over continuous spaces, Journal of Global Optimization, vol. 11(4), pp. 341-359, 1997. doi: 10.1023/A:1008202821328

[5] M. Graeser, T. Knopp, et al. *Towards Picogram Detection of Superparamagnetic Iron-Oxide Particles Using a Gradiometric Receive Coil.* Scientific Reports, 7, 6872, doi: 10.1038/s41598-017-06992-5

[6] D. Meeker. Finite element method magnetics, 2018, January 30. Retrieved from http://www.femm.info/wiki/Documentation/

Sample Temperature Control in a Three-Dimensional Magnetic Particle Spectrometer

X. Chen[a]*, A. Behrends[a], A. Neumann[a], and T. M. Buzug [a]

[a] *Institute of Medical Engineering, University of Lübeck, Germany*
* *Corresponding author, email:{chen,buzug}@imt.uni-luebeck.de*

Magnetic Particle Imaging (MPI) is a novel imaging modality that uses various static and oscillating magnetic fields to image the spatial distribution of superparamagnetic iron oxide nanoparticles (SPIONs) with high sensitivity and no ionizing radiation. A Magnetic Particle Spectrometer (MPS) is used to measure the characteristics of SPIONs and achieve the system matrix of the imaging devices. A three-dimensional MPS has been presented lately including its first measurement results. In this paper, a temperature control setup in the MPS is introduced and its feasibility of controlling the sample temperature is demonstrated.

I. Introduction

In 2005 Bernhard Gleich and Jürgen Weizenecker introduced MPI as a novel imaging technology, it provides sub-millimeter spatial resolution and fast acquisition time for medical imaging [1, 2, 3]. An MPS can measure the characteristics of SPIONs and estimate their usability in different application [4]. Moreover, it can emulate the magnetic field inside an MPI imaging device for fast acquisition of the system matrix [5, 6].

Lately, a three-dimensional MPS has been introduced [7]. However, during measurement the heat dissipated from the transmit coils influences the temperature of the sample. Since the magnetization of the SPIONs is sensitive to the temperature [8], it is necessary to stabilize the temperature during measurement. On the other hand, if the response of SPIONs can be measured under different temperatures, it is also possible to estimate their temperature in-vivo using color MPI [9]. Therefore, a temperature control setup has been designed and implemented to manipulate the sample temperature.

II. Material and Methods

The MPS used here to build the temperature control setup has a bore size of 26 mm diameter, which is also the inner diameter of the central transmit coil. Two cylindrical pipes-one with 25 mm outer diameter and 1 mm thickness, the other with 20 mm outer diameter and 1 mm thickness-are concentrically placed inside the bore. This forms a 1.5 mm gap between the pipes. The space inside the inner pipe is the sample chamber, which has a diameter of 18 mm. As shown in Fig. 1, two fixtures with inlet and outlet fix the two pipes in their position. Additionally, the fixtures can be fastened to the frame of the transmit coils.

The 1.5 mm gap between the pipes is for water to flow. When the water with a certain temperature flows between the pipes,

the heat dissipated from the water transfers to the sample chamber to reach a thermal equilibrium. Therefore, the change of the water temperature thus enables the control of the sample temperature. At the same time, the water acts as an isolation shell to prevent the heat transfer between the transmit coils and the sample chamber.

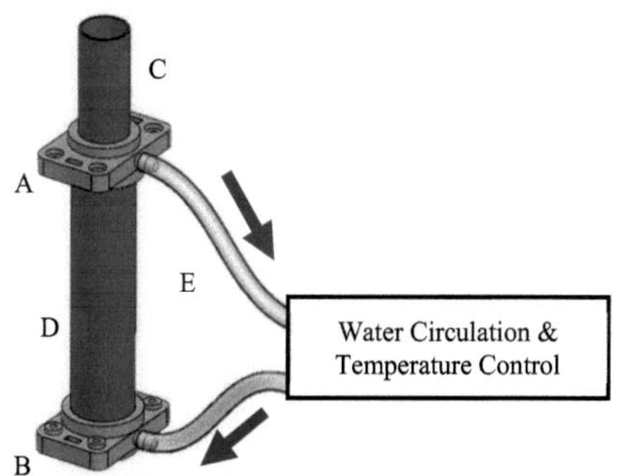

Figure 1: *Demonstration of temperature control setup. A: Fixture with outlet, B: Fixture with inlet, C: Inner pipe, D: Outer pipe, E: Water tube. The arrows show the direction of the water flow.*

A pump (18 W, TSSS, Changshu, China) is used to circulate water through the system. An immersion heater (300 W, Relags, Tuntenhausen, Germany) can heat the water in a reservoir, and two Peltier elements (60 W, Kimilar, Shenzhen, China) are used for cooling the water. The heating and cooling equipment are connected to a thermostat (ITC 310T, Inkbird, Shenzhen, China) equipped with a dual relay. The included sensor measures the water temperature in the reservoir. When the measured temperature is different from the set temperature in the thermostat, the heating/cooling equipment will turn on to bring the water to the set temperature. Temperature hysteresis can be set to avoid flickering of the switch.

For the experiment, a sample vial filled with water substituting a SPION sample is placed inside the sample chamber. Three fiber-optic temperature sensors (PRB-400, Osensa, Burnaby, Canada) are used to measure the temperature of the sample, the transmit coil and the water in the reservoir. The temperature hysteresis is set to 1 °C. The temperature of the water in the reservoir is changed by manually setting the thermostat. Starting from 25 °C, the water temperature is increased in steps of 5 °C to 40 °C. Then, it is decreased in steps of 2 °C to 32 °C. In the end, the water temperature is quickly increased to 55 °C.

III. Results

As seen from Fig. 2, the sample temperature changes according to the temperature of the water, i.e. an equilibrium state inside the sample chamber can be reached. It takes about 12 min to increase the sample temperature in 5 °C steps, and it takes longer for higher temperatures. For decreasing the sample temperature in steps of 2 °C, it needs about 7 min and it takes longer for lower temperatures.

The temperature control setup is able to change the sample temperature from 32°C to 55°C, though it takes a longer time. The sudden increase and decrease of the coil temperature at about 50 to 60 min are due to the turning off and on of the cooling of the transmit coils. There is only a slight increase of the sample temperature when there is a big increase in temperature of the transmit coils, thus the influence of the transmit coils is limited by the water isolation shell.

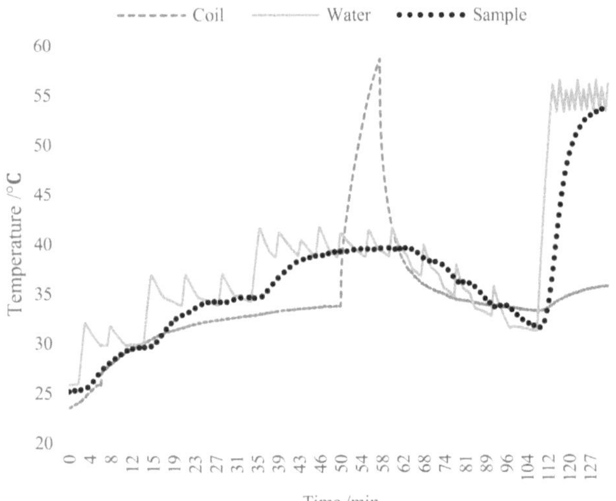

Figure 2: *Plot of temperature vs time. The dashed line is the temperature of the transmit coil, the solid line is the temperature of the water in the reservoir, the dotted line is the temperature of the sample.*

IV. Discussion

In Fig. 2, the water temperature fluctuates at each set temperature level. The overheating/overcooling is due to the low sample rate of the thermostat, in other words, the measured temperature from the built-in sensor has a certain time lag. The later adjustment of temperature is due to the 1°C temperature hysteresis set in advance.

The reason for rapidly changing the coil temperature is to change the heat transfer direction between the water isolation shell and the transmit coils, in order to analyze the feasibility of the temperature control. As long as the heat transferred from the transmit coils to the water isolation shell is less than the heat dissipated from the water to the environment plus the maximum power of the cooling equipment, the temperature of the sample can still be controlled.

As seen in Fig. 2, there is a deviation between the sample temperature and the water temperature at 55°C. This is because of the high dissipation from the water to the environment, an equilibrium is slowly reached.

V. Conclusions

The introduced temperature control setup is capable of changing the thermal equilibrium state inside the sample chamber, in order to manipulate the sample temperature. However, at higher temperature the equilibrium is slowly reached. The water isolation shell is able to limit the influence from the transmit coils.

ACKNOWLEDGEMENTS

This work was supported by the Federal Ministry of Education and Research, Germany (BMBF) under grant 13GW0069A.

AUTHOR'S STATEMENT

Conflict of interest: Authors state no conflict of interest.

REFERENCES

[1] B. Gleich and J. Weizenecker. Tomographic imaging using the nonlinear response of magnetic particles. *Nature*, 435(7046):1214-1217, 2005. doi: 10.1038/nature03808.

[2] T. Knopp and T. M. Buzug. *Magnetic Particle Imaging: An Introduction to Imaging Principles and Scanner Instrumentation.* Springer, Berlin/Heidelberg, 2012. doi: 10.1007/978-3-642-04199-0.

[3] J. Weizenecker, J. Borgert, and B. Gleich. A simulation study on the resolution and sensitivity of magnetic particle imaging. *Physics in Medicine and Biology*, 52(21):6363-6374, 2007. doi: 10.1088/0031-9155/52/21/001.

[4] S. Biederer, T. Knopp, T. F. Sattel, K. Lüdtke-Buzug, B. Gleich, J. Weizenecker, J. Borgert, and T. M. Buzug. Magnetization response spectroscopy of superparamagnetic nanoparticles for magnetic particle imaging. *Journal of Physics D: Applied Physics*, 42(20):205007, 2009. doi: 10.1088/0022-3727/42/20/205007.

[5] M. Grüttner, M. Graeser, S. Biederer, T. F. Sattel, H. Wojtczyk, W. Tenner, T. Knopp, B. Gleich, J. Borgert, and T. M. Buzug. 1D-image reconstruction for magnetic particle imaging using a hybrid system function. In: *Nuclear Science Symposium and Medical Imaging Conference (NSS/MIC)*, 2545-2548, 2011. doi: 10.1109/NSSMIC.2011.6152687.

[6] A. von Gladiss, M. Graeser, P. Szwargulski, T. Knopp, and T. M. Buzug. Hybrid system calibration for multidimensional magnetic particle imaging. *Physics in Medicine and Biology.* 62(9):3392-3406, 2017. doi: 10.1088/1361-6560/aa5340.

[7] X. Chen, M. Graeser, A. Behrends, A. von Gladiss, and T. M. Buzug. First measurement and SNR results of a 3D magnetic particle spectrometer. *International Journal on Magnetic Particle Imaging*, 4(1), 2018. doi: 10.18416/IJMPI.2018.1810001.

[8] S. Draack, T. Viereck, C. Kuhlmann, M. Schilling, and F. Ludwig. Temperature-dependent MPS measurements. *International Journal on Magnetic Particle Imaging, 3*(1), 2017. doi:10.18416/ijmpi.2017.1703018.

[9] J. B. Weaver, A. M. Rauwerdink, and E. W. Hansen, Magnetic nanoparticle temperature estimation. *Medical Physics*, 36(5):1822–1829, 2009. doi: 10.1118/1.3106342.

Monitoring Iron Oxide Nanoparticle Uptake in Plants with Magnetic Particle Spectroscopy

A.C.S. Samia[*]

[a] *Department of Chemistry, Case Western Reserve University, Cleveland, OH 44106, USA*
[*] *Corresponding author, email:* _anna.samia@case.edu_

Abstract: Magnetic particle spectroscopy (MPS) offers a promising approach to monitor the uptake and distribution of iron oxide nanoparticles (IONPs) in plants. In our study, we exposed garden cress (Lepidium sativum) plants to EDTA-capped IONPs and observed an enhancement in biomass and chlorophyll production compared to plants treated with a commercial Fe-EDTA fertilizer. Moreover, we could demonstrate that the IONP uptake and tissue distribution (with plants grown in hydrophonic media) can be quantitatively monitored using MPS, and the results of the analysis are consistent with findings from the more laborious atomic absorption spectroscopy method that is conventionally used to study plant uptake.

I. Introduction

Although iron is one of Earth's most abundant elements, its availability to plants remains an agricultural challenge, particularly in high pH environments. At high pH, iron forms insoluble ferric oxide-hydroxides making it inaccessible to plants. It is estimated that about 30% of the world's cropland is too alkaline for optimal plant growth, and some staple crops, like rice, are particularly susceptible to iron deficiency, thereby necessitating the need for continued research in developing iron-based fertilizers (1).

Iron deficiency in plants known as chlorosis is visibly manifested in the yellowing of plant leaves, which if left untreated can lead to eventual plant death. The standard approach to treat iron chlorosis is to apply iron fertilizers, specifically in chelated iron forms that help maintain iron availability for plant uptake. Chelated iron fertilizers like Fe-EDTA (ethylenediaminetetraacetic acid) remains available for longer periods than non-chelated iron analogs. Alternatively, recent studies have demonstrated the potential of using iron oxide nanoparticles (IONPs) as fertilizers to address iron deficiency in plants. While some studies demonstrate a significant enhancement in plant growth upon treatment with IONPs, other investigations provide conflicting results (1). This phenomenon can be largely attributed to the wide variations in experimental parameters pertaining to IONP size, shape, surface coating, plant type, and growth conditions. Moreover, most IONP plant uptake studies have utilized atomic absorption spectroscopic (AAS) methods, which involve laborious strong acid digestion sample processing, with the inability to distinguish between intact IONP versus leached iron ion plant uptake. To address these challenges, our group has developed a synthetic approach to produce highly stable IONPs that mimic the chelating ligands found in commercial chelated iron fertilizers, which enabled us to promote effective plant uptake and IONP translocation. Moreover, we have effectively demonstrated that the plant uptake process and IONP translocation in different plant tissues can be effectively monitored using magnetic particle spectroscopy (MPS), which is a zero-dimensional magnetic particle imaging (MPI) scanner without spatial resolution that is used to characterizer MPI tracers (2-3). Here we used MPS to monitor the absorption and translocation of different sized (10 nm and 20 nm) EDTA-coated iron oxide nanoparticles (IONP-EDTA) in garden cress (*Lepidium sativum*) plants. Garden cress (GC) was picked for its short growth cycle and its nutritional value. We evaluated the IONP effects on plant biomass, growth, and chlorophyll production, in comparison to effects of plant exposure with a commercial Fe-EDTA fertilizer. Our MPS studies were validated by AAS and we could demonstrate that this method is a reliable, sensitive, and effective analytical tool for the study and development of IONP based fertilizers.

II. Material and Methods

The Fe-EDTA fertilizer used was purchased from Greenway, Biotech Inc. The iron (III) chloride, oleic acid, trimethylamine N-oxide, and 1-octadecene chemicals used in the synthesis of the IONPs were obtained from Sigma Aldrich and used as received. The EDTA ligand was purchased from Gelest, Inc. Garden cress (GC) seeds were purchased from Sprout House, LLC.

II.I IONP Synthesis and Characterization

Spherical IONPs with average sizes of 10 and 20 nm were separately synthesized using a previously reported thermal decomposition approach (3). The as-prepared IONPs have wüstite phase and were subsequently oxidized to magnetite using trimethylamine N-oxide. To introduce EDTA ligands, a ligand exchange process using silane-EDTA was performed on the oxidized oleic acid-capped magnetite IONPs. The particle size and shape distribution of the IONPs were evaluated using a JEOL 1200CX transmission electron microscope (TEM) operated at 80kV. The hydrodynamic diameter and zeta-potential of the IONP-EDTA samples were characterized using a ZetaPALS particle size analyzer (Brookhaven). The powder X-ray diffraction patterns of the IONPs were collected using a Rigaku MiniFlex x-ray powder diffractometer using Cu Kα radiation (γ = 0.154 nm). The total Fe concentration in each sample was measured using a fast sequential atomic absorption spectrophotometer (AAS) Varian 220FS AA.

II.II IONP Plant Uptake and Translocation Studies with MPS.

The GC seeds were sprouted in water to mimic hydrophonic conditions and after 5 days, the germinated seeds were incubated with the synthesized IONP-EDTA samples (500 Fe ppm total) for an additional 5 days. Water and Fe-EDTA (500 Fe ppm total) were used as control groups. The daily changes in IONP plant uptake in solution was evaluated using a custom built x-space MPS that exposed the IONPs to a sinusoidal magnetic field with a frequency of 16.8 kHz and 20 mT field amplitude (3). After 5 days of IONP-EDTA or Fe-EDTA exposure, the plants were collected, thoroughly washed, and dried under vacuum to measure the plant biomass and tissue growth. The plant tissues were also sampled for chlorophyll analysis using an ethanol extraction method. Similarly, some of the sampled tissue sections were evaluated using MPS to compare the relative IONP distribution in the leaf, stem, and root components and the results were compared with AAS analysis.

III. Results

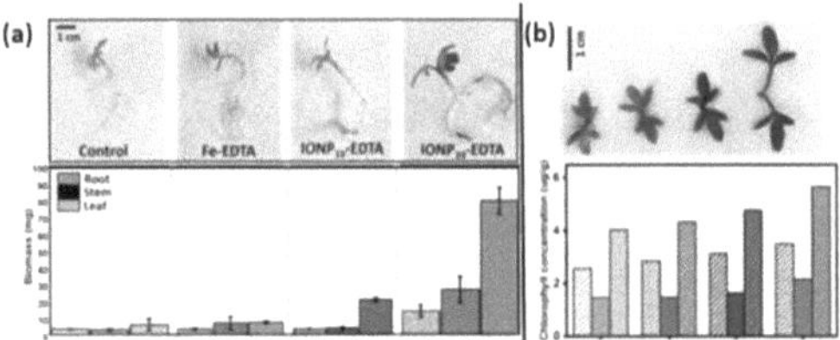

Figure 1: a. *(top) Garden cress plants exposed to different IONP-EDTA and Fe-EDTA treatments, and the corresponding average biomass of the collected root, stem, and leaf tissues (bottom).* ***b.*** *(top) Close-up image of the leaves collected from the treated plants and their corresponding extracted chlorophyll content (bottom).*

TEM analysis confirms the production of monodisperse spherical IONPs with an average diameter of 10 and 20 nm, respectively. Powder XRD reveals the magnetite phase, and DLS measurements show an average hydrodynamic radius of 14 nm and 24 nm, respectively, for the corresponding ligand exchanged IONP-EDTA. Phenotypic observations on the GC plants after 5 days of IONP-EDTA exposure revealed significantly enhanced plant growth upon treatment with 20 nm IONP-EDTA in comparison to both Fe-EDTA and 10 nm IONP-EDTA plant exposure (Fig. 1a). This observation matched the chlorophyll analysis (Fig. 1b). On the other hand, the daily uptake of the IONPs and its plant tissue distribution could be successfully monitored using

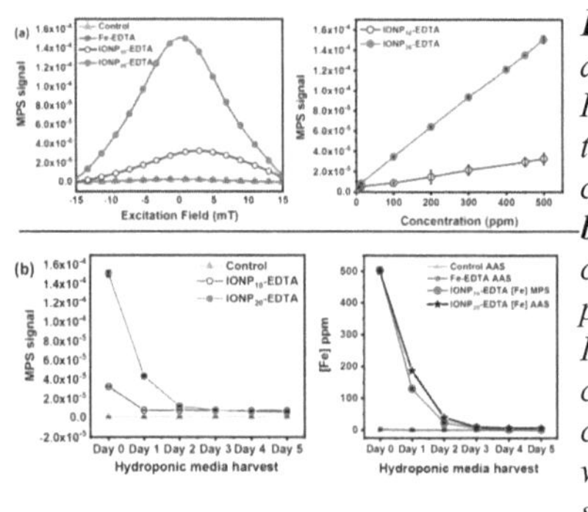

Figure 2: a. *(left) MPS data obtained from the IONP-EDTA samples and their corresponding calibration plots (right).* ***b.*** *(left) MPS data collected at different time points to monitor daily IONP uptake, and the corresponding comparison of results with AAS analysis, showing good correlation (right).*

MPS (Fig. 2a). The results from MPS studies matched with the Fe analysis performed using AAS (Fig.2b).

IV. Discussion

This study demonstrates the great potential of MPS as a reliable analytical method to accurately monitor IONP plant uptake and translocation, which can be exploited for the development of optimized fertilizers and also in the phytotoxic studies involving engineered NPs. Moreover, the study shows the great potential of IONPs as iron fertilizer additives. The large directed concentration of iron contained within the nanoparticle structure could enable the significant reduction of the total amount of fertilizers needed, while slowing down the iron release rate for controlled iron plant uptake; owing to the protected and stable structure afforded by optimized capping ligands. The slow but sustainable iron release mechanism from engineered IONPs can in turn decrease the risk for formation of damaging oxygen radical species to the plants and associated organisms.

V. Conclusions

In summary, the work presented could effectively demonstrate the compatibility of the MPS method in studying the uptake process of IONPs in plants. Additionally, the study showcases a significant enhancement effect on the phenotypic traits of the garden cress plants when treated with IONPs vs the traditional Fe-chelated fertilizers. These results suggest the potential of IONPs as fertilizer additives for the cultivation of healthier food crops.

ACKNOWLEDGEMENT

This work was supported by a NSF-CAREER Grant (DMR-1253358) from the Solid State and Materials Chemistry Program

REFERENCES

[1] D.J. Burke, N. Pietrasiak, S.F. Situ, E.C. Abenojar, M. Porche, P. Kraj, Y, Lakliang, and A.C.S. Samia "Iron oxide and titanium dioxide nanoparticle effects on plant performance and root associated microbes" *Int. J. Mol. Sci.* 16:23630-23650., 2015. doi:10.3390/ijms161023630

[2] Z. Zhang, D.B. Reeves, I.M. Perreard, W.C. Kett, K.E. Griswold, B. Gimi, and J.B. Weaver. Molecular sensing with magnetic particle spectroscopy of nanoparticle Brownian motion. *Biosens. Bioelec.* 50: 441-446, 2013. doi: 10.1016/j.bios.2013.06.049.

[3] L.M. Bauer, S.F. Situ, M.A. Griswold, and A.C.S. Samia. High-performance iron oxide nanoparticles for magnetic particle imaging – guided hyperthermia (hMPI). *Nanoscale* 8: 12162-12169, 2016. doi: 10.1039/C6NR01877G.

Generalizing ELISA Spectroscopic Methods Using Antibody Targeted Nanoparticles.

S.W. Gordon-Wylie[a*], D.B. Ness[c], Y. Shi[b], S.G. Diamond[a], S.K. Mirza[a], and J.B. Weaver[a,b,c]

[a] *Thayer School of Engineering, Dartmouth College, Hanover, USA*
[b] *Department of Physics, Dartmouth College, Hanover, USA*
[c] *Department of Radiology, Dartmouth Hitchcock Medical Center, Lebanon, USA*
[*] *Corresponding author, email: scott.w.gordon@dartmouth.edu*

Abstract: Iron oxide based magnetic nanoparticles (NPs) hold great promise as passive sensors for in-vivo applications. We have developed methods of measuring protein biomarker concentrations using aptamer or antibody derivatized NPs that can be used in vivo. We use Brownian rotation induced relaxation effects of the derivatized NPs to measure biomarker concentrations based on a proportional increase in the number of NPs linked together as the concentration of the biomarker target increases. We demonstrate using polyclonal antibodies the measurement of the pain/inflammation marker IL-6 and show detection limits in the 10 pM range using our current spectrometer.

I. Introduction

I.I. General Considerations

We are adapting magnetic spectroscopy of nanoparticle Brownian rotation (1) to measure the concentrations of a wider array of biomarker molecules more simply. We call the technology *in vivo* ELISA because of its similarity to ELISA optical methods. We have previously used aptamers for targeting nanoparticles (NPs) primarily because the conjugation is simple and robust. Limitations of aptamers are short lifetimes in vivo due to enzymatic digestion, and comparatively few high affinity aptamers exist compared to a wide range of possible biomarkers. In comparison, there are antibodies for almost all biological proteins and antibodies that are robust over time *in vivo*. Polyclonal antibodies are a mix of antibodies that bind all possible regions on the target molecule and are the most widely available. Monoclonal antibodies are refined from polyclonal antibodies and bind a specific region of the targeted molecule. Pairs of monoclonal antibodies exist for sandwich ELISA applications but they are not nearly as common as polyclonal antibodies. We have demonstrated that polyclonal antibodies can used with our spectroscopic methods to measure the concentration of almost any molecule. We demonstrate using IL-6, a common cytokine that generally induces innate immune responses for bacterial infections among other stimuli. The general inflammatory response results in upregulation of IL-6 as well. Pain, especially chronic pain, generally involves inflammatory response so IL-6 is an excellent marker for pain as well. Ultimately the application is for in-vivo diagnostics.

I.II. The spectrometer

The spectrometer uses a small AC magnetic field (10 mT) applied sequentially at different driving frequencies with a small constant DC field (1 mT) oriented perpendicular to the alternating field to direct the alternating NP magnetization to the pickup coil (oriented along the DC field), see Fig. 1.

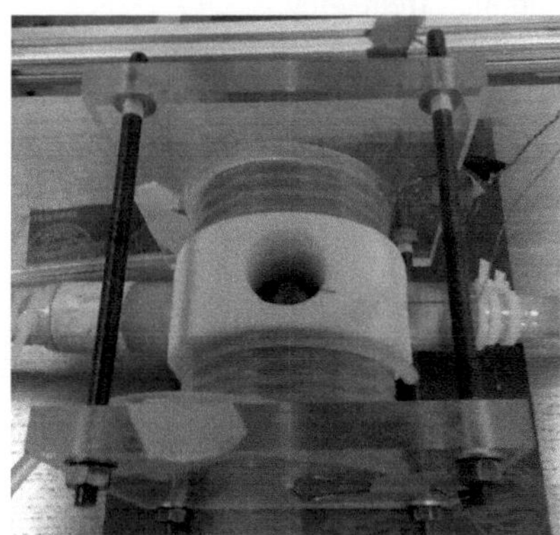

Figure 1: *Spectrometer used to measure harmonic ratios for the NP experiments. The large coils wrapped in translucent cooling tubing are the AC drive coils. The receive coil is wrapped around the small sample in the middle and is perpendicular to the AC coils. The DC field is oriented perpendicular to the field of view.*

At each AC frequency, the ratio of the 4th harmonic to the 2nd harmonic is used as a concentration independent metric of rotational freedom. The perpendicular receive-coils minimize the feed-through from the drive field. Speaking generally, an increase in rotational freedom (less aggregated) drives the harmonic ratio up while a decrease in freedom (more aggregated) drives the harmonic ratio down.

II. Material and Methods

BNF Starch 100 nm nanoparticles were obtained from Micromod already derivatized with streptavidin. Streptavidin loading proved to be important, and therefore was confirmed relative to vendor specifications using an in-house titration protocol. The concentration of antibodies must be much larger than the number of streptavidin binding sites; for the antibodies we purchased, the ideal number of biotin binding sites per NP was about 150-200. More than this favors too much crosslinking during conjugation. Less than this means too few antibodies are attached to the particle. When necessary streptavidin binding sites were blocked with 10 kDa mPEG-Biotin.

Antibody/Protein pairs were purchased from R&D Biotechne, Abcam or Peprotech.

NP derivatization was performed in the presence of BSA, using serial addition of small aliquots of dilute NP solution to an excess of concentrated biotinylated-AB solution. Purification was by magnetic separation. Under favorable conditions the excess of antibody can be reused.

Derivatized NPs were then challenged with various amounts of protein in a 0.1% BSA/PBS 1X buffer. The response was developed overnight at 4 deg C, or over 4-6 hours at room temperature. NPs were then measured at 30 deg C using the spectrometer shown in Fig 1. and described elsewhere (2).

III. Results

Typical spectra are shown in Fig. 2 as a plot of harmonic ratio versus applied frequency.

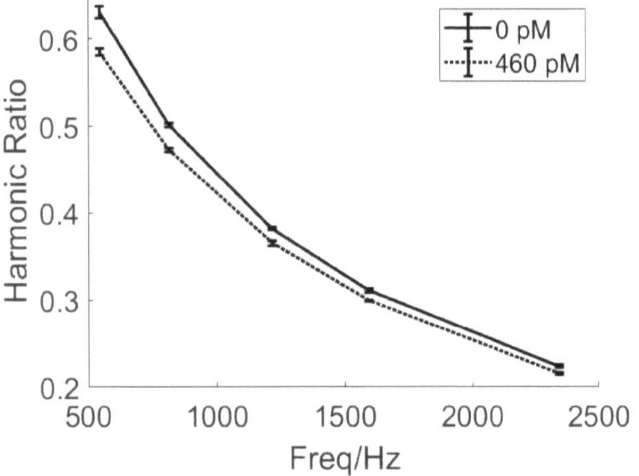

Figure 1: Typical protein challenge results: The dark line is a control spectrum for IL-6 antibody tagged NPs, the dotted line is for the same stock solution after challenge with IL-6 protein to a final concentration of 460 pM

In order to determine an approximate detection limit, statistical significance measures were used with a 0.05 significance level. Table 1 shows calculated p-values using each of the five applied frequencies averaged over two different sets of solutions & challenges.

Table 1: Sensitivity to IL-6: p-values for representing the probability that the IL-6 spectra are significantly different from the distribution of reference spectra. Insignificant entries are highlighted in gray.

Challenge/pM	76	15	7	1.5	0.75	0.45
p-value	10^{-7}	0.020	0.047	0.832	0.514	0.533

From which we infer a detection limit of about 10 pM for this set of experiments.

IV. Discussion

Obtaining significant results for a specific antibody/protein pair, in this case for IL-6, is extremely encouraging. As we work to extend this result into a true platform technology the challenge is in optimizing the ability of the bound antibody to recognize the protein in such a way that the net result is to form a bridge between NPs. Simply binding protein to the surface of the NP leads to only very small changes in signal. For IL-6 we were able to use a simple polyclonal AB mixture effectively. For other targets, such as Granzyme B, a simple polyclonal mixture has so far yielded a lower gain (basically % of aggregates formed on challenge) than for the IL6 system. Boosting the gain using polyclonals from other cell lines, or using monoclonal antibodies is where things stand currently.

V. Conclusions

Polyclonal antibodies can be used to target NPs for magnetic nanoparticle spectroscopic biomarker concentration estimates termed *in vivo* ELISA. Detection of IL6 using antibody tagged NPs in combination with measurement of Brownian motion induced rotational relaxation rate effects has been accomplished with a detection limit of ~10 pM using our current spectrometer. Extension of these results into a full platform technology for detecting any biomarker and, in particular pain and inflammation markers, *in vivo* is currently being developed.

ACKNOWLEDGEMENTS
Funding from NIH/NIBIB under grant 1R21EB021456.

AUTHOR'S STATEMENT
SD has interest in Lodestone Inc and SM has interest in PEER Inc.

REFERENCES
[1] Zhang X, Reeves DB, Perreard IM, Kett WC, Griswold KE, Gimi B, Weaver JB. Molecular sensing with magnetic nanoparticles using magnetic spectroscopy of nanoparticle Brownian motion. Biosensors and Bioelectronics 2013, 50(0): 441-446.
[2] Khurshid H, Shi Y, Berwin BL, Weaver JB. Evaluating blood clot progression using magnetic particle spectroscopy. Medical physics 2018, 45(7): 3258-3262.

synomag®: The New High-Performance Tracer for Magnetic Particle Imaging

P. Vogel [a], T. Kampf [a,b,*], M.A. Rückert [a], C. Grüttner [c], A. Kowalski [c], H. Teller [c], and V.C. Behr [a]

[a] *Experimental Physics 5 (Biophysics), University of Würzburg, 97074 Würzburg, Germany*
[b] *Diagnostic and Interventional Neuroradiology, University Hospital Würzburg, 97080 Würzburg, Germany*
[c] *micromod Partikeltechnologie GmbH, 18119 Rostock, Germany*
[*] *Corresponding author, email: Thomas.Kampf@physik.uni-wuerzburg.de*

Abstract: The success of tracer-based tomographic methods, such as Magnetic Particle Imaging (MPI), depends on two major factors: scanner and tracer. Within the last years several hardware enhancements have been presented improving temporal and spatial resolution for MPI systems, but there was still a lack of efficient commercially available tracers. Here we report on synomag® particles as a new tracer tailored for MPI, which shows almost three-times higher signal intensities in a Traveling Wave MPI scanner than Resovist®.

I. Introduction

Magnetic Particle Imaging (MPI) is a promising imaging modality for multiple applications in biology, chemistry and medicine [1, 2]. It is based on the nonlinear response of superparamagnetic iron-oxide nanoparticles (SPIONs) to time varying magnetic fields. As a tracer-based imaging modality, the performance and success of MPI systems strongly depend on the hardware and the tracer itself. Since several enhancements in hardware design and development have been shown in the last years [2], only few novel approaches in tracer development with a high gain can be found [3, 4].

In this study, a novel high-performance tracer for MPI (synomag®, micromod, Germany) is characterized and compared to the established tracer Resovist® (Bayer, Germany) using Traveling Wave MPI (TWMPI) [5].

II. Material and Methods

II.I High Performance tracer

The new synomag®-particles are multi-core particles featuring a nanoflower substructure of iron oxide crystallites (Fig. 1) along with an excellent biocompatibility. The particles are synthesized by a polyol method via thermal decomposition of a suitable iron precursor [10, 11].

II.II Traveling Wave MPI

The TWMPI scanner is an alternative MPI scanner approach [5] offering a high flexibility in gradient strength [6], temporal resolution [7] and scanning modes [8, 9].

For comparison, synomag® and Resovist® were measured under same conditions: for generating all data sets, 2D-slice-scanning mode (SSM) is used running at frequencies f_1=1050 Hz and f_2=12150 Hz and scanning a FOV of 65 mm

in length and 29 mm in diameter with a gradient strength of 1.5 T/m were performed. The total acquisition time was 200 ms with 10 averages. For signal-to-noise (SNR) determination, the datasets were Fourier transformed and the magnitude of the harmonic at 47550 Hz (first left-handed sideband-harmonic of the forth higher harmonic of f_2: $4 \cdot f_2 - f_1$) was taken. For reconstruction a standard Wiener filter with an appropriate point-spread-function (PSF) is applied to the re-gridded raw-images [8].

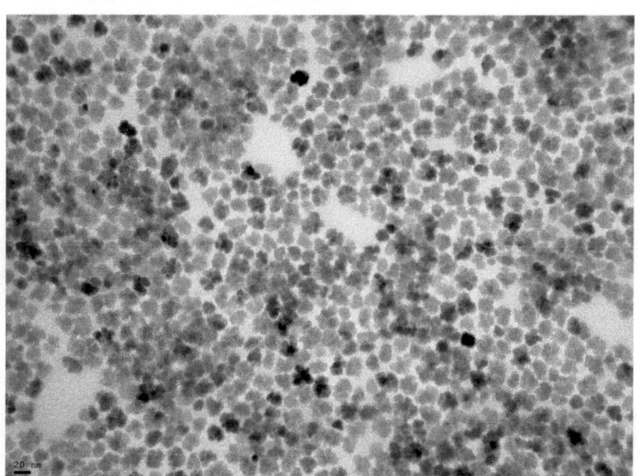

Figure 1: *TEM of synomag® particles.*

III. Results

In Tab. 1 an overview about the results of the measured samples is given. The samples were prepared with several dilutions and measured in multiple volume sizes. For comparison, the iron mass of every particle system is normalized to the measured SNR (based on the originating concentration). By determining an average value of the SNR/µg Fe, the signal strength of synomag® is 172 % higher than that of Resovist®.

Table 1: *Overview about the values from different particle samples: synomag® (micromod, Germany, conc. 17 mg Fe/ml) and Resovist® (Bayer, Germany, conc. 27.5 mg Fe/ml).*
** The variation of the SNR values can be a result of pipetting small volumes.*
*** The SNR value is taken from the magnitude of the Fourier transformed at frequency 47.55 kHz.*

Sample	Dilution factor	Volume [µl]	Iron mass [µg]	SNR (**)	SNR /µg Fe
synomag	1:10	79	134	3200	23.8
synomag	1:10	10	17	392	23.1
synomag	1:100	5	0.9	12	13.6
synomag	1:100	10	1.7	29	17.1
synomag	1:100	74	12.6	216	17.1
synomag	1:1000	90	1.5	9.2	6.0*
Resovist	1:10	89	245	1422	5.8
Resovist	1:100	2	0.6	3.2	5.8
Resovist	1:100	5	1.4	7.9	5.7
Resovist	1:100	10	2.8	16	5.7
Resovist	1:100	73	20	120	6.0
Resovist	1:1000	100	2.8	16	5.8

In Fig. 2 a selection of raw-images (left) and reconstructed images (right) for both tracers is given. In all cases the signal is strong enough to reconstruct all points clearly. The width of the PSF for synomag® is smaller because of a higher iron concentration on the one side, but also because of a higher SNR over the total spectrum resulting in a better resolution.

This sets the stage for the application specific surface design of synomag® particles meeting the requirements for further pre-clinical investigations.

AUTHOR'S STATEMENT
Research funding: The author states no funding involved. Conflict of interest: Authors state no conflict of interest.

REFERENCES
[1] B. Gleich and J. Weizenecker. Tomographic imaging using the nonlinear response of magnetic particles. *Nature*, 435(7046):1217-1217, 2005. doi: 10.1038/nature03808.
[2] T. Knopp, et al., Magnetic Particle Imaging: From Proof of Principle to Preclinical Applications, *Physics in Medicine & Biology*, vol. 62(14):R124. 2017.
[3] R. Ferguson, et al., Optimizing magnetite nanoparticles for mass sensitivity in magnetic particle imaging, *Med. Phys*, vol. 38(3), pp. 1619-26, 2011.
[4] F. Ludwig, et al., Characterization of magnetic nanoparticle systems with respect to their MPI performance, *Biomed Tech (Berl)*, vol. 58(6), pp. 535-45, 2013. Doi:10.1515/bmt-2013-0013.
[5] P. Vogel, et al., Traveling Wave Magnetic Particle Imaging, *IEEE TMI*, vol. 33(2), pp. 400-7, 2014. Doi: 10.1109/TMI.2013.2285472
[6] M.A. Rückert, et al., Adaptive hardware lens for TWMPI, *Proc. on IWMPI #8 (Hamburg)*, T12, 2018.
[7] P. Vogel, et al., Superspeed Traveling Wave Magnetic Particle Imaging,, *IEEE Trans. Magn.*, vol. 51(2): 6501603, 2015. DOI: 10.1109/TMAG.2014.2322897.
[8] P. Vogel & S. Lother, et al., MRI meets MPI: a bimodal MPI-MRI-tomograph, *IEEE TMI*, vol. 33(10), pp. 1954-9, 2014. DOI: 10.1109/TMI.2014.2327515.
[9] P. Vogel, et al., Real-time 3D Dynamic Rotating Slice-Scanning Mode for TWMPI, *IJMPI*, vol. 3(2):1706001, 2017. Doi:10.18416/ijmpi.2017.1706001.
[10] L. Lartigue, et al., Cooperative organization in iron oxide multi-core nanoparticles potentiates their efficiency as heating mediators and MRI contrast agents, *ACS Nano*, 6(12): 10935.10949, 2012.
[11] P. Lit. Bender, et al., Relating Magnetic Properties and High Hyperthermia Performance of Iron Oxide Nanoflowers. *J. Phys. Chem. C*, 2018. 122(5): p. 3068-3077.

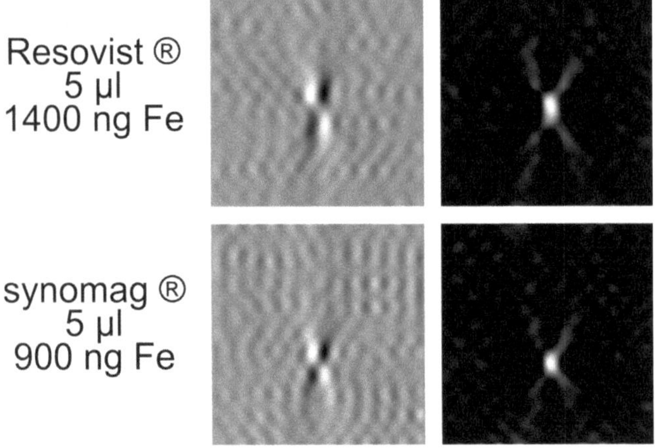

Figure 2: *Results of the reconstructed images:* **left:** *the point-spread-function (raw-image).* **Right:** *the reconstructed images.*

IV. Conclusions

The superior performance of synomag® particles with an almost three-times higher signal intensity compared to Resovist® using TWMPI technology is reported.

Long-term stable multimodal solid-state measurement phantoms for quantitative magnetic particle imaging

L. Wöckel[a], O. Kosch[b], J. Wells[b], F. Wiekhorst[b], K.-H. Herrmann[c], J.R. Reichenbach[c], S. Günther[d], C. Grüttner[e], and S. Dutz [a]*

[a] *Institut für Biomedizinische Technik und Informatik, Technische Universität Ilmenau, Germany*
[b] *Physikalisch-Technische Bundesanstalt Berlin, Germany*
[c] *Institute of Diagnostic and Interventional Radiology (IDIR), Friedrich Schiller University Jena, Germany*
[d] *Institute of Fluid Mechanics, Technische Universität Dresden, Germany*
[e] *micromod Partikeltechnologie GmbH, Rostock, Germany*
**Corresponding author, email: silvio.dutz@tu-ilmenau.de*

Magnetic particle imaging (MPI) is a tomographic imaging method to determine the spatial distribution of magnetic nanoparticles (MNP) within a defined volume. To evaluate the spatio-temporal resolution and the sensitivity of existing MPI scanners, we developed MPI phantoms with defined structures. To achieve long term stability of the measurement objects, we developed a method to incorporate commercially available MNP into a synthetic polymer with iron concentrations up to 200 mmol/l. The properties of polymer matrix embedded MNP were tested by magnetic particle spectroscopy (MPS) and the phantoms could successfully be visualized by MPI, computed tomography (CT) and magnetic resonance imaging (MRI).

I. Introduction

Magnetic Particle Imaging (MPI) is based on the spectral response of magnetic nanoparticles (MNP) to an oscillating magnetic excitation field. In combination with a static gradient field, spatial encoding of an MNP distribution in a volume is given. With detection limits in the nanomolar range [1] of MNP and due to its high spatio-temporal resolution, MPI is suitable for clinical applications like tumor detection or cell labeling [2]. To assess the potential and capability of different MPI scanner designs and architectures defined reference phantoms for imaging studies are required. Currently, most phantoms for MPI are based on nanoparticle dispersions filled in thin capillaries or containers [3]. The disadvantages of these phantoms are adhesion of the MNP to the walls of the capillaries and particle-particle interactions, often leading to agglomeration processes of MNP. As a consequence, the long-term stability is limited and such phantoms are not suitable for MPI scanner assessments. To overcome this disadvantage we developed long-term stable phantoms for MPI. Since MPI only detects MNP, we used MRI and µCT to gain information of the overall geometry of the phantoms.II. Materials and Methods

II.I Preparation of Ferrogels

For phantom preparation, the MNP have to be transferred from aqueous suspension into a synthetic matrix. Therefore, commercially available MNP (perimag®, micromod Partikeltechnologie GmbH) were dispersed into long-term stable matrix material (ELASTOSIL®, Wacker Chemie AG) with concentrations up to 200 mmol/L using an ethanol transfer protocol as described before [4].

II.II Construction of Phantoms

Our 3D printed phantoms consist of a mold with eight, radially arranged notches (2 x 2 mm^2 rectangular cross section, 5.4 mm length) into which approximately 24 µL MNP elastosil mixture were filled.

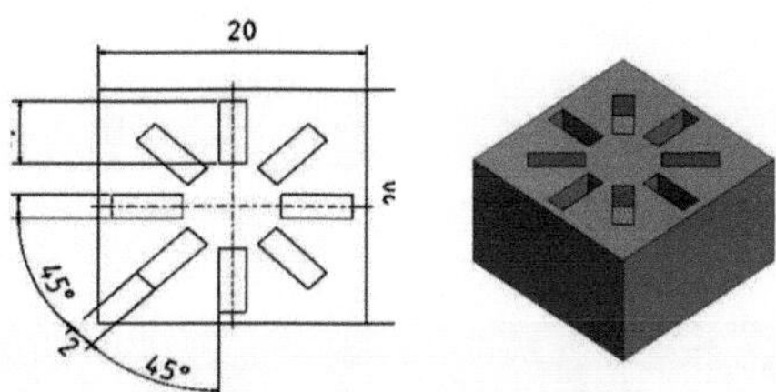

Figure 1: *Left: Sketch of the mold, Right: 3D-CAD model.*

II.III Characterization

The influence of immobilization of the MNP in the elastosil matrix on the MPI performance was investigated by magnetic particle spectroscopy (MPS). For the measurements, we used a commercial MPS spectrometer (MPS-3, Bruker) operating at an excitation frequency of 25 kHz and an amplitude of 25 mT. We analyzed changes in the amplitudes of the lower odd harmonics of the MPS spectrum between original MNP suspension and after elastosil matrix embedding. Finally, the phantoms were imaged by MPI (MPI 25/20FF, Bruker, Ettlingen, Germany), MRI (9.4T BioSpec 94/20 USR, Bruker, Ettlingen, Germany), and μCT (TomoTU, TU Dresden, Germany).

III. Results

The concentration independent harmonic ratio between 5th and 3rd harmonic (A5/A3) of the MPS spectra exhibited a decrease after embedding the MNP into elastosil compared to the MNP suspension. Repeated measurements over a period of one year revealed nearly no changes of the MPS performance of the spectra of the MNP in elastosil (Figure 2). One year after preparation, a loss of A5/A3 of less than 1% was observed, demonstrating the excellent long-term stability of the mixture and its very stable dynamic magnetic properties. Thus, the combination perimag® and elastosil is very promising in terms of long-term stability and signal performance and was used to prepare the phantoms.

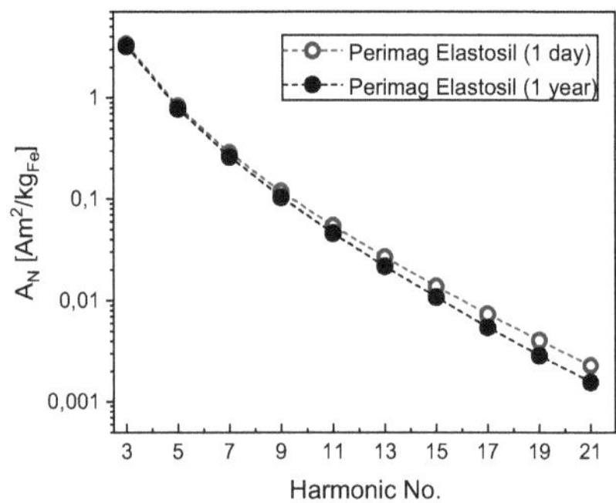

Figure 2: *MPS spectra of perimag® embedded in elastosil, measured at 25 mT, normalized to iron amount, measured 1 day after preparation and the same samples remeasured after storage of one year; lines serve only as a guide to the eye.*

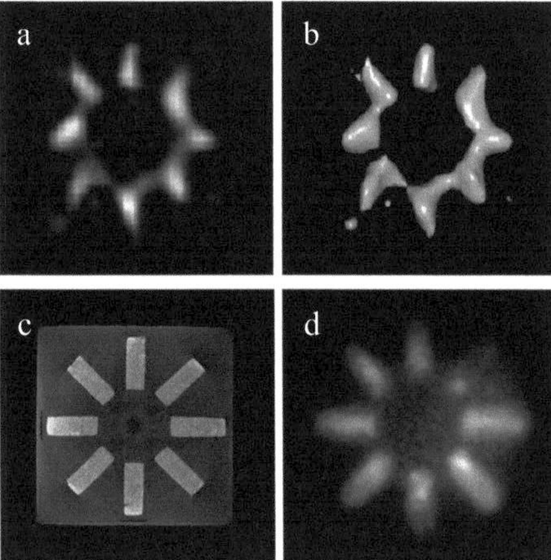

Figure 3: *Multimodal imaging of the phantom. Shown are MPI intensity image (a) and surface rendered image (b) as well as the reconstructed images from μCT (c) and MRI, ZTE sequence (d).*

Next, the MNP elastosil phantoms were imaged with MPI, MRI and μCT (Figure 3). The MPI reconstructions show the entire geometry of the phantom. In the μCT image, MNP elastosil matrix and 3D printed mold are clearly distinguishable. A rough picture of the geometry of the phantom can also be imaged in MRI.

IV. Discussion

With the establishment of an ethanol transfer process for embedding the MNP in a synthetic polymer matrix, we are able to provide long-term stable MNP phantoms for MPI imaging applications. The MPS spectra of the MNP elastosil matrix show a decrease of harmonics after immobilization of the MNP in the synthetic matrix, which first of all suppresses the Brownian rotation of the MNP and additionally may lead to a reduced dynamic response caused by MNP interactions. The MPI images are influenced by immobilization in a similar way, leading to a reduced reconstruction quality.

V. Conclusions

In this study, a long-term stable (more than one year) MNP synthetic polymer matrix for preparation of measurement phantoms for magnetic particle imaging is presented. The observed decrease of tracer performance found after the MNP transfer into ethanol and embedding into elastosil is compensated by the superior MPI signal intensity of perimag® together with the excellent long-term stability of the MNP elastosil matrix. From this material, long-term stable measurement phantoms for multimodal imaging were prepared, which were imaged sucessfully by means of MPI, μCT, and MRI.

ACKNOWLEDGEMENTS

This work was supported by Deutsche Forschungsgemeinschaft (DFG) in the frame of the project quantMPI (DU 1293/6-1 and TR 408/9-1).

AUTHOR'S STATEMENT

Research funding: The author state no funding involved. Conflict of interest: Authors state no conflict of interest. Informed consent: Informed consent has been obtained from all individuals included in this study. Ethical approval: The research related to human use complies with all the relevant national regulations, institutional policies and was performed in accordance with the tenets of the Helsinki Declaration, and has been approved by the authors' institutional review board or equivalent committee.

REFERENCES

[1] M. Graeser et al. Human-sized Magnetic Particle Imaging for Brain Applications. arXiv:1810.07987 (**2018**).

[2] H. Paysen, J. Wells, O. Kosch, U. Steinhoff, L. Trahms, T. Schaeffter, F. Wiekhorst. Towards quantitative magnetic particle imaging: A comparison with magnetic particle spectroscopy. *AIP Advances* 8: 056712 (**2018**).

[3] T. Knopp, T. M. Buzug. Magnetic Particle Imaging: An Introduction to Imaging Principles and Scanner Instrumentation. *Springer-Verlag Berlin Heidelberg* (**2012**).

[4] L. Wöckel, J. Wells, O. Kosch, S. Lyer, C. Alexiou, C. Grüttner, F. Wiekhorst, S. Dutz. Long-term stable measurement phantoms for magnetic particle imaging. *J. Magn. Magn. Mater.* 471: 1–7 (**2019**).

Confounding Effects of Temperature and Viscosity Towards Relaxation Mapping

M. Utkur[a,b*] and E. U. Saritas[a,b,c]

[a] *Department of Electrical and Electronics Engineering, Bilkent University, Ankara, Turkey*
[b] *National Magnetic Resonance Research Center (UMRAM), Bilkent University, Ankara, Turkey*
[c] *Neuroscience Program, Sabuncu Brain Research Center, Bilkent University, Ankara, Turkey*
[*] *Corresponding author, email: mustafa.utkur@bilkent.edu.tr*

Abstract: Potential functional imaging applications of magnetic particle imaging (MPI) include viscosity mapping and temperature mapping. However, these two environmental factors can have confounding effects on the MPI signal. We recently proposed a technique to map the relaxation constant directly from the MPI signal. In this work, we apply this technique to investigate the confounding effect of temperature and viscosity on the relaxation map, using experiments performed on our in-house magnetic fluid hyperthermia (MFH) and magnetic particle spectrometer (MPS) setups.

I. Introduction

Magnetic particle imaging (MPI) cell tracking applications have demonstrated that the nanoparticle response alters inside a cell [1,2], possibly due to increased intracellular viscosity [3]. Recently, a few methods were proposed for measuring viscosity with MPI, for example, through the harmonic ratio of nanoparticle's magnetization curve [3], through the nanoparticle delays induced by relaxation [4], or via a multi-contrast reconstruction [5]. However, these techniques may be susceptible to errors as the viscosity of the medium is also dependent on temperature.

The effect of temperature on the MPI signal was previously investigated for therapeutic purposes [6]. A multi-color MPI technique was also proposed for temperature mapping [7]. Integrating temperature and viscosity mapping to separate these two confounding effects would be beneficial for diagnostic and therapeutic purposes.

Previously, we have proposed a technique to map the nanoparticle relaxation time constant via estimating it by recovering the mirror symmetry of the underlying nanoparticle signal, without any calibration or prior information [8, 9]. Recently, we have extended this technique to show that it can be used for viscosity mapping in imaging experiments [10]. In this work, we investigate the confounding effects of temperature and viscosity for our relaxation-based viscosity mapping technique.

II. Material and Methods

II.I. Theory

The relaxation behaviors of nanoparticles are governed by Brownian and Néel relaxation mechanisms, where the alignment of nanoparticle magnetization occurs externally and internally, respectively. The zero-field relaxation time constants for these two mechanisms are given as [11].

$$\tau_B = \frac{3V_H\eta}{k_bT} \quad (1) \qquad \tau_N = \tau_0 e^{\frac{KV_C}{k_bT}} \quad (2)$$

Here, V_H is hydrodynamic volume, η is viscosity, k_b is the Boltzmann constant, T is temperature, K is anisotropy constant, V_C is the core volume of nanoparticle, and τ_0 is the attempt time [11]. Previously, the relaxation-delayed signal in x-space MPI was modeled with [12]:

$$s_{received}(t) = s_{ideal(t)} * \frac{1}{\tau}e^{-\frac{t}{\tau}} \quad (3)$$

τ is the relaxation time constant and $s_{ideal}(t)$ is the nanoparticle signal without relaxation. In this phenomenological model, τ does not directly correspond to τ_B or τ_N, but is a combination of the two. We have previously proposed a relaxation mapping technique that can directly estimate τ from the MPI signal [8, 9]. Here, we utilize the same technique for the magnetic particle spectrometer (MPS) experiments, to determine the simultaneous effects of viscosity and temperature on τ.

II.II. Experimental Setup

Our in-house magnetic fluid hyperthermia (MFH) and MPS setups are shown in Fig. 1. We have targeted seven different temperature values (see Table 1). The samples were heated up from 20 °C to 50 °C using the MFH setup. Once a targeted temperature was reached, the sample was briefly moved to the MPS setup for measurement, and promptly returned back to the MFH setup. This transfer was performed manually.

The MFH setup is composed of a water-cooled excitation coil with 3 layers of 6 turns each, made out of a 6-mm diameter hollow copper tube with 1-mm wall thickness. The magnetic field was calibrated using a sniffer coil. Heating was achieved at 147 kHz and 15 mT. A signal generator (GW Instek MFG2260) was utilized to generate the excitation signal, which was then amplified with a power amplifier (AE Techron 7224). The temperature of the nanoparticles was monitored with a fiber optic temperature probe (Reflex-4) throughout the experiments to ensure that there was no significant heat loss during sample transfer between MFH and MPS setups. MPS measurements were performed on our in-house setup [8] at 1.1 kHz and 15 mT.

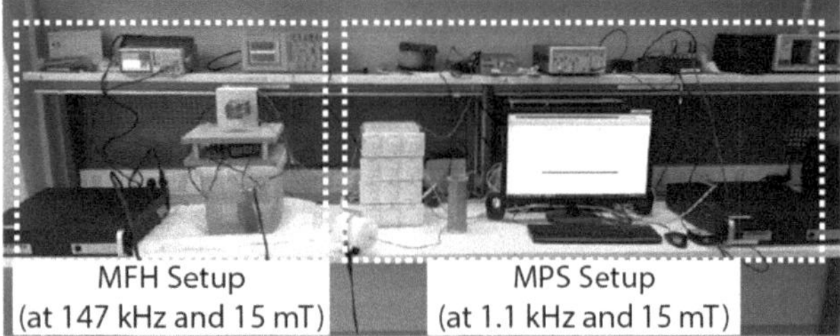

Figure 1: *Our in-house MFH and MPS setups. The nanoparticles are heated up at 147 kHz and 15 mT with the MFH setup (left). The MPS signals are acquired at 1.1 kHz and 15 mT (right).*

II.III. Sample Preparation

Four different glycerol/water mixtures were prepared with the same total volume of 500 μL, and the same nanoparticle amount of 378 μL of undiluted Perimag nanoparticles (Micromod GmbH) at 230 mmol Fe/L to avoid any concentration bias. The resulting glycerol percentages were 0% (i.e., water only), 8.8%, 16.8%, and 24.4% by volume. Table 1 lists the corresponding viscosity levels. Here, the values at 20 °C, 30 °C, 40 °C, and 50 °C were taken from [13], and the remaining values were interpolated. Similar viscosity values are highlighted with identical shading.

Table 1: *Viscosity of glycerol by volume at different temperatures.*

Glycerol	Viscosity (mPa·s)						
(%)	20°C	25°C	30°C	35°C	40°C	45°C	50°C
0	1.00	0.90	0.80	0.73	0.66	0.60	0.55
8.8	1.25	1.12	1.00	0.90	0.80	0.73	0.66
16.8	1.60	1.42	1.25	1.12	1.00	0.90	0.80
24.4	2.10	1.83	1.60	1.42	1.25	1.12	1.00

III. Results & Discussion

The estimated relaxation time constants at seven different temperatures are shown in Fig. 2 for the fixed sample case (left) and fixed viscosity case (right). The fixed-viscosity case was plotted incorporating the information in Table 1. At a fixed temperature, τ decreases as viscosity increases, which is consistent with our previous work at 1.1 kHz [8]. More importantly, τ decreases with increasing temperature, as expected from Eqs. 1 and 2. This decrease has different slopes for the fixed sample vs. the fixed viscosity cases, highlighting the need to separate the effects of temperature and viscosity. If the nanoparticles enter a high viscosity

medium *in vivo* (e.g., cancerous tissue) and then heated up via MFH, τ will decrease more than what one would expect with the temperature change alone. This would cause an overestimation in the temperature map. Note that this problem is not specific to our method, but can potentially hinder all multi-color MPI temperature mapping techniques.

Experimentally estimated τ values display different trends under different drive field parameters [8]. For example, τ may increase or decrease with viscosity, depending on the amplitude/frequency of the drive field. While this behavior is not well understood, it could be exploited to extract both viscosity and temperature information, e.g., via estimating τ from two different measurements at different drive field amplitudes or frequencies.

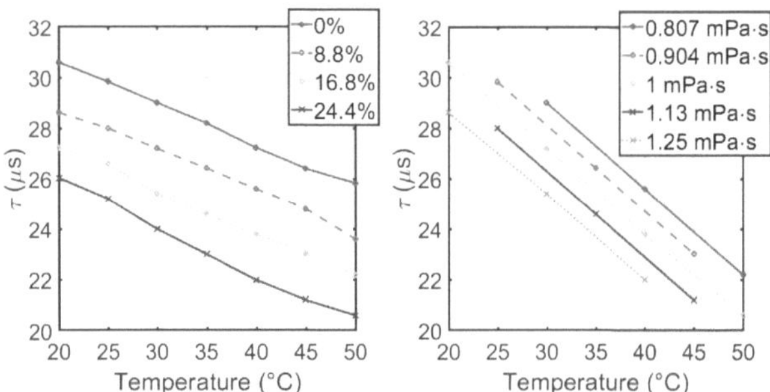

Figure 2: *τ vs. temperature. The same data is displayed in two different formats: fixed sample case at four different glycerol percentages (left) and fixed viscosity case, using Table 1 (right).*

V. Conclusions

In this work, we have demonstrated the confounding effects of viscosity and temperature on our relaxation mapping technique. If the viscosity of the medium *in vivo* is different than what one expects, this can cause erroneous temperature estimations. Therefore, these two effects need to be separated via incorporating additional measurements.

AUTHOR'S STATEMENT
Research funding: This work was supported by the Scientific and Technological Research Council of Turkey (TUBITAK 115E677). Conflict of interest: Authors state no conflict of interest.

REFERENCES
[1] D. E. Markov et. al., Human erythrocytes as nanoparticle carriers for magnetic particle imaging. Phys. Med. Biol., 55(21):6461–6473, 2010. doi:10.1088/0031-9155/55/21/008.
[2] J. Rahmer et. al., Nanoparticle encapsulation in red blood cells enables blood-pool magnetic particle imaging hours after injection. Phys. Med. Biol., 58(12):3965–3977, 2013. doi:10.1088/0031-9155/58/12/3965.
[3] A. M. Rauwerdink and J. B. Weaver. Viscous effects on nanoparticle magnetization harmonics. J. Magn. Magn. Mater. 322(6):609-613,2010, doi:10.1016/j.jmmm.2009.10.024.
[4] T. Viereck et. al., Dual-frequency magnetic particle imaging of the Brownian particle contribution. J. Magn. Magn. Mater., 427:156-161, 2017. doi:10.1016/j.jmmm.2016.11.003.
[5] M. Möddel et. al., Viscosity quantification using multi-contrast magnetic particle imaging. New J. Phys., 20(083001), 2018. doi:10.1088/1367-2630/aad44b.
[6] K. Murase et. al., Usefulness of Magnetic Particle Imaging for Predicting the Therapeutic Effect of Magnetic Hyperthermia. OJMI, 5(2), 2015. doi:10.4236/ojmi.2015.52013.
[7] C. Stehning et. al., Simultaneous magnetic particle imaging (MPI) and temperature mapping using multi-color MPI. IJMPI, 2(2), 2016. doi:10.18416/ijmpi.2016.1612001.
[8] M. Utkur et. al., Relaxation-based viscosity mapping for magnetic particle imaging. Phys. Med. Biol., 62(9):3422, 2016, doi:10.1088/1361-6560/62/9/3422.
[9] Y. Muslu et. al., Calibration-Free Relaxation-Based Multi-Color Magnetic Particle Imaging. IEEE TMI, 37(8):1920–1931, 2018. doi:10.1109/TMI.2018.2818261.
[10] M. Utkur et. al., Viscosity Mapping through Relaxation Effects for Functional Magnetic Particle Imaging. IWMPI (Hamburg), 2018.
[11] R. M. Ferguson et. al., Size-Dependent Relaxation Properties of Monodisperse Magnetite Nanoparticles Measured Over Seven Decades of Frequency by AC Susceptometry. IEEE Trans. Magn., 49(7):3441–3444, 2013. doi:10.1109/TMAG.2013.2239621.
[12] L. R. Croft et. al., Relaxation in X-space magnetic particle imaging. IEEE TMI, 31(12):2335-2342, 2012, doi:10.1109/TMI.2012.2217979.
[13] J. B. Segur and H.E. Oberstar. Viscosity of Glycerol and Its Aqueous Solutions. Ind. Eng. Chem. Res., 43(9):2117–2120, 1951. doi:10.1021/ie50501a040.

Improved depth sensitivity by separation of excitation and detection coils

M.M. van de Loosdrecht[a*], **H.J.G. Krooshoop**[a], **and B. ten Haken**[a]

[a] *Magnetic Detection and Imaging group, Faculty of Science and Technology, University of Twente, Enschede, the Netherlands*
[*] *Corresponding author, email: m.m.vandeloosdrecht@utwente.nl*

A laparoscopic probe for magnetic sentinel node procedures has been developed. Superparamagnetic iron oxide nanoparticles (SPIONs) are used as a tracer. They are selectively detected by Differential Magnetometry (DiffMag). Excitation and detection coils are separated. To make this possible, we developed active compensation, which removes influence of the excitation field. Separation of coils leads to improved depth sensitivity, from 20 mm with our handheld probe to 80 mm with our novel laparoscopic probe. As stated by Biot-Savart law, we win a factor distance to the third power by separating the excitation and detection part of the system.

I. Introduction

A novel laparoscopic probe for magnetic sentinel node procedures has been developed, as shown in Fig. 1. This procedure is used to determine if a tumor has metastasized via the lymphatic system [1], enabling personalized patient care. To find lymph nodes that have the highest chance on containing metastases – sentinel nodes – we make use of superparamagnetic iron oxide nanoparticles (SPIONs) as a tracer.

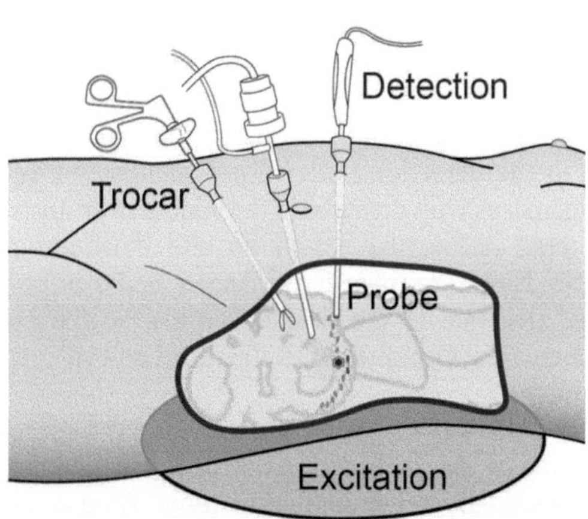

Figure 1: *Novel laparoscopic probe for magnetic sentinel node biopsy. Excitation and detection part of the system are separated to improve depth sensitivity.*

To selectively detect SPIONs in the diamagnetic human body we make use of Differential Magnetometry (DiffMag). DiffMag utilizes nonlinear properties of SPIONs, similar to Magnetic Particle Imaging (MPI) and Magnetic Particle Spectroscopy (MPS). The main differences are that we use a smaller AC amplitude (± 1 mT, depending on prototype and location) and measure in the time domain instead of harmonics spectra. In DiffMag, the excitation field consists of two parts: a continuous AC field and DC offsets. The total excitation sequence consists of four parts: no DC offset (u_0), a positive DC offset (u_+), no DC offset (u_0) and a negative DC offset (u_-). Due to nonlinearity of SPIONs, the amplitude of the detected signal is lower when a positive or negative DC offset is applied. The difference in amplitude between blocks with and without DC offsets is defined as DiffMag counts:

$$DiffMag\ counts = \frac{1}{2}[(u_0 - u_+) + (u_0 - u_-)]$$

Similar to MPI and MPS, DiffMag makes use of excitation and detection coils. A handheld probe was developed that contains both excitation and detection coils for use in open surgery [2]. However, in laparoscopic surgery, the diameter of the probe is restricted by the use of standard trocars. The depth sensitivity of a coil is determined by the diameter of the coil, according to Biot-Savart law. As a result, making the handheld probe smaller would result in inadequate depth sensitivity, making it impossible to find sentinel nodes in laparoscopic surgery.

II. Material and Methods

II.I. Setup

The problem of limited depth sensitivity can be solved by separation of the excitation and detection part of the system. The excitation coils will be large and placed underneath the patient, as shown in Fig. 1. The detection coils can be small enough to fit through standard laparoscopic trocars (12 mm).

The main challenge after separating excitation and detection coils is movement of the detection coils with respect to the excitation coils, leading to a changing mutual inductance. The detector signal will be obscured by the changing excitation field, making it impossible to detect the tiny magnetic signature of SPIONs.

To solve this problem, we developed active compensation. Compensation coils are used to couple in extra field. This field is actively adjusted to match imbalance of the probe. This imbalance of the probe is caused both by the excitation field and by materials with a linear magnetic susceptibility in the mT field range, such as tissue and surgical steel. Active compensation is only possible because we make use of DiffMag. Due to the extra field coupled in by the compensation coils, the amplitude of the measured signal changes. However, the difference in amplitude – DiffMag counts – remain exactly the same.

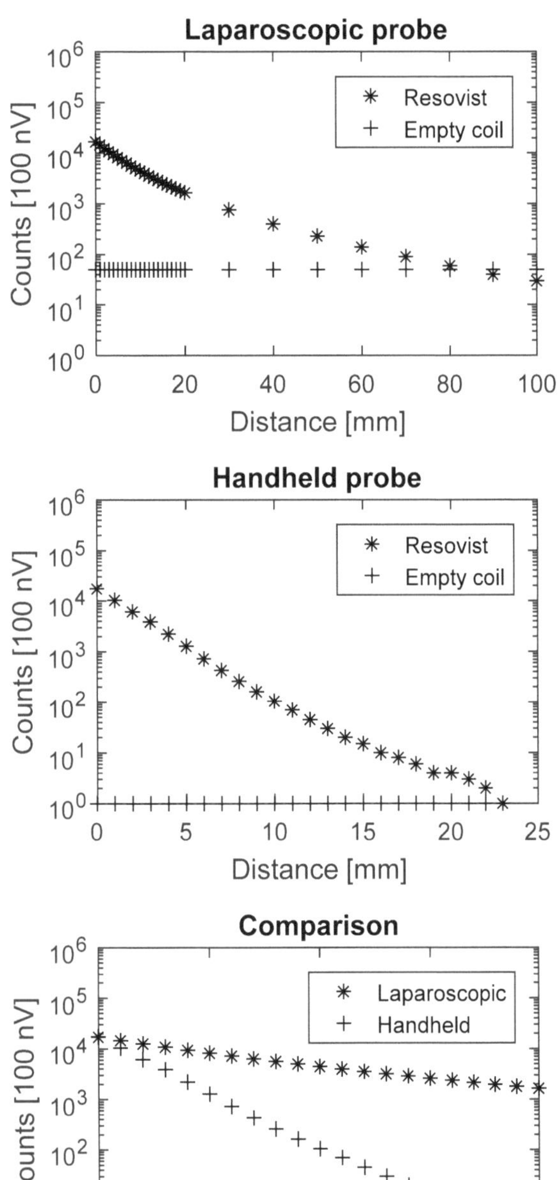

Figure 2: *Measurement results for our laparoscopic and handheld probe at various distances to the probe.*

II.II. Material

A Resovist® (Bayer Schering Pharma GmbH) sample of ± 1.5 mL containing ± 45 mg Fe was used in all measurements.

II.III. Measurements

The sample was measured at various distances to the probe with our laparoscopic probe and our handheld probe. For the laparoscopic probe, with separated excitation and detection coils, the sample was placed at a set location in the excitation field (at the central axis through the coil, 3 cm above excitation coil surface). The probe containing the detection coils was first positioned directly on top of the sample. Next, a robotic arm (Meca500, Mecademic) was used to move the probe upwards. For the first 20 mm this was done in steps of 1 mm, and after 20 mm in steps of 10 mm to a total distance of 100 mm. For the handheld probe, the probe was placed on top of the sample and then moved upwards in steps of 1 mm to a total distance of 20 mm.

III. Results

Measurement results are shown in Fig. 2. It is shown that SPIONs can be measured 20 mm deep with our handheld probe and 80 mm deep with our laparoscopic probe.

IV. Discussion

Increase in depth sensitivity from 20 to 80 mm is a result of separation of the excitation and detection part of the system. Decrease of a magnetic field over distance is described by Biot-Savart law. How rapid the field decreases is influenced by both the diameter of the coils and the distance to the sample. Biot-Savart law states that the magnetic field created by a circular coil decreases with distance to the third power. In the handheld probe, measuring nodes that lie deeper in tissue means an increased distance to the excitation coils as well as to the detection coils. Consequently, the measured signal decreases with distance to the sixth power. In our novel laparoscopic probe, the excitation and detection part are separated. Therefore, measuring deeper nodes only leads to increased distance to the detection coils, so the measured signal decreases with distance to the third power.

V. Conclusions

Our solution of separating excitation and detection coils leads to a fundamentally better depth sensitivity. As stated by Biot-Savart law we win a factor distance to the third power when the diameter of the probe remains constant.

ACKNOWLEDGEMENTS

Financial support from the Netherlands Organization for Scientific Research (NWO), under the research program Magnetic Sensing for Laparoscopy (MagLap) with project number 14322 is gratefully acknowledged.

REFERENCES

[1] A. E. Giuliano and A. Gangi, "Sentinel node biopsy and improved patient care," Breast J., vol. 21, no. 1, 2015.

[2] S. Waanders, M. Visscher, R. R. Wildeboer, T. O. B. Oderkerk, H. J. G. Krooshoop, and B. Ten Haken, "A handheld SPIO-based sentinel lymph node mapping device using differential magnetometry.," Phys. Med. Biol., vol. 61, no. 22, pp. 8120–8134, Nov. 2016.

Bruker – Lunch Session

Jochen Franke

Product Manager Magnetic Particle Imaging, System Engineering & Integration
Bruker BioSpin MRI, Germany

Achievements of the MPI community – Time is of the essence

Take a break and enjoy lunch with us! We will give you a quick overview of the recent outstanding scientific achievements in the field of MPI. From real-time applications to image guided actuation, Jochen Franke will provide you a vivid summary of the latest results gathered on the Bruker MPI system.

Bruker is glad to relentlessly drive innovation for scientists, while our close collaboration with the very dynamic MPI community is the key success factor empowering MPI as one of the most promising imaging techniques for new spatially encoded theranostics approaches.

As time is of the essence, get inspired by our life science community recent achievements. Continue pioneering the fascinating field of Magnetic Particle Imaging technology together with us. Let's pave new ways to personalized medicine and revolutionize clinical diagnostic and therapeutic routines.

Session 08: Instrumentation II

Feasibility of a spatial resolution enhancement by a passive dual coil resonator (pDCR) insert for large bore MPI systems

S.D. Reinartz*[#][b], D. Pantke[#][a], A. Mogarkar[a], F. Mueller[a] and V. Schulz[a]

[a] *Physics of Molecular Imaging Systems, RWTH Aachen University, Aachen, Germany*
[b] *Department of Diagnostic and Interventional Radiology, Uniklinikum RWTH Aachen, Aachen, Germany*
* *Corresponding author, email: {sebastian.reinartz;volkmar.schulz}@pmi.rwth-aachen.de*
[#] *equally contributing authors*

Abstract: Signal-to-noise amplification is one of the key items to establish MPI as a clinical tool. Instead of using a dedicated receive coil, our approach is to use of a purely passive dual coil resonator (pDCR), which is placed in the direction of the x-axis in the MPI scanner bore (Bruker, Ettlingen). The pDCR is tuned to a high resonance frequency ($\gg$ 25 kHz) to avoid direct coupling with the drive fields. The measurement of the corresponding spectra at incrementally increased amplitudes of the drive fields showed a new peak at high harmonics at approx. 650 kHz as well as a general increase of the particle signal and background noise. No relevant warming was observed (10 mT, 2 seconds scan time)

I. Introduction

Signal-to-noise ratio (SNR) enhancement in MPI is one of the most important and active topics, e.g. in order to differentiate structures from background noise [1, 2]. To achieve this, special receiving coils in combination with low-noise amplifiers are usually used to capture the MPI signal with the highest SNR. One of the biggest challenges with the additional local receive coils is to minimize the inductive coupling between the MPI drive field coils and the local receive coil to reduce drifting of background signal. Unfortunately, lower particle concentrations still ended up in images with low spatial resolution [3] as higher harmonic signals disappear in the noise level of the receiver. In many applications, improved details of the object to be examined with high resolution are required. For this purpose, we propose a novel purely passive dual coil resonator (pDCR) according to the principle of a Lenz lens [4, 5], first developed for our Bruker MPI scanner. The pDCR is inserted into the scanner bore without any electrical connection to the MPI system. The intrinsic function of the pDCR is to increase the inductive coupling between the object and the x-channel of the MPI system at higher frequencies (Fig. 1a). In addition to the investigations of the gain in spatial resolution, and possible thermal effects were also investigated.

II. Material and Methods

Design: A coaxial cylinder construction (Fig. 1b) with an inner diameter of 50 mm and an outer diameter of 108 mm was 3D printed (Fig. 1c). On each cylinder, 20 turns of a 1.5mm thick insulated Litz wire were continuously wound with identical sense of winding and electrically connected by means of a capacitor (C = 0.726 nF). Thus, the setup was

tuned to a resonant frequency of ~596 kHz. The frequency was selected to be on the right edge of the receive chain's resonance peak. This pDCR fits into the bore of the preclinical MPI (Bruker, Ettlingen, Fig 1b) along its x-axis and is placed in the center of the field of view (FOV). This reduces the effective scanner bore to 40 mm in diameter, taking into account the wall thickness of 5mm.

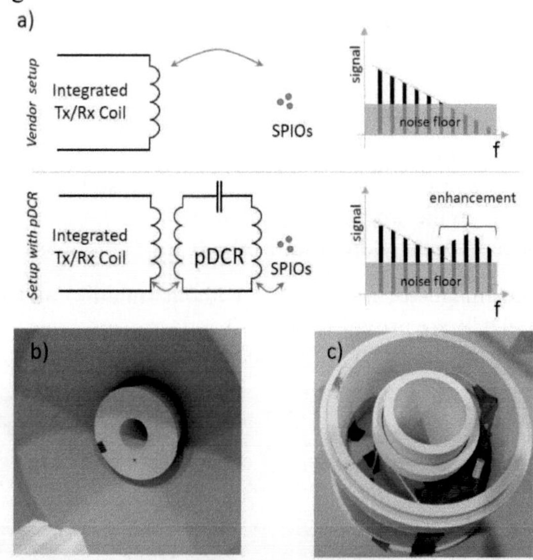

Figure 1: *a) Schematics of the pDCR with signal enhancement due to increased coupling of the high frequency components of the SPIO signal with the integrated Tx/Rx coil. b) pDCR inserted into the Bruker MPI system. c) 3D printed pDCR.*

Application: A phial for acquiring system matrices with a sample of 2 mm³ filled with Perimag 25 mg/ml (micromod, Germany) was investigated with and without the pDCR. The drive field strengths of 1-10 mT were increased incrementally in 1 mT steps in all excitation channels. The standard excitation frequencies of the drive fields were used, the number of averages was set to 100, which ended up in approx. 2 seconds measurement time per image. Immediately afterwards, heating of the Litz wires and the capacitor was checked manually. Object measurements were subtracted from background measurements.

III. Results

In each of the ten drive field strengths of the x-channel, a new peak was visible in the background corrected spectra, stable at approx. 650 kHz (Fig. 2). Furthermore, a plateau-like increase of the spectrum until the right edge of the new resonance peak was observed as well, increasing particle signal and background noise.

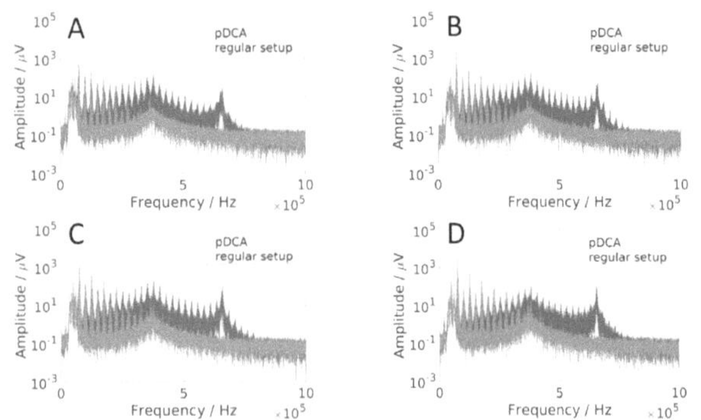

Figure 2: *Spectra without pDCR (light grey- standard setting) and with pDCR (dark grey) for A=7mT, B=8mT, C=9mT and D=10mT drive field amplitude of a 2 mm³ Perimag® 25mg/ml sample, (micromod, Germany).*

The SNR was increased for every drive field amplitude by 0.11/0.05 (7 mT), 0.12/0.04 (8 mT), 0.13/0.04 (9 mT), and 0.07/0.04 (10 mT). A considerable net gain can be observed depending on the frequency, particularly in the region of the resonance frequency, in mean 2.50 ± 0.5.

Phantom images of a letter "C" without (middle) and with (right) pDCR are provided in Fig. 3.

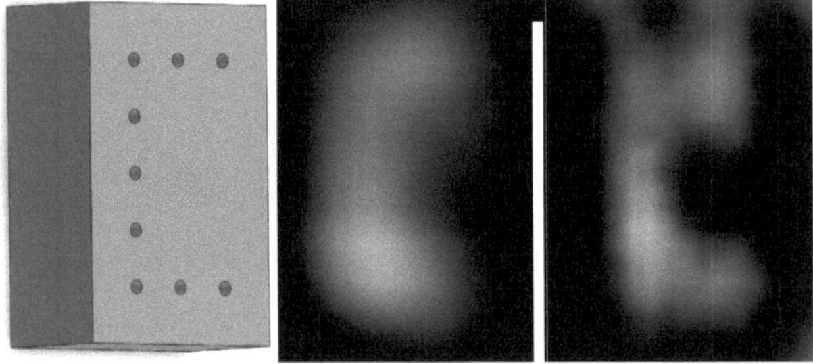

Figure 3*: Example letter "C": Left: CAD Phantom sketch, composed of several drillings filled with Perimag. Middle: image without pDCR. Right: image with pDCR (An improved resolution and increased signal intensity can be observed, but also increased level of noise. (Reconstruction: Frequencies: 1.25MHz, iterations 2).*

A slight, just palpable warming could be detected in all experiments only at 9 and 10mT field strength.

IV. Discussion

This simple design of the pDCR theoretically causes the MPI signal to dominantly couple into the inner coil of the pDCR which induces current. Due to electronic connection, the associated current also flows through the large turns of the pDCR and thus emits another B-field, which corresponds to the amplified MPI signal. The low-noise amplifier of the x-channel of the MPI device now registers a superposition of the original MPI signal and the amplified signal from the pDCR. This can be seen in the presented measurements.

The net gain of the received signal potentially leads to an enhanced image spatial resolution as mostly higher frequencies are amplified. The resonance peak of ~596 kHz (free space) is shifted to about 650 kHz. This shift is very likely caused by the coupling of the pDCR with the MPI scanner's transmit and receive coils.

Detailed investigations of the overall pDCR concept on the spatial resolution and SNR will be presented during the conference.

V. Conclusions

In this paper, the proof of concept of a selective MPI signal amplification by a purely passive double coil resonator (pDCR) has been demonstrated. A phantom image indicates the clear gain in SNR and image resolution. So far, no substantial heating was observed. Further investigations on gain in spatial resolution and SNR are needed.

ACKNOWLEDGEMENTS

We thank our colleagues from the department of "Physics of Molecular Imaging Systems" who provided knowledge and expertise that greatly assisted the research.

AUTHOR'S STATEMENT

Research funding: The author state no funding involved. Conflict of interest: Authors state no conflict of interest.

REFERENCES

1. Weizenecker, J., J. Borgert, and B. Gleich, *A simulation study on the resolution and sensitivity of magnetic particle imaging.* Phys Med Biol, 2007. **52**(21): p. 6363-74. DOI: 10.1088/0031-9155/52/21/001
2. Borgert, J., et al., *Fundamentals and applications of magnetic particle imaging.* J Cardiovasc Comput Tomogr, 2012. **6**(3): p. 149-53. DOI: 10.1016/j.jcct.2012.04.007
3. Graeser, M., et al., *Towards Picogram Detection of Superparamagnetic Iron-Oxide Particles Using a Gradiometric Receive Coil.* Sci Rep, 2017. **7**(1): p. 6872. DOI: 10.1038/s41598-017-06992-5
4. Schoenmaker, J., K. Pirota, and J. Teixeira, *Magnetic flux amplification by Lenz lenses.* Review of Scientific Instruments, 2013. **84**(8): p. 085120. DOI: 10.1063/1.4819234
5. Wiltshire, M., et al., *Microstructured magnetic materials for RF flux guides in magnetic resonance imaging.* Science, 2001. **291**(5505): p. 849-851. DOI: 10.1126/science.291.5505.849

Towards a Single-Sided FFL MPI Scanner for *in vivo* Breast Cancer Imaging

E. Mason [a] **and A. Tonyushkin** [b*]

[a] *Harvard-MIT Health Sciences & Technology, Cambridge, MA, USA*
[b] *Physics Department, University of Massachusetts Boston, Boston, MA, USA*
[*] *Corresponding author, email: alexey.tonyushkin@umb.edu*

MPI has shown great promise to surpass existing in vivo imaging modalities in many clinical applications. However, one of the challenges to MPI being translated into clinical practice has been the ability to scale up the selection field coils to surround a human body while being able to generate and drive a sufficiently strong magnetic field gradient. These requirements impose safety concerns as well as prohibitively high power consumption in devices with large cylindrical volume. Therefore, we consider alternative topologies such as a single-sided geometry in which all the hardware is located on one side of the imaging volume to allow imaging regions of interest in humans, e.g., breast cancer. Here, we present our progress in developing such a single-sided field-free line MPI scanner.

I. Introduction

A single-sided MPI scanner [1,2] could be an essential technology to translate the MPI modality into the human domain. This will enable diagnosis of specific pathologies, such as cancer. MPI cancer imaging relies on passive or active nanoparticle accumulation by tumor tissue, such that the nanoparticles serve as tumor markers [3,4]. In this work, we assume sufficiently specific and sensitive accumulation to correlate presence of superparamagnetic ion-oxide nanoparticles (SPIOs) with tumor tissue and absence of SPIOs with healthy tissue. Specifically, the geometry of the single-sided scanner is suitable for the breast cancer imaging through SPIO uptake by tumor [4] or lymph nodes [5]. Breast cancer is the most common type of cancer in women worldwide [6]. The current standard screening method is x-ray mammography that has particularly low sensitivity and specificity in dense breast tissue. Mammography also involves significant patient discomfort. Other screening techniques include MRI, ultrasound, and CT. However, they can only be used as supplemental techniques due to being too expensive, time consuming, or utilizing ionizing radiation. Thus, it is important to develop a new safe, ultra-sensitive, and robust screening technique.

We present our progress toward the development of a novel single-sided MPI scanner suitable for *in vivo* breast cancer imaging in humans. The single-sided device has all the hardware on one side of the imaging volume; therefore, such a device can be used equally well on small animals and humans for multidimensional diagnostic imaging and as a magnetic particle spectrometer (MPS) [7]. In our approach, we develop a single-sided MPI system with a more promising field topology, namely, field-free line (FFL) [8,9] as opposed to the originally implemented field-free point

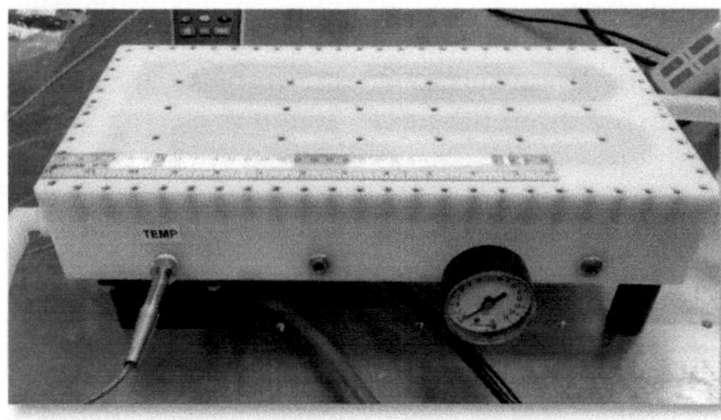

Figure 1: *Single-sided FFL selection-drive coil set in the enclosure with the temperature and pressure sensors.*

(FFP) [1] geometry, for a potential gain in SNR, more robust image reconstruction, and larger field of view.

II. Material and Methods

Fig. 1 shows the complete coil structure in the enclosure with the embedded temperature and water pressure sensors. The system is designed to hold high DC and AC currents, handle large magnetic forces, and incorporates water cooling to address high power dissipation both due to coil losses and eddy currents in the coil structure. The final prototype was manufactured by Resonance Research, Inc. (Billerica, MA).

Fig. 2 shows the simulation model of the coils and the simulated contour field plots at the reference current $I = 150$ A. In this prototype device, we incorporated the minimum number of elongated electromagnetic coils required to encode the image. The top coils are used to create a stationary selection gradient magnetic field, as well as to shift the FFL in the xy-plane by altering the relative current in the coils. The bottom coil, located in the middle as shown in Fig. 2A, is used primarily as a coil to generate the

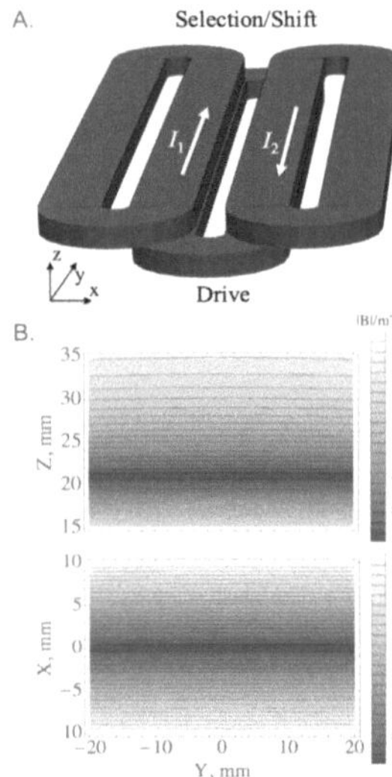

Figure 2: A. Selection-drive structure design composed of three coils. B. The magnetic field simulations showing the FFL in the zy- and xy-planes. Notably, the FFL is straight over more than 4 cm of length.

drive field. Each electromagnetic coil is 30 cm long (5.5:1 aspect ratio) and consists of 8 pancake-like elements with 26 windings of rectangular copper wire. The maximum magnetic fields at the surface in the *iso*-plane are measured to be 0.62 mT/A from the top coils and 0.2 mT/A from the bottom coil. The measured static height of the FFL above the device's surface is h=17 mm +/- 1 mm. The measured gradient strength is 15 mT/m/A, which gives gradient G = 1.5 T/m at I=100 A.

III. Results and Discussion

The data and the corresponding experimental arrangments showing the Rx coil and the sample placed on top of the surface coil are given in Fig. 3.

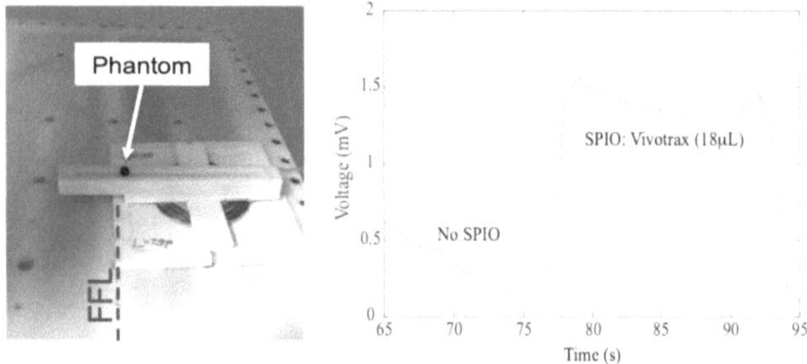

Figure 3: Experimental setup and the 3rd harmonic signal from the undiluted 0.1 mg Fe point sample of VivoTrax showing SNR=30.

In the magnetic particle detection experiment, a point-source bulb phantom of 18 µL undiluted VivoTrax SPIO (Magnetic Insight, Alameda, CA) was used. The phantom was placed in a holder in the symmetry (FFL) plane at the overall height of 1 cm above the surface (see Fig. 3). The drive coil was driven at a carrier frequency of f_0=23 kHz and a current amplitude of I=14.2 A, which was pulsed with 1.2% duty cycle. The received signal was notch filtered to reject the drive frequency component and tuned to the 3rd harmonic. The time series 3rd harmonic data with and without the sample show SNR=30 (see Fig. 3), which, in principle, allows ~10 times further dilution of the sample without any upgrades to the apparatus.

In order to be able to perform imaging in 3-D, we will implement *xy*-plane shifting of the FFL and combine it with the depth adjustment and mechanical rotation of the imaging object. While the next generation scanner may have mechanically rotated coils, for simplicity, our prototype scanner has a stationary coil structure. For the image encoding, we will implement a mechanical turntable and utilize a standard filtered back-projection reconstruction technique.

IV. Conclusions

To date, we have built a first prototype of a single-sided coil assembly with the FFL geometry that consists of all the required coils in a unilateral configuration. The measured magnetic field corroborates the simulations. We further validated our device by demonstrating magnetic particle signal detection using a point-source phantom. Further work aims to develop a fully functional multidimensional scanner based on single-sided geometry, which will serve as a proof-of-concept device for a single-sided scanner with the potential applications in breast cancer imaging.

ACKNOWLEDGEMENTS

We thank Dr. L. Wald for hosting at MGH/Martinos Center for Biomedical Imaging.

AUTHOR'S STATEMENT

Research funding: University of Massachusetts President Office through OTCV Award and Joseph P. Healey Research Grant from UMass Boston. Authors state no conflict of interest.

REFERENCES

[1] T. F. Sattel, T. Knopp, S. Biederer, et al. Single-sided device for magnetic particle imaging. *J. Phys. D: Appl. Phys.*, 42(1):1–5, 2009. doi:10.1088/0022-3727/42/2/022001.

[2] C. Kaethner, M. Ahlborg, K. Gräfe, et al. Asymmetric Scanner Design for Interventional Scenarios in Magnetic Particle Imaging. *IEEE Trans. Magn.*, 51(2):6501904, 2015. doi:10.1109/TMAG.2014.2337931.

[3] H. Maeda, et al. Tumor vascular permeability and the EPR effect in macromolecular therapeutics: A review, *J. Control. Release*, vol. 65, pp. 271–284, 2000.

[4] X. X.-H. Peng, et al. Targeted magnetic iron oxide nanoparticles for tumor imaging and therapy. *Int. J. Nanomedicine*, 3(3): 311–321, 2008.

[5] D. Finas, K. Baumann, L. Sydow, et al. Detection and distribution of superparamagnetic nanoparticles in lymphatic tissue in a breast cancer model for magnetic particle imaging, *Biomed. Tech.* 57, 81–83, 2012. doi:10.1515/bmt-2012-4158.

[6] R.L. Siegel, K.D. Miller, A. Jemal, Cancer statistics, *Cancer J. Clin.* 67, 7–30, 2017. doi:10.3322/caac.21387.

[7] E. Mason, C. Z. Cooley, E. Mattingly, et al. A Magnetic Particle Detector for Margin Assessment in Breast-Conserving Surgery, in 8th IWMPI, 2018, Hamburg, Germany.

[8] A. Tonyushkin. Single-sided field-free line generator magnet for multidimensional magnetic particle imaging, *IEEE Trans. Magn.*, 53(9):5300506, 2017. doi:10.1109/TMAG.2017.2718485.

[9] A. Tonyushkin. Single-sided hybrid selection coils for field-free line magnetic particle imaging. *Int. J. Magn. Particle Imag.*, 3(1): 1703009, 2017. doi:10.18416/ijmpi.2017.1703009.

Dynamic Imaging with a 3D Single-Sided MPI Scanner

A. von Gladiss[a*], Y. Blancke Soares[a], T. M. Buzug[a] and K. Gräfe[a]

[a] *Institute of Medical Engineering, University of Luebeck, Luebeck, Germany*
[*] *Corresponding author, email: {gladiss,buzug,graefe}@imt.uni-luebeck.de*

A single-sided Magnetic Particle Imaging (MPI) scanner has been used for 2D and 3D imaging of static phantoms. In order to exploit its full potential in preclinical and clinical use, the dynamic movement of a two dot phantom has been acquired and reconstructed. This work presents the first dynamic 3D images of a moving phantom that was acquired in a 3D single-sided MPI scanner.

I. Introduction

Magnetic Particle Imaging (MPI) is an emerging medical imaging modality and tailored for clinical application. It features a very high temporal resolution, exquisite sensitivity, the potential of submillimeter spatial resolution and does not use ionizing radiation. It uses superparamagnetic nanoparticles as tracer material such as Resovist (Bayer-Schering, Berlin, Germany) that has already been used clinically as contrast agent in magnetic resonance imaging.

MPI has first been presented in 2005 [1]. In 2009, the beating heart of a mouse has been imaged in real time without triggering techniques [2]. MPI scanners with different bore geometries have been investigated for clinical and preclinical use [3, 4]. A single-sided approach has been introduced in 2009 [5]. Here, both the signal generation and acquisition components are located on one side of the patient allowing for an unlimited patient access.

The single-sided scanner (see Fig. 1) has been designed for imaging of tracer material that accumulates in the sentinel lymph node (SLN) of the human axilla. In case of breast cancer, the SLN might need to be removed for investigating metastasis [6]. Current imaging techniques lack spatial resolution or apply radionuclides for localizing the SLN. MPI may provide a harmless and more precise alternative.

After 1D and 2D imaging with the single-sided MPI scanner [5, 7], 3D images have been presented in 2018 [8]. So far, static phantoms have been imaged focusing on spatial resolution and sensitivity. In this work, a phantom is moved manually during the measurement exploiting the temporal resolution of the single-sided scanner in 3D.

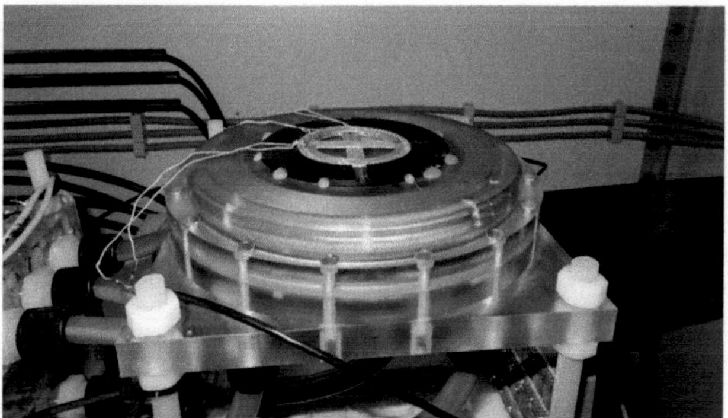

Figure 1: *A single-sided MPI scanner features unlimited access to the patient, as the hardware components are located on one side.*

II. Material and Methods

II.I. System Matrix Measurement

A field of view (FOV) of 16 mm x 32 mm x 32 mm has been discretized into 8 x 16 x 16 voxels resulting in a voxel size of 2 mm x 2 mm x 2 mm. A system matrix has been measured using a particle sample of 8 μl of undiluted Resovist. The receive signal has been averaged 200 times.

II.II. Phantom Measurement

Two dots of a phantom with a centre to centre distance of 7 mm have been filled with each 8 μl of undiluted Resovist (see Fig. 2). The phantom has been placed onto the scanner surface (x = 0). During the acquisition, the phantom has been moved manually in the yz-plane of the scanner, that is parallel to the scanner surface. The receive signal has been averaged 10 times resulting in an acquisition time of 393 ms per imaging frame.

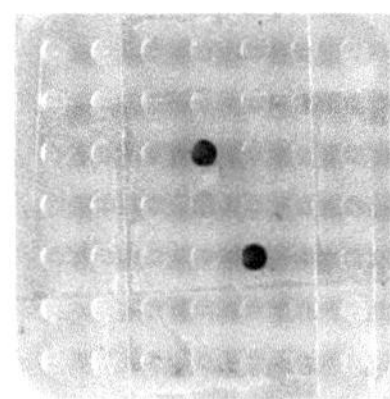

Figure 2: *Two dots of the phantom with a centre to centre distance of 7 mm have been filled with 8 µl of undiluted Resovist.*

II.III. Reconstruction

The measurement data have been reconstructed using the system matrix using a regularized Kaczmarz algorithm (number of iterations: 10, regularization factor: 0.1) [9]. The frequency components between 50 kHz and 1 MHz exceeding an SNR threshold of 30 have been selected for reconstruction.

III. Results

Fig. 3 shows the reconstruction results of the moving phantom shown in Fig. 2 as projection images. The phantom shifts over time in the yz-plane on top of the scanner (x = 0). During the acquisition, one dot of the phantom leaves the FOV. A frame rate of 2.5 frames per second (fps) has been reached.

The reconstruction time per frame was about 3.2 s using Matlab without optimization techniques as parallel computing or system matrix compression.

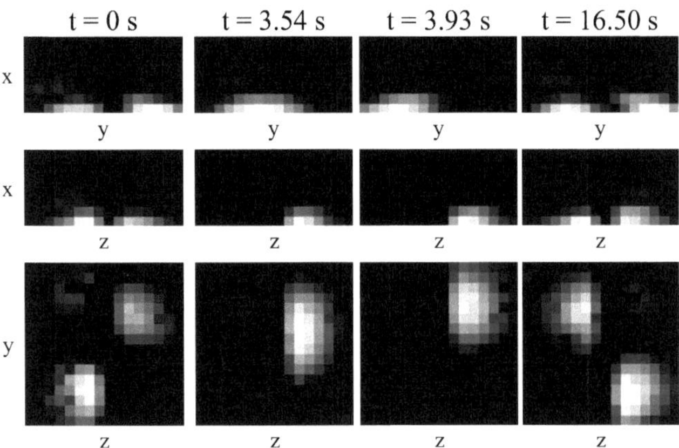

Figure 3: *Reconstruction results of the moving phantom. Projection images of 4 acquisition frames are visualized. The FOV is 16 mm x 32 mm x 32 mm. The phantom moves in the yz-plane on top of the scanner surface (x = 0).*

IV. Discussion

Averaging the receive signal over 10 trajectory periods provides a sufficient SNR of the measurements for reconstructing the phantom shown in Fig. 2. The frame rate may be increased by both applying a moving average algorithm and decreasing the number of averages.

The phantom has been moved in the yz-plane on top of the scanner surface. Here, the sensitivity of the scanner is highest. Further investigations will show if the number of averages

has to be increased when moving an object in 3D and thus, increasing the distance to the scanner surface.

The reconstruction time using Matlab with 3.2 s per frame needs to be decreased in order to allow for online reconstruction and visualization of measurement data. A fast implementation and system matrix compression may allow for a reconstruction time in ms range. A reconstruction time of 39 ms per frame should be reached as this corresponds to the trajectory period. Then, the single-sided scanner may reach its full potential in terms of temporal resolution.

V. Conclusions

It has been shown that the single-sided MPI scanner can acquire data of a moving phantom while scanning a volume. The data have been reconstructed featuring a frame rate of 2.5 fps. The frame rate may even increase.

The spatial resolution, sensitivity and temporal resolution of the single-sided MPI scanner have been investigated. It may provide a valuable modality in clinical diagnostics.

ACKNOWLEDGEMENTS

The authors thankfully acknowledge the financial support by the German Research Foundation (DFG, grant numbers BU 1436/7-1 and BU 1436/9-1) and the Federal Ministry of Education and Research (BMBF, grant numbers 13GW0230B and 01DL17010A).

AUTHOR'S STATEMENT

The authors state no conflict of interest.

REFERENCES

[1] Gleich et al. Tomographic imaging using the nonlinear response of magnetic particles. *Nature*, 2005. doi: 10.1038/nature03808.
[2] Weizenecker et al. Three-dimensional real-time in vivo magnetic particle imaging. *Phys. Med. Biol.*, 2009. doi: 10.1088/0031-9155/54/5/L01.
[3] Rahmer et al. 3D line imaging on a clinical magnetic particle imaging demonstrator. *IWMPI*, 2015. doi: 10.1109/IWMPI.2015.7107029.
[4] Sattel et al. Open coil arrangement for interventional magnetic particle imaging. *ISMRM*, 2010.
[5] Sattel et al. Single-sided device for magnetic particle imaging. *J. Phys. D*, 2009. doi: 10.1088/0022-3727/42/2/022001.
[6] Finas et al. SPIO Detection and Distribution in Biological Tissue - A Murine MPI-SLNB Breast Cancer Model, *IEEE Trans. Magn.*, 2015. doi: 10.1109/TMAG.2014.2358272.
[7] Gräfe et al. 2D Images Recorded With a Single-Sided Magnetic Particle Imaging Scanner. *IEEE Trans. Magn.*, 2016. doi: 10.1109/TMI.2015.2507187.
[8] Gräfe et al. First Phantom Measurements with a 3D Single Sided MPI Scanner. *IWMPI*, 2018.
[9] Knopp et al. Weighted iterative reconstruction for magnetic particle imaging. *Phys. Med. Biol.*, 2010. doi: 10.1088/0031-9155/55/6/003.

Flow of Magnetic Nanoparticles detected by 2nd Harmonic Responses using HTS SQUID Array

S. Tanaka*, M. Kabasawa and K. Hayashi

Department of Environmental and Life Sciences, Toyohashi University of Technology, Toyohashi, Japan
** Corresponding author, email: tanakas@ens.tut.ac.jp*

Abstract: We have developed a high-Tc superconducting (HTS) three-channel Superconducting Quantum Interference Device (SQUID) array. The signal from Magnetic nano-particles (MNPs) in motion was measured by the three channel SQUID array in a DC bias magnetic field and an AC modulation magnetic field. The dependence of the SQUID signal on the angle of the MNP flow to the baseline of the SQUID array was measured and discussed. The results suggest that the signal peak values are highly dependent on the angle.

I. Introduction

There are several methods available to investigate brain functions, such as MPI [1, 2], f-MRI, EEG, MEG and NIRS. Each method has advantages of either space resolution, time resolution, device size or cost. One promising candidate for brain activity investigation is using a highly sensitive magnetic sensor, high-Tc Superconducting Quantum Interference Device (SQUID). We proposed a method of the investigation using a small SQUID array and magnetic nanoparticles (MNPs) [3]. The advantage of this method is low cost and high spatial sensitivity with high speed. We employed a method detecting a second harmonic response when applying an AC modulation magnetic field and a DC bias field [4]. A $YBa_2Cu_3O_{7-y}$ (YBCO) thin film was used to make a three-channel SQUID array, which consists of three direct coupled SQUID magnetometers on a 10 mm × 10 mm substrate, was designed and fabricated for the research [3]. The SQUID array was mounted on a sapphire thermal conduction rod in vacuum and cooled to 77 K by liquid nitrogen. Resovist (Fe_2O_3, 28mg/ml), which is a commercially available MNP, was used as a sample. In this paper we will discuss the dependence of the signal waveform on the angle of the MNP flow to the baseline of the SQUID array.

II. Experimental

The experimental setup for the measurement of the MNPs motion in a thin tube is shown in Fig. 1. DC and AC Helmholtz-type coils were located on the top of the cryostat, where a Teflon (fluorocarbon) thin tube with an inner diameter of 0.8 mm was threaded at the center of the coils. The lift-off distance between the center of the tube and the sensitive surface of the SQUID array was 2 mm. MNPs sample of 0.23 µl, which iron content was 6.23 µg was used. A DC magnetic field of 1.85 mT_{P-P}/μ_0 and an AC modulation field of 2.16 mT_{P-P}/μ_0@79 Hz were applied.

The sample in the tube, which was oriented at different angles from 0 to 90 degrees was moved above the SQUID.

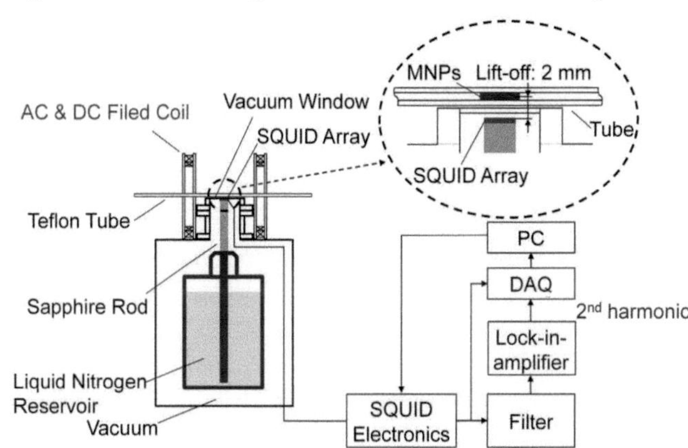

Figure 1: *Experimental setup. The sample moved above Ch3, Ch2 and Ch1 at different angles from 0 to 90 degrees.*

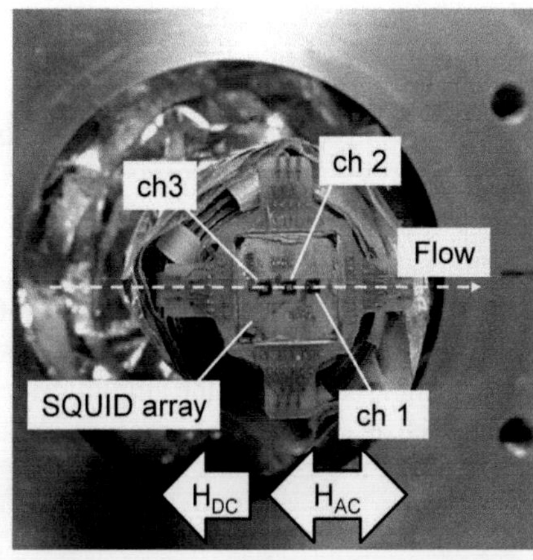

Figure 2: *Top view of SQUID array. Three magnetometers are in-line with a separation of 2.3 mm. The pick-up loop consists of a 1 mm × 1 mm square loop*

Three directly coupled SQUID magnetometers were designed and fabricated on a single chip as a SQUID array. They were made from a sputtered YBCO thin film with a thickness of 200 nm on a 10 mm × 10 mm SrTiO₃ bi-crystal substrate.

The detail of the SQUID array mounted on a cryostat is shown in Fig. 2. Three magnetometers are in-line with a separation of 2.3 mm. The pick-up loop consists of a 1 mm × 1 mm square loop with a width of 200 µm; the size of a SQUID washer slit is 5 µm × 60 µm, which corresponds to an inductance of 35.5 pH.

III. Results

Fig. 3 shows the typical second harmonic signal wave-forms. In this case, the MNPs sample (0.23 µl, original concentration 28mg/ml) was moved at an angle of 30 degrees as shown in an inset of the figure.

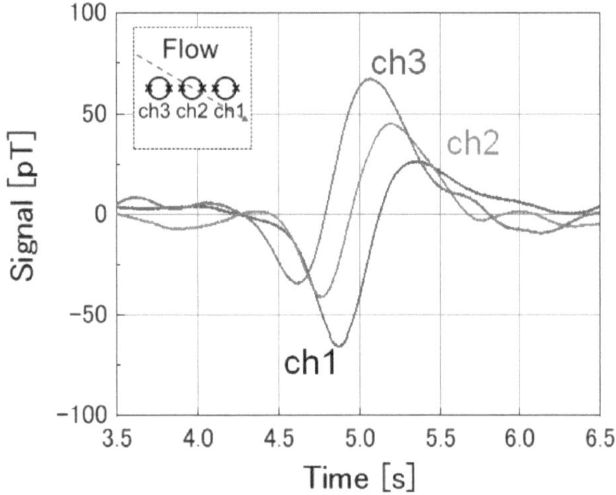

Figure 3: *Time trace signal of the SQUID array with an angle of 30degrees. Each positive and negative peak value on a channel is different except for ch2.*

Each positive and negative peak value on a channel is different except for ch2. While the positive peak of ch3 is larger than the negative one, the negative peak of ch1 is larger than the positive one. Successively the angler dependence was systematically measured at different angles of 0, 30, 45 and 90 degrees.

The speed of the sample was calculated as 28.6 mm/s from the time trace. Fig.4 shows each peak of the waveform. The amplitudes of positive and negative peaks of ch2 are almost the same at each angle. However, the amplitudes of positive and negative peaks of ch1 and ch3 are three to five times different at any of the angles used.

We note that some signal in ch2 at 90 degrees is due to the misalignment between the tube and the SQUID, since the signal intensity in ch2 at 90 degree must be theoretically zero.

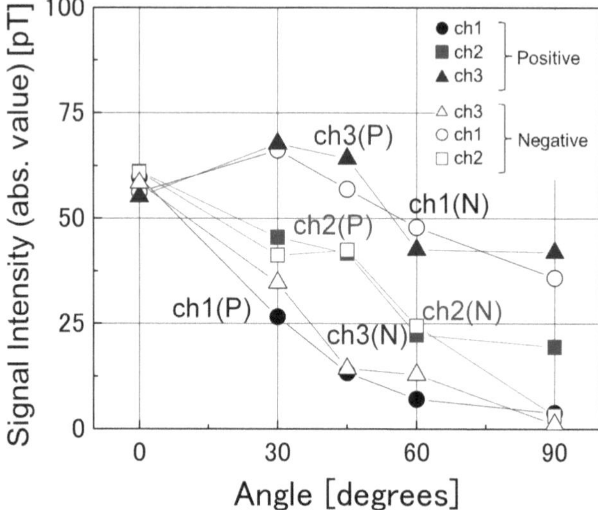

Figure 4: *Angler dependence vs SQUID signal amplitude measured at 0, 30, 45 and 90 degrees. Solid symbols show amplitude of positive peaks; open symbols show negative ones.*

IV. Discussion

This information of amplitudes can be used for the identification of the sample flow because the peak values have dependence of the angles.

V. Conclusions

A high-Tc SQUID array was developed and used for the detection of a small volume of water diluted MNPs sample in motion as a preliminary study on bio-applications. In the measurement, it was demonstrated that the signal from each SQUID magnetometer was dependent on its position and the movement of the MNP sample. In the near future we expect to be able to show a detailed map of the flow pass by increasing the number of array channels.

REFERENCES

[1] B. Gleich and J. Weizenecker. Tomographic imaging using the nonlinear response of magnetic particles. *Nature*, 435(7046):1217-1217, 2005. doi: 10.1038/nature03808.

[2] T. Knopp and T. M. Buzug. *Magnetic Particle Imaging: An Introduction to Imaging Principles and Scanner Instrumentation.* Springer, Berlin/Heidelberg, 2012. doi: 10.1007/978-3-642-04199-0.

[3] S. Tanaka, T. Matsuo, K. Kobayashi, M. Kabasawa, T. Ohtani and S. Ariyoshi. Measurement of Magnetic Nanoparticles by Small HTS SQUID Array. *IEEE Trans. Appl. Supercond.,* 2792405_1-6, 2018. doi: 10.1109/TASC.2018. 2792405.

[4] S. Tanaka, T. Oishi, T. Suzuki, T. Ohtani and S. Ariyoshi. Imaging of Magnetic Nanoparticles using second harmonic signals. *IEEE Trans. on Magnetics*, 99, 1-4, 2015. doi: 10.1109/TMAG.201

A Rabbit Sized Field-Free-Line Magnetic-Particle-Imaging Scanner – Past, Present, and Future

J. Stelzner[a]*, K. Gräfe[a], A. von Gladiss[a], J. Beuke[a], and T.M. Buzug[a]*

[a] Institute of Medical Engineering, Universität zu Lübeck, Lübeck, Germany
** Corresponding author, email: {stelzner,buzug}@imt.uni-luebeck.de*

A Magnetic Particle Imaging device is being developed that has an accessible inner diameter of 180 mm and uses the spatial encoding concept of field-free-line imaging. In this work, the properties of the imaging system are described in terms of geometry, magnetic, and electrical parameters. Furthermore, all modules of the scanner are briefly described.

I. Introduction

A project is presented that is aiming for the construction of a Magnetic Particle Imaging (MPI) setup that is capable of accommodating animals with the scale of a mini pig or a New Zealand rabbit [1].

MPI is an imaging modality that is based on the detection of higher harmonics when an oscillating magnetic field is applied on a superparamagnetic tracer. By adding an inhomogeneous selection field simultaneously, spatial encoding is achieved to facilitate medical imaging. There are basically two types of selection fields: One that uses a field-free point (FFP) and another with a field-free line (FFL) [2]. While FFL imaging enables a higher sensitivity than an FFP system with the same measurement-field size and gradient strength due to a more complex field topology, there are also challenges arising.

II. Material and Methods

II.I Main Properties of the Scanner

As the MPI scanner is aiming for preclinical purposes involving animals in the size of a rabbit, the cylindrical bore diameter was chosen to be 180 mm in diameter. The inner bore is surrounded by the drive-field generator (DFG) that consists of a curved Helmholtz coil-pair for the particle excitation in horizontal direction and another one for the excitation in vertical direction. The next outer layer is a copper shield separating the DFG on its inside from selection-field generator (SFG) on its outside. The SFG involves three main components: On the inner layer of the SFG, there is the axial gradient generator (AGG), a solenoid aligned with the bore axis that changes its winding direction on half way to generate a static magnetic field with a main gradient in axial direction. The next field-generator element is a magnetic quadrupole, which extends on two layers to reach the desired field properties and surrounds the before mentioned AGG. The combination of the latter two

components is sufficient to generate an FFL. The outermost field-generator component is another two-layer quadrupole and enables the scanner setup to rotate the FFL. Fig. 1 shows a CAD model and Fig. 2 a photograph of the field generator.

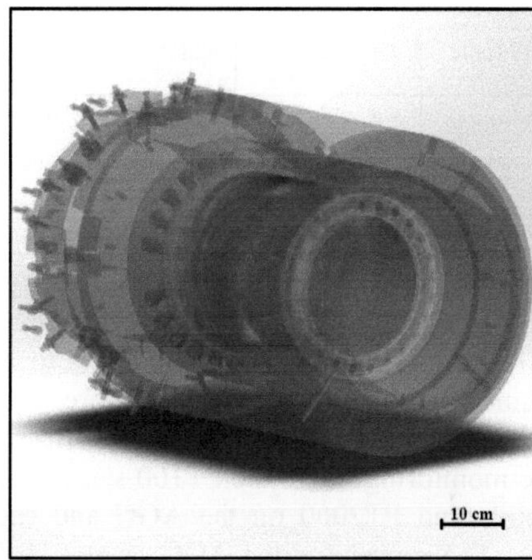

Figure 1: The CAD model of the field generator. The visible coil inside generates the vertical component of the drive field.

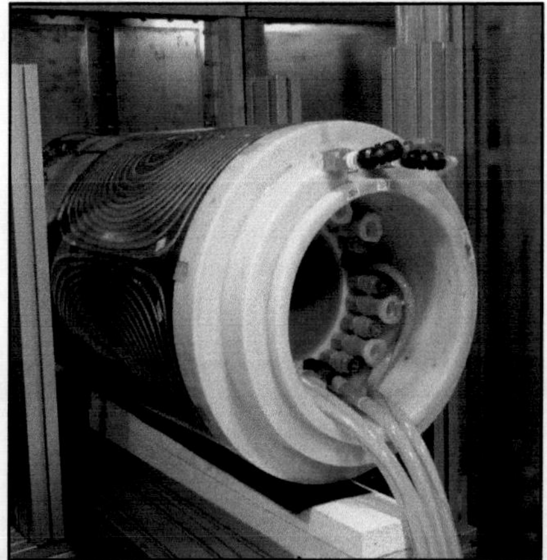

Figure 2: The regarded field generator with oil-cooling tubes.

The intended magnetic field parameters for the setup are 15 mT$_{peak}$ for the drive field amplitude $\mu_0\hat{H}$ and 0.8 T/m for the magnetic-field gradient G. Thus, the target FOV has a diameter d of 37.5 mm enabling, for instance, imaging of the heart or the liver of a potential animal model without exceeding common safety limitations [3].

II.I. Electrical Properties of the Scanner

The inner part of the DFG is able to generate a magnetic flux density of 44 µT/A. To create a magnetic field of 15 mT$_{peak}$, a current of 342 A$_{peak}$ or 171 A$_{RMS}$ respectively is required. Using litz-wire for the DFG, involving 10000 strands with a diameter of 63 µm each, there is a current density of 3.1 A/mm². Since the outer part of the DFG is further away from the center, a higher current must be applied. Table 1 lists the characteristic parameters.

Table 1: *Characteristic Target Values of the Field Generator*

Component	Magnetic Field	Current	Power Requirement
Inner DFG	15 mT$_{peak}$	171 A$_{RMS}$	0.5 kW
Outer DFG	15 mT$_{peak}$	306 A$_{RMS}$	1.8 kW
AGG	0.8 T/m	751 A$_{DC}$	12.2 kW
Inner Quadrupole	0.4 T/m	428 A$_{RMS}$	7.3 kW
Outer Quadrupole	0.4 T/m	479 A$_{RMS}$	9.9 kW

To obtain optimum field properties for minimum electrical power, the design of each magnetic field generating component was designed thoroughly [4]. However, due to the high power consumption, which amounts to more than 30 kW, liquid cooling is utilized. Therefore, the DFG is cooled with oil as the SFG is cooled with water. For temperature monitoring, there are PT100 sensors on each of the DFG coils and PT2000 on the AGG and each of the quadrupoles. The power for the AGG is provided by four SM 6000 power supplies (*Delta Electronics*, Taiwan). The Quadrupoles are driven by 2 AE Techron 7796 amplifiers (*AE Techron*, USA), each. For each DFG coil, there is one AE Techron 7796. In between, a custom made two-channel analogue bandpass filter and a capacitive matching network is used [5, 6].

III. Results

First results have been published amongst others in 2016 [7], where a continuous operation with 1 kA$_{peak}$ could be achieved to generate a 22 mT$_{peak}$ drive field by the inner DFG coil. Within that work, an amplitude spectrum was recorded that clearly indicates a change when using small amounts of undiluted Resovist.

Measurements of the magnetic field were presented to validate foregoing simulations. Superposition has pictured the selection- and drive-field shape inside the FOV [8, 9]. Also, an alternative receive coil-topology based on oppositely tilted solenoids, which is tailored for the presented scanner, showed promising enhancement of the received amplitude spectrum [10].

IV. Discussion and Conclusions

A medium bore MPI-FFL scanner system was designed and constructed to study the technical challenges on the way to clinical MPI. First experiments reveal the problems to cope with high voltages and currents as well as heat load in the scaling process. Further, the system still faces various challenges according undesirable coupling effects, avoidance of ground loops, disturbance by the system periphery, and a reliable operation at target power supply.

ACKNOWLEDGEMENTS

The authors thankfully acknowledge the financial support by the Federal Ministry of Education and Research (BMBF, grant number 13N11090), the European Union and the State Schleswig-Holstein (Programme for the Future – Economy, grant number 122-10-004). Moreover, the authors thank all project alumni, especially Gael Bringout for his remarkable groundwork.

AUTHOR'S STATEMENT
The authors state no conflict of interest.

REFERENCES

[1] J. Weizenecker, B. Gleich, and J. Borgert. Magnetic particle imaging using a field free line. Journal of Physics D: Applied Physics, 41(10):2–4, 2008. doi: 10.1088/0022-3727/41/10/105009.

[2] G. Bringout, J. Stelzner, M. Ahlborg, A. Behrends, K. Bente, C. Debbeler, A. von Gladiß, K. Gräfe, M. Graeser, C. Kaethner, S. Kaufmann, K. Lüdtke-Buzug, H.Medimagh,W. Tenner, M.Weber, and T. M. Buzug. Concept of a rabbit-sized ffl-scanner. In *5th International Workshop on Magnetic Particle Imaging*, 49, 2015. DOI: 10.1109/IWMPI.2015.7107032.

[3] G. Bringout, H. Wojtczyk, M. Grüttner, M. Graeser, W. Tenner, J. Hägele, F. M. Vogt, J. Barkhausen and T. M. Buzug. Safety Aspects for a Pre-clinical Magnetic Particle Imaging Scanner, *Springer Proceedings in Physics*, 355-359, 2012, DOI: 10.1007/978-3-642-24133 8_57.

[4] G. Bringout and T. M. Buzug. Coil design for magnetic particle imaging: Application for a preclinical scanner. *IEEE Transactions on Magnetics*, 51(2):5100808, 2015. doi: 10.1109/TMAG.2014.2344917.

[5] T. M. Buzug, G. Bringout, M. Erbe, K. Gräfe, M. Graeser, M. Grüttner, A. Halkola, T. F. Sattel, W. Tenner, H. Wojtczyk, J. Haegele, F. M. Vogt, J. Barkhausen and K. Lüdtke-Buzug. Magnetic particle imaging: Introduction to imaging and hardware realization, *Zeitschrift für Medizinische Physik*, 22(4), 323-334, 2012, DOI: 10.1016/j.zemedi.2012.07.004.

[6] A. Behrends, M. Graeser, J. Stelzner, and T. M. Buzug. Signal Chain Optimization in Magnetic Particle Imaging, *Deutsche Gesellschaft für Biomedizinische Technik Jahrestagung*, 526--529, 2014, DOI: 10.1515/bmt-2014-5008.

[7] J. Stelzner, G. Bringout, A. von Gladiss, H. Medimagh, M. Ahlborg, T. F. Sattel, and T. M. Buzug. First Spectrum Measurements with a Rabbit-Sized FFL-Scanner, In: International Workshop on Magnetic Particle Imaging, 138, 2016.

[8] J. Stelzner and T. M. Buzug. Magnetic-Field Measurement and Simulation of a Field-Free Line Magnetic-Particle Scanner, *Current Directions in Biomedical Engineering*, 3(2), 837 -- 840, 2017, DOI: https://doi.org/10.1515/cdbme-2017-0191.

[9] A. Bakenecker, T. Friedrich, A. von Gladiss, M. Graeser, J. Stelzner, and T. M. Buzug. Experimental Validation of the Selection Field of a Rabbit Sized FFL Scanner, In *7th International Workshop on Magnetic Particle Imaging*, 41, 2017.

[10] J. Stelzner, M. Weber, and T. M. Buzug. A Receive Coil Topology Based on Oppositely Tilted Solenoids for a Predefined Drive Field, In: International Workshop on Magnetic Particle Imaging, 81-82, 2018.

Author Index

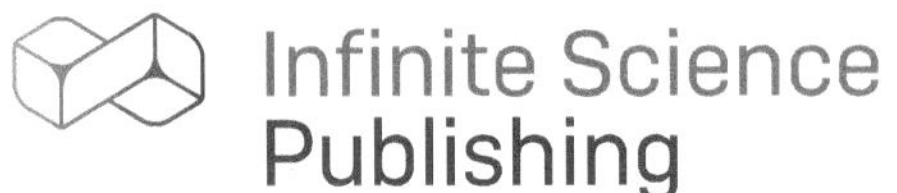